Tumors
of the
Bones and Joints

Atlas
of
Tumor Pathology

Jose Costa

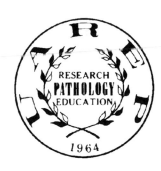

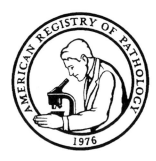

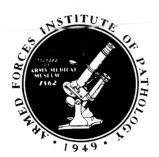

ATLAS OF TUMOR PATHOLOGY

Third Series
Fascicle 8

TUMORS OF THE
BONES AND JOINTS

by

ROBERT E. FECHNER, M. D.
Professor of Pathology
University of Virginia
Health Sciences Center, Box 214
Charlottesville, Virginia 22908

and

STACEY E. MILLS, M. D.
Professor of Pathology
University of Virginia
Health Sciences Center, Box 214
Charlottesville, Virginia 22908

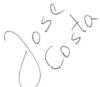

Published by the
ARMED FORCES INSTITUTE OF PATHOLOGY
Washington, D.C.

Under the Auspices of
UNIVERSITIES ASSOCIATED FOR RESEARCH AND EDUCATION IN PATHOLOGY, INC.
Bethesda, Maryland
1993

Accepted for Publication
1992

Available from the American Registry of Pathology
Armed Forces Institute of Pathology
Washington, D.C. 20306-6000
ISSN 0160-6344
ISBN 1-881041-08-5

ATLAS OF TUMOR PATHOLOGY

EDITOR
JUAN ROSAI, M.D.
Department of Pathology
Memorial Sloan-Kettering Cancer Center
New York, New York 10021-6007

ASSOCIATE EDITOR
LESLIE H. SOBIN, M.D.
Armed Forces Institute of Pathology
Washington, D.C. 20306-6000

EDITORS' NOTE

The Atlas of Tumor Pathology has a long and distinguished history. It was first conceived at a Cancer Research Meeting held in St. Louis in September 1947 as an attempt to standardize the nomenclature of neoplastic diseases. The first series was sponsored by the National Academy of Sciences-National Research Council. The organization of this Sisyphean effort was entrusted to the Subcommittee on Oncology of the Committee on Pathology, and Dr. Arthur Purdy Stout was the first editor-in-chief. Many of the illustrations were provided by the Medical Illustration Service of the Armed Forces Institute of Pathology, the type was set by the Government Printing Office, and the final printing was done at the Armed Forces Institute of Pathology (hence the colloquial appellation "AFIP Fascicles"). The American Registry of Pathology purchased the Fascicles from the Government Printing Office and sold them virtually at cost. Over a period of 20 years, approximately 15,000 copies each of nearly 40 Fascicles were produced. The worldwide impact that these publications have had over the years has largely surpassed the original goal. They quickly became among the most influential publications on tumor pathology ever written, primarily because of their overall high quality but also because their low cost made them easily accessible to pathologists and other students of oncology the world over.

Upon completion of the first series, the National Academy of Sciences-National Research Council handed further pursuit of the project over to the newly created Universities Associated for Research and Education in Pathology (UAREP). A second series was started, generously supported by grants from the AFIP, the National Cancer Institute, and the American Cancer Society. Dr. Harlan I. Firminger became the editor-in-chief and was succeeded by Dr. William H. Hartmann. The second series Fascicles were produced as bound volumes instead of loose leaflets. They featured a more comprehensive coverage of the subjects, to the extent that the Fascicles could no longer be regarded as "atlases" but rather as monographs describing and illustrating in detail the tumors and tumor-like conditions of the various organs and systems.

Once the second series was completed, with a success that matched that of the first, UAREP and AFIP decided to embark on a third series. A new editor-in-chief and an associate editor were selected, and a distinguished editorial board was appointed. The mandate for the third series remains the same as for the previous ones, i.e., to oversee the production of an eminently practical publication with surgical pathologists as its primary audience, but also aimed at other workers in oncology. The main purposes of this series are to promote a consistent, unified, and biologically sound nomenclature; to guide the surgical pathologist in the diagnosis of the various tumors and tumor-like lesions; and to provide relevant histogenetic, pathogenetic, and clinicopathologic information on these entities. Just as the second series included data obtained from ultrastructural (and, in the more recent Fascicles, immunohistochemical) examination, the third series will, in addition, incorporate pertinent information obtained with the newer molecular biology techniques. As in the past, a continuous attempt will be made to correlate, whenever possible, the nomenclature used in the Fascicles with that proposed by the World Health Organization's International Histological Classification of Tumors. The format of the third series has been changed in order to incorporate additional items and to ensure a consistency of style throughout. This includes the dropping of the 's possessive in eponymic terms, in accordance with the WHO and the International Nomenclature of Diseases. Close cooperation between the various authors and their respective liaisons from the editorial board will be emphasized to minimize unnecessary repetition and discrepancies in the text and illustrations.

To its everlasting credit, the participation and commitment of the AFIP to this venture is even more substantial and encompassing than in previous series. It now extends to virtually all scientific, technical, and financial aspects of the production.

The task confronting the organizations and individuals involved in the third series is even more daunting than in the preceding efforts because of the ever-increasing complexity of the matter at hand. It is hoped that this combined effort—of which, needless to say, that represented by the authors is first and foremost—will result in a series worthy of its two illustrious predecessors and will be a suitable introduction to the tumor pathology of the twenty-first century.

Juan Rosai, M.D.
Leslie H. Sobin, M.D.

ACKNOWLEDGMENTS

We gratefully acknowledge the expert editorial assistance of Nancy J. Kriigel and Linda M. Mills, the photographic expertise of Ursula W. Miller, and the artistic talents of Linda Berry.

The authors extend their special thanks to the following physicians who, since the publication of the prior edition, generously provided material from their own files:

Dr. L. V. Ackerman
Stony Brook, New York

Dr. H. D. Alpern
Cooperstown, New York

Dr. F. B. Askin
Baltimore, Maryland

Dr. A. G. Ayala
Houston, Texas

Dr. K. W. Barwick
Jacksonville, Florida

Dr. R. M. Belding
Barre, Vermont

Dr. R. D. Brunning
Minneapolis, Minnesota

Dr. T. E. Casey
New Orleans, Louisiana

Dr. P. E. Gates
Barre, Vermont

Dr. A. Greenspan
Sacramento, California

Dr. T. E. Keats
Charlottesville, Virginia

Dr. M. J. Klein
New York City, New York

Dr. M. Kyriakos
St. Louis, Missouri

Dr. R. W. McKenna
Dallas, Texas

Dr. T. L. Pope Jr.
Winston-Salem, North Carolina

Dr. J. A. Richman
Cooperstown, New York

Dr. T. W. Westgaard
Sandefjord, Norway

Dr. J. T. Wolfe III
Jacksonville, Florida

Dr. L. E. Wold
Rochester, Minnesota

TUMORS OF THE BONES AND JOINTS

Jose Costa

Contents

Table 3
LODWICK RADIOLOGIC GRADING SYSTEM*

Grade	Radiologic Features
IA	Geographic destruction with sclerotic rim and partial or no cortical destruction
IB	Geographic destruction with no sclerotic margin, or cortical shell expanded more than 1 cm
IC	Geographic destruction with complete cortical penetration
II	Geographic combined with moth-eaten and/or permeative destruction
III	Moth-eaten and/or permeative destruction only

* from Hudson (21).

Table 4
SIMPLIFIED RADIOLOGIC GRADING OF BONE TUMORS*

Grade	Radiologic Features
Low grade, nonaggressive	Geographic destruction with sclerotic rim
Medium grade, moderately aggressive	Geographic destruction, no sclerotic rim, and/or cortex "expanded" more than 1 cm or completely penetrated
High grade, very aggressive	Moth-eaten and/or permeative destruction only

* from Hudson (21).

The *single lamellar reaction* consists of a sheet of woven bone that appears radiographically as a single radiodense line 1 to 2 mm from the cortical surface. It may merge with the cortex at its peripheral margins (26). This reaction is typical of benign processes and is often seen with osteomyelitis, eosinophilic granuloma, and, occasionally, other benign tumors (26). Eventually, the space between the cortex and the periosteum is filled in with reactive bone to produce a solid periosteal reaction.

The *lamellated reaction*, also called "onion-skinning," is created by concentric planes of periosteal new bone, separated by a loose, vascular connective tissue (26). When associated with a malignant tumor, the spaces between the layers of bone may become secondarily colonized with malignant cells, but the layers do not form in response to "waves" of subperiosteal tumor growth (26). Lamellated periosteal reactions are seen with primary osseous sarcomas including Ewing sarcoma and osteosarcoma as well as in some benign bone tumors, osteomyelitis, stress fracture, and even as a transient feature of normal growth (20,26).

The *parallel spiculated*, "hair on end," or "sunburst" reaction is characteristic of extremely rapid growth. Although resembling lines of periosteal bone radiographically, there is a honey-comb-like compartmentalization when sectioned parallel to the surface of the underlying bone (26). The spaces between the trabeculae of bone are filled, at least initially, with loose, vascular connective tissue that may be replaced with tumor. This form of periosteal reaction is not typically seen with benign tumors, but is more characteristic of malignancy or certain inflammatory processes (26).

The periosteal reactions described above are of the uninterrupted or continuous type. Their pattern is a reflection of the rate of periosteal reaction and the nature of the inciting lesion, neoplastic or reactive. When the periosteal reaction is broken so that it forms a cuff on either side of a central defect, the possibility of a sarcoma becomes far more likely. The defect may be due to destruction of the periosteal rim by tumor or pressure by tumor on the periosteum leading to osteoclastic resorption of bone (26).

The *buttress* is the interrupted version of the solid periosteal reaction. It may be seen at the margin of a periosteal shell surrounding a surface lesion such as a periosteal chondroma or an expanding intramedullary lesion such as an aneurysmal bone cyst. Alternately, a buttress may be created by the central destruction of a previously solid periosteal reaction. The latter pattern should suggest malignant transformation of a preexisting benign process (26).

PERIOSTEAL REACTIONS
CONTINUOUS   INTERRUPTED

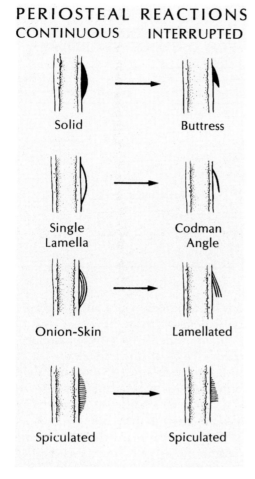

Solid   Buttress

Single Lamella   Codman Angle

Onion-Skin   Lamellated

Spiculated   Spiculated

Figure 4
PATTERNS OF PERIOSTEAL REACTION
Schematic representation of periosteal reactions. The arrows indicate that continuous periosteal reactions may be interrupted, due to destruction of the periosteal reaction by tumor invasion or pressure by the tumor leading to resorption of the reactive bone. (Modified from fig. 2 from Ragsdale BD, Madewell JE, Sweet DE. Radiologic and pathologic analysis of solitary bone lesions. Part II: Periosteal reactions. Radiol Clin North Am 1981;19:749-83.)

The *Codman angle* is the interrupted counterpart of the single lamellar reaction. Codman angles are usually indicative of extracortical extension by a rapidly growing, frequently malignant process. They may be seen in rapidly growing but benign lesions such as aneurysmal bone cyst, or in reactive processes such as osteomyelitis and subperiosteal hematoma (18). Codman angles are usually free of tumor, although they may be infiltrated secondarily through their open end or by transcortical growth (26).

The *interrupted lamellated reaction* and the *interrupted spiculated reaction* may result from the rapid extraosseous extension of a mass that was also characterized by a rapid intraosseous growth phase. These reactions may also be seen in response to primarily juxtacortical lesions such as parosteal osteosarcoma. The distinction between solid, lamellated, and spiculated reactions may be difficult on clinical radiographs due to loss of detail as a result of density summation (26).

Is the Joint Space Involved?

The articular cartilage provides an extremely effective barrier to tumor growth, at least at the macroscopic and radiographic level. Extension into the joint space is uncommon and usually occurs by lateral growth around the articular cartilage. Transarticular involvement is more consistent with an inflammatory, rather than neoplastic process.

Is the Lesion Multifocal?

The presence of multiple, radiographically discrete lesions in a single bone is uncommon, and, depending on the radiographic characteristics, should suggest a number of diagnostic possibilities. Multiple "punched out" defects at varying stages of development are characteristic of eosinophilic granuloma. Multifocal involvement, particularly of a single bone by radiographically similar tumors, is common in epithelioid hemangioendothelioma. Inflammatory processes are rarely multifocal. The reactive "brown tumor" of hyperparathyroidism is frequently multifocal, and, of course, multiple myeloma and metastatic disease are typically multifocal. Malignant osseous tumors with occasional multifocal involvement include osteosarcoma and Ewing sarcoma.

Is the Tumor of Uniform Appearance?

The recognition of radiographic variability is important for radiographic interpretation and for directing subsequent biopsies. The variation may be due to a preexisting and presumably premalignant process or represent a variation in the composition of a single lesion. Close cooperation between radiologist, surgeon, and pathologist is necessary to document the existence of the various patterns and their potential relationship based on the radiograph, direct the biopsies to each of the areas seen, and correlate the histologic features with the location of each biopsy. This team approach will prevent errors in diagnosis or the need for rebiopsy.

STAGING OF BONE TUMORS

Currently, at least two different, well-developed staging systems are being applied to osseous neoplasms. The first, using the common TNM approach, was developed by the American Joint Commission on Cancer, and proposed for bone tumors by the International Union Against Cancer in 1987 (32). The system applies to all primary, intramedullary malignant tumors except multiple myeloma. Parosteal or juxtacortical malignancies do not fit well into this system. The categories of T (tumor), N (nodes), and M (metastases) are based on a combination of physical examination and imaging techniques.

The primary tumor is classified as T_x if it cannot be assessed, T_0 if there is no evidence of primary tumor, T_1 if the tumor is confined within the cortex, and T_2 if it invades beyond the cortex. The regional lymph nodes are classified as N_x if they cannot be assessed, N_0 if there are no detectable metastases, and N_1 if there are nodal metastases. Distant metastases (M) are classified as M_x if they cannot be assessed, M_0 if none is detectable, and M_1 if they are present.

Histologic grading applies to all tumors except for Ewing sarcoma and primary lymphoma of bone. These neoplasms are defined as G_4 (see below). The histopathologic grading is categorized as G_x if a grade cannot be assessed, G_1 for well-differentiated tumors, G_2 for moderately differentiated tumors, G_3 for poorly differentiated tumors, and G_4 for undifferentiated neoplasms. These stages are based on tumor extent, microscopic grade, lymph node status, and presence or absence of distant metastases (Table 5).

A second staging system, developed by Enneking et al. (30) and adapted by the American Joint Committee Task Force on Bone Tumors, may be applied to both osseous and soft tissue neoplasms (31). Unlike the TNM system, this approach can also be applied to extramedullary osseous neoplasms. This system is based on the histologic grade of the tumor, as well as the biologic behavior of different tumor types before chemotherapy. The correlation of stage and sur-

Table 5

TNM STAGING SYSTEM FOR OSSEOUS NEOPLASMS

Stage	Grade	Tumor	Node	Metastasis
Stage IA	$G_{1,2}$	T_1	N_0	M_0
Stage IB	$G_{1,2}$	T_2	N_0	M_0
Stage IIA	$G_{3,4}$	T_1	N_0	M_0
Stage IIB	$G_{3,4}$	T_2	N_0	M_0
Stage III	Not defined			
Stage IVA	Any G	Any T	N_1	M_0
Stage IVB	Any G	Any T	Any N	M_1

vival has been validated in a pilot study of cases from several institutions (30).

The tumor grade is not purely histologic, but is determined by several components that influence both prognosis and response to treatment, including assessment of biologic aggressiveness, assessment of radiographic aggressiveness, and the presence of additional findings such as skip lesions. There are three grades: G_0 – benign; G_1 – low grade malignant; and G_2 – high grade malignant. G_1 tumors have limited metastatic potential and include intraosseous well-differentiated osteosarcoma and common giant cell tumor. Radiographically, G_1 tumors have the appearance of an indolent, slowly enlarging lesion. G_2 tumors are typically malignant with great local aggressiveness and high metastatic potential before chemotherapy. Examples include Ewing sarcoma, conventional osteosarcoma, grade 3 chondrosarcoma, and malignant fibrous histiocytoma. Radiographically, there is a highly destructive, permeative appearance. G_2 tumors also have a propensity for skip areas and occasional regional metastases.

Further classification in this system relates to whether the neoplasm has involved more than one "compartment." Intraosseous tumors that are confined to the intramedullary portion of the bone, without breaching the cortex, are referred to as intracompartmental (T_1). If the tumor has extended beyond the cortex to invade the joint or soft tissues, it is considered extracompartmental (T_2). Lesions that arise from the external cortical surface, such as parosteal sarcoma, are classified as T_1 lesions, unless they show evidence of inward invasion to involve the medullary cavity, or outward into the muscle or fascia. At that point, they are considered to be T_2 lesions. The presence or absence of metastases is also assessed in this system. Pulmonary metastases are the most common, but regional lymph node metastases are ominous findings as well.

The three major stages of the Enneking system are listed in Table 6. The first two are based on the grade and degree of extracompartmental extension.

Table 6

"ENNEKING" STAGING SYSTEM

Stage	Grade	Site
IA	G_1 (low)	T_1
IB	G_1 (low)	T_2
IIA	G_2 (high)	T_1
IIB	G_2 (high)	T_2
III	metastases (any G)	metastases (any T)

REFERENCES

The Structure of the Normal Bone

1. Delaisse JM, Boyde A, Maconnachie E, et al. The effects of inhibitors of cysteine-proteinases and collagenase on the resorptive activity of isolated osteoclasts. Bone 1987;8:305–13.
2. Eriksen EF. Normal and pathological remodeling of human trabecular bone: three dimensional reconstruction of the remodeling sequence in normals and in metabolic bone disease. Endocr Rev 1986;7:379–408.
3. Lian JB, Gundberg CM. Osteocalcin. Biochemical considerations and clinical applications. Clin Orthop 1988;226:267–91.
4. Talmage RV, Grubb SA. A laboratory model demonstrating osteocyte-osteoblast control of plasma calcium concentrations. Table model for plasma calcium control. Clin Orthop 1977;122:299–306.
5. Teitelbaum SL, Bullough PG. The pathophysiology of bone and joint disease. Am J Pathol 1979;96:283–354.

The Examination and Processing of Osseous Neoplasms

6. Anderson C. Manual for the examination of bone. Boca Raton, Fla: CRC Press, 1982;36–8.
7. Fechner RE, Huvos AG, Mirra JM, Spjut HJ, Unni KK. A symposium on the pathology of bone tumors. Pathol Annu 1984;19(Pt 1):125–94.
8. Fornasier VL. Fine detail radiography in the examination of tissue. Hum Pathol 1975;6:623–31.
9. Hajdu SI, Melamed MR. Limitations of aspiration cytology in the diagnosis of primary neoplasms. Acta Cytol 1984;28:337–45.
10. Hill P. Local recurrence in primary osteosarcoma of the femur. Br J Surg 1973;60:40–1.
11. Luna LG. Manual of histologic staining methods of the Armed Forces Institute of Pathology. 3rd ed. New York: McGraw-Hill, 1968:8–11, 44–5.
12. McKenna RJ, Schwinn CP, Soong KY, Higinbotham NL. Sarcomata of the osteogenic series (osteosarcoma, fibrosarcoma, chondrosarcoma, parosteal osteogenic sarcoma, and sarcomata arising in abnormal bone). An analysis of 552 cases. J Bone Joint Surg [Am] 1966;48:1–26.
13. Raymond AK, Chawla SP, Carrasco CH, et al. Osteosarcoma chemotherapy effect: a prognostic factor. Semin Diagn Pathol 1987;4:212–36.
14. Raymond AK, Ayala AG. Specimen management after osteosarcoma chemotherapy. In: Unni KK, ed. Bone tumors. New York: Churchill Livingstone, 1988:157–81.
15. Rosai J. Ackerman's surgical pathology. 7th ed. St. Louis: CV Mosby, 1989:1864,1882.
16. Schmidt WA. Principles and techniques of surgical pathology. Menlo Park, Calif: Addison-Wesley, 1983: 588–617.
17. Weatherby RP, Unni KK. Practical aspects of handling orthopedic specimens in the surgical pathology laboratory. Pathol Annu 1982;17(Pt 2):1–31.

Radiography of Osseous Neoplasms

18. Edeiken J, Hodes PJ. New bone production and periosteal reaction. In: Roentgen diagnosis of diseases of bone, 2nd ed., Vol. 1. Baltimore: Williams and Wilkins, 1973;39–54.
19. Ewing J. A review and classification of bone sarcomas. Arch Surg 1922;4:485–533.
20. Hancox NM, Hay JD, Holden WS, Moss PD, Whitehead AS. The radiological "double contour" effect in the long bones of newly born infants. Arch Dis Child 1951;26:543–8.
21. Hudson TM. Radiologic-pathologic correlation of musculoskeletal lesions. Baltimore: Williams & Wilkins, 1987;1–7.
22. Lodwick GS. A systemic approach to the roentgen diagnosis of bone tumors. In: MD Anderson Hospital and Tumor Institute: Tumors of bone and soft tissue. Chicago: Yearbook Medical Publishers, 1965:49–68.
23. Lodwick GS, Wilson AJ, Farrell C, Virtama P, Dittrich F. Determining growth rates of focal lesions of bone from radiographs. Radiology 1980;134:577–83.
24. Madewell JE, Ragsdale BD, Sweet DE. Radiologic and pathologic analysis of solitary bone lesions. Part I: Internal margins. Radiol Clin North Am 1981;19:715–48.
25. Murphy WA Jr. Imaging bone tumors in the 1990s. Cancer 1991;67:1169–76.
26. Ragsdale BD, Madewell JE, Sweet DE. Radiographic and pathologic analysis of solitary bone lesions. Part II: Periosteal reactions. Radiol Clin North Am 1981; 19:749–83.
27. Rosenthal DI, Schiller AL, Mankin HJ. Chondrosarcoma: correlation of radiological and histological grade. Radiology 1984;150:21–6.
28. Sweet DE, Madewell JE, Ragsdale BD. Radiologic and pathologic analysis of solitary bone lesions. Part III: Matrix patterns. Radiol Clin North Am 1981;19:785–814.
29. Taconis WK, Mulder JD. Fibrosarcoma and malignant fibrous histiocytoma of long bones: radiographic features and grading. Skeletal Radiol 1984;11:237–45.

Staging of Bone Tumors

30. Enneking WF, Spanier SS, Goodman MA. A system for the surgical staging of musculoskeletal sarcoma. Clin Orthop 1980;153:106–20.
31. Enneking WF. A system of staging musculoskeletal neoplasms. Clin Orthop 1986;204:9–24.
32. Hermanek P, Sobin LH, eds. TNM classification of malignant tumours. 4th ed. Berlin; New York: Springer-Verlag, 1987:7–9.

SARCOMAS ARISING IN BENIGN NEOPLASMS OR NON-NEOPLASTIC CONDITIONS

Most osseous neoplasms arise in bone lacking detectable prior abnormalities. There are, however, certain preexisting conditions, including both benign neoplasms and non-neoplastic processes, that are associated with the development of an osseous sarcoma. Sarcomas associated with benign neoplasms are discussed in chapters dealing with the appropriate sarcoma or the benign precursor. Sarcomas arising from non-neoplastic conditions (Table 7) are discussed here. Premalignant conditions in bone have been reviewed in detail by Unni and Dahlin (23).

SARCOMA ARISING IN PAGET DISEASE

Definition. A sarcoma of skeletal origin arising in a bone demonstrated radiographically or microscopically to contain preexisting Paget disease. Sarcomas arising in unaffected bones of patients with Paget disease are not part of this group.

General Features. The development of sarcomas in bones affected by Paget disease (osteitis deformans) is well recognized. Most Paget sarcomas are osteosarcomas (84 percent); the remainder are malignant fibrous histiocytomas and, occasionally, fibrosarcomas. The overall frequency of sarcomatous change is low (1 percent), and probably in direct proportion to the severity of the underlying disease. Paget sarcomas are uncommon in monostotic disease and may occur in up to 10 percent of patients with severe, polyostotic involvement. Because Paget disease is relatively common, Paget sarcomas account for about 3 percent of all osteosarcomas (23).

Clinical Features. In two large series (11,26) with a total of 103 Paget sarcomas, patient age ranged from 31 to 92 years, with a median of approximately 60 years. There was a slight male predominance (57 percent). Of patients with osteosarcoma over 21 years of age, 14 percent had tumors that developed in bones affected by Paget

Table 7

OTHER CONDITIONS ASSOCIATED WITH SUBSEQUENT OSSEOUS SARCOMAS

Precursor Condition	Sarcoma
Radiation	Osteosarcoma, MFH,* others
Paget disease	Osteosarcoma, MFH, others
Bone infarct	MFH, osteosarcoma, others
Fibrous dysplasia	Osteosarcoma, MFH
Prosthesis	Ewing sarcoma, MFH, osteosarcoma, angiosarcoma, lymphoma
Osteogenesis imperfecta	Osteosarcoma
Chronic osteomyelitis	Angiosarcoma, myeloma, lymphoma, osteosarcoma, fibrosarcoma[+]
Familial retinoblastoma	Osteosarcoma
von Recklinghausen disease	MFH, fibrosarcoma
Simple cyst	MFH, osteosarcoma
Aneurysmal bone cyst	Osteosarcoma

*Malignant fibrous histiocytoma
[+]Many older reports of fibrosarcoma are more likely MFH

disease. In patients over 40 years of age, the frequency rose to 20 percent.

Progressively increasing pain, often associated with a palpable mass was the most common complaint. Typically the pain was of less than 1 year's duration (mean, 5.6 months). Pathologic fractures occurred in only about 16 to 22 percent of cases. Serum alkaline phosphatase levels were above normal in 85 percent of patients and, in about half of patients, reflected a rise above previous premalignant levels associated with their Paget disease. "Explosive" increases in alkaline phosphatase were not demonstrable. Distant metastases were present at the time of diagnosis in 29 percent of patients in one series (26).

Sites. The skeletal distribution of osteosarcoma arising in Paget disease tends to parallel the distribution of uncomplicated Paget disease. The large tubular bones of the appendicular skeleton and the flat bones of the axial skeleton are involved with equal frequency, in contrast to the marked predilection for the long bones seen in primary osteosarcoma (11). In a series of 65 cases reported from Memorial Hospital, 37 percent involved the pelvic bones, 25 percent the leg, 23 percent the arm, and 14 percent the craniofacial bones. Involvement of the spine was uncommon, despite the relatively common occurrence of Paget disease in this location (4,11,26).

Radiographic Appearance. Lytic, sclerotic (fig. 5), and mixed patterns are seen. In the series from Memorial Hospital, tumors with a lytic appearance were the most common (64 percent), followed by sclerotic lesions (18 percent) (11). Periosteal reaction is less common than with sarcomas arising de novo (26).

Gross Findings. The gross appearance is similar to that of conventional high-grade intraosseous osteosarcoma or malignant fibrous histiocytoma, except for the changes of Paget disease in the surrounding bone (fig. 6).

Microscopic Findings. Most Paget sarcomas are histologically conventional, high-grade intramedullary osteosarcomas (figs. 7, 8). Fibrohistiocytic, osteoblastic, fibroblastic, and chondroblastic patterns of differentiation are all commonly observed. Telangiectatic and small cell variants are rare (26). Less frequently, Paget sarcomas may have microscopic features of malignant fibrous histiocytoma or fibrosarcoma.

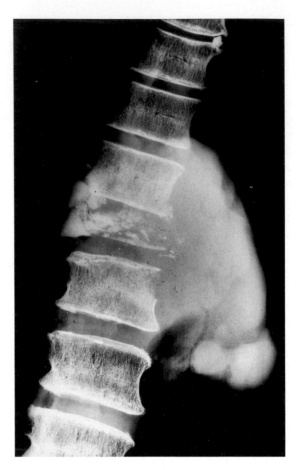

Figure 5
SARCOMA ARISING IN PAGET DISEASE OF BONE
Some vertebra have dense bone indicating Paget disease. A heavily mineralized osteosarcoma has arisen from one vertebral body and almost destroyed it. (Courtesy of Dr. K.W. Barwick, Jacksonville, FL.) (Figures 5 and 6 are from the same patient.)

Treatment and Prognosis. Therapeutic options for sarcomas arising in Paget disease are identical to those for their primary counterparts. Unfortunately, many of the patients have unresectable local or metastatic tumor at the time of presentation. The 5-year survival historically has been only about 5 to 8 percent. This is due, at least in part, to the tendency for flat bone involvement. Axial disease is far more difficult to surgically resect, and may remain clinically undetectable longer than a sarcoma involving an extremity. Poor prognosis of Paget sarcoma may also be the result of a delay in diagnosis due to masking of the lesion, symptomatically, by the pain associated with the Paget disease; more

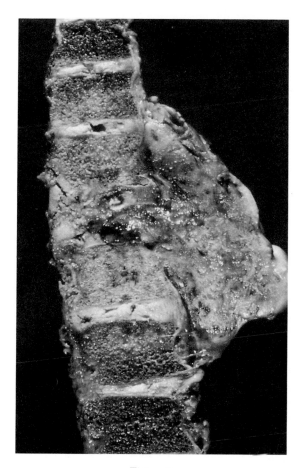

Figure 6
SARCOMA ARISING IN PAGET DISEASE
Coarse trabeculations are seen in vertebral bodies adjacent to the osteosarcoma. (Courtesy of Dr. K.W. Barwick, Jacksonville, FL.)

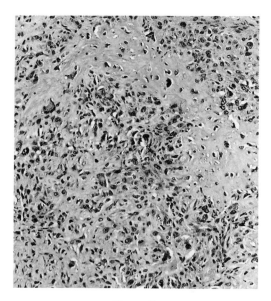

Figure 7
OSTEOSARCOMA ARISING IN PAGET DISEASE
A conventional, high-grade intramedullary osteosarcoma is present in a patient with vertebral Paget disease. (Figures 7 and 8 are from the same patient.)

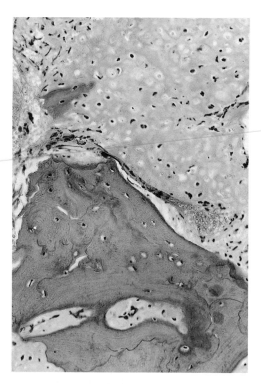

Figure 8
OSTEOSARCOMA ARISING IN PAGET DISEASE
Amorphous osteoid pattern of osteosarcoma (top) is adjacent to abnormal bone of Paget disease with irregular cement lines.

frequent metastases because of the highly vascular nature of the underlying disease; and the older age of the patients.

POSTRADIATION SARCOMA OF BONE

Definition. To be considered a postradiation or radiation-related sarcoma, the neoplasm should meet several criteria first proposed by Cahan et al. (6) and later modified by Arlen et al. (1). There must be microscopic or roentgenographic evidence that any precursor lesion was benign or, if malignant, was devoid of osteoblastic activity; radiation must have been given and the sarcoma documented to arise in the irradiated field; and a relatively long latent period must have elapsed between the radiation and the subsequent clinical appearance of the sarcoma. Cahan et al. initially suggested 5 years, but Arlen et al. proposed at least 3 to 4 years as a more realistic minimal interval. Finally, all sarcomas must be documented histologically.

General Features. The development of sarcomas in irradiated bones is uncommon, but well documented. Their occurrence should limit the use of radiation for the treatment of benign osseous lesions, and is a factor when considering treatment options for extraosseous lesions located adjacent to bones, such as breast carcinomas.

Tountas et al. (21) reviewed postradiation sarcomas of bone from the prechemotherapy era and showed a direct correlation between the amount of radiation absorbed and the incidence of a subsequent sarcoma. In patients receiving the usual therapeutic dose of up to 7000 rads, the incidence of postradiation sarcoma is approximately 0.2 percent. In patients receiving 20,000 rads, an obviously unusual circumstance, the incidence of subsequent sarcoma rises to over 20 percent. Patients receiving radiation below 1000 rads have an incidence of postradiation sarcoma that is approximately the incidence of de novo sarcoma. This suggests that there is a minimal threshold that must be exceeded (27).

There is suggestive evidence that patients treated with cytotoxic chemotherapy without radiation are at increased risk for developing sarcomas of bone as well (22). It remains to be seen whether patients treated with combined radiation therapy and chemotherapy have a higher risk of developing sarcomas in the irradiated field. There is one report of a 10-year-old who had four synchronous osteosarcomas in the fibula and tibia 8 years after radiation and chemotherapy for rhabdomyosarcoma of the calf (20).

Weatherby et al. (25) reviewed the Mayo Clinic experience with 78 postradiation sarcomas. The average latent period was 14.3 years. Osteosarcoma was the most common histologic type, accounting for 49 percent of the cases. Malignant fibrous histiocytomas and fibrosarcomas accounted for an additional 41 percent. The remainder were chondrosarcomas, with single cases of metastasizing chondroblastoma, lymphoma, and Ewing sarcoma. At Memorial Hospital 15.4 percent of skeletal malignant fibrosarcomas and 5.5 percent of osteosarcomas were postradiation tumors (12).

Clinical Features. Age at the time of diagnosis ranged from 9 to 77 years (mean, 45 years) in the series of 78 patients from the Mayo Clinic, with a slight female predominance (62 percent) (25). This was believed to be due to the relatively large number of postradiation sarcomas developing after radiation therapy for carcinomas of the breast, cervix, and endometrium.

Symptoms were similar to those of patients developing sarcoma without prior radiation. Pain and swelling, usually of abrupt onset, were common in contrast to the long and asymptomatic latent period following radiation.

Sites. Virtually any bone in the body may be involved. The axial skeleton, because of its closer association with the viscera receiving radiation, is more commonly affected than the extremities (22). The sacrum, pelvis, cranium, and shoulder girdle are common sites.

Radiographic Appearance. Roentgenograms usually indicate a malignant lesion, but sometimes malignant changes are obscured by the effect of the prior radiation. In patients who have received radiation for the treatment of a visceral carcinoma the radiographic diagnosis is often metastatic carcinoma (25).

Gross and Microscopic Findings. The tumors are indistinguishable from sarcomas arising de novo.

Treatment and Prognosis. Treatment regimens for postradiation sarcoma are identical to those for their "spontaneous" counterparts. Complete surgical excision, when possible, coupled with radiation and prophylactic chemotherapy are the therapeutic mainstays. In the series of 78 postradiation sarcomas of all types (predominantly osteosarcomas) reported by Weatherby et al. (25), 64 patients were eligible for 5-year survival calculations. For the 27 patients with sarcomas of the extremities, the 5-year survival was 30 percent and the 10-year survival was 26 percent. Twenty-four patients had sarcomas of the spine, pelvis, and shoulder girdle. All but 1 of these patients was dead of tumor in 4 years or less, and 17 died within 1 year. The remaining 13 patients eligible for follow-up had sarcomas of the skull and jaw bones. The 5-year survival in this group was 31 percent and 3 of the 4 survivors had sarcomas of the mandible. Postradiation sarcomas seem to have approximately the same prognosis as their "spontaneous" counterparts.

SARCOMAS ASSOCIATED WITH BONE INFARCTS

Bone infarcts are relatively common lesions, typically occurring in the metaphyseal region of the long bones, often around the knee. They seldom warrant biopsy, and are therefore infrequently encountered by pathologists, apart from avascular necrosis of the femoral head, which can be considered a form of acute or subacute infarction. A variety of conditions predispose to the development of bone infarcts including alcoholism; steroid therapy; renal dialysis; compressed air exposure such as occurs in caisson workers and divers; Legg-Perthes disease; hemoglobinopathies, especially sickle cell disease and trait; Gaucher disease; chronic pancreatitis; gout; and hereditary bone dysplasia (16).

General Features. The development of a sarcoma in a preexistent bone infarct is rare. Frierson et al. (9) noted that only about 31 malignant fibrous histiocytomas had been described in association with bone infarcts as of 1986, with few additional, sporadic case reports (10). More than 90 percent of patients with infarct-related sarcomas have evidence of multiple infarcts (16). The radiographic appearance of infarcts and an associated malignancy are illustrated on page 165.

Clinical Features. Patients range in age from 16 to 80 (median, 54) years (16). Males are affected twice as often as females, due in part to the increased incidence of occupationally related infarcts. Because of the association of infarcts with sickle cell disease and trait, black patients have accounted for 29 percent of cases. Complaints are nonspecific and typically consist of progressively worsening pain, with or without an associated mass (16). The interval between the development of the bone infarct and the subsequent sarcoma, when known, is usually a decade or more. In many instances, however, the asymptomatic, preexistent infarct is discovered at the same time as the sarcoma.

Sites. Most lesions center around the knee and proximal femur. Occasionally the humerus or radius may be involved (16). Metaphyseal lesions are by far the most common, followed by diaphyseal involvement and, rarely, epiphyseal lesions.

Radiographic Appearance. Chronic bone infarcts typically appear as irregular, but sharply demarcated intramedullary densities. The increased radiographic density is due to a combination of dystrophic calcification in areas of necrosis, as well as an increased amount of reactive bone surrounding the necrotic component. Serpiginous rims of calcification at the periphery of the infarct may focally mimic the "popcorn" calcifications of cartilage, but are of considerably greater size. Typically, multiple infarcts are present, involving, for example, both sides of a knee joint.

Areas of associated sarcoma appear as irregular zones of lytic destruction. As the majority are malignant fibrous histiocytomas, matrix production is not commonly seen radiographically.

Gross Appearance. Bone infarcts appear as sharply demarcated, serpiginous or ring-like areas of dense, yellow-tan tissue. Infarct-associated tumors have ranged in size from 5 to 15 cm (16). The sarcomatous component has the typical appearance of its de novo counterpart. Hemorrhage and necrosis are usually obvious, and cortical destruction or permeation is common.

Microscopic Appearance. Frierson et al. (9) demonstrated an interesting spatial arrangement to a bone infarct and its associated sarcoma. The sarcomatous component became increasingly more cellular and microscopically bizarre as one moved outward from the central, relatively acellular zone of infarction. These findings suggest that the sarcoma arises from a malignant transformation of the reparative, predominantly fibroblastic tissue located at the periphery of an infarct. Otherwise, sarcomas in bone infarcts display the typical microscopic features of malignant fibrous histiocytomas, high-grade intramedullary osteosarcomas, or, perhaps, fibrosarcomas.

Treatment and Prognosis. Sarcomas arising in bone infarcts are clearly high-grade, aggressive neoplasms. Mirra (16) noted that of 21 patients with follow-up, 57 percent died of disease from 6 to 48 (mean, 18) months after diagnosis. The principles of surgical intervention, chemotherapy, and radiation therapy applied to de novo osseous sarcomas are appropriate for the treatment of these secondary neoplasms.

SARCOMAS ARISING AT SITES OF PROSTHESES

There have been scattered reports of malignant fibrous histiocytoma, Ewing sarcoma, "hemangioendothelioma," osteosarcoma, and lymphoma arising at the sites of previously placed orthopedic prostheses (2,5,8,14,15,18,19). Because of the demonstrated carcinogenic effect, at least in animals, of some metals employed in these devices, this finding would appear to be of some concern. However, given the extreme rarity of sarcoma development in this setting, and the 300,000 to 400,000 total joint replacements performed annually worldwide, it is unlikely that a cause-effect relationship will be clearly demonstrated. In some cases, there was longstanding osteomyelitis, and this may also be a factor in the development of malignancy.

Patients with sarcomas in the sites of prostheses have ranged from children to elderly adults. The interval between insertion of the prosthesis and development of the sarcoma has spanned several years to decades. Most prostheses, however, had been present for greater than 10 years (14,19). Rare malignancies arising only a short time after prosthesis placement probably represent neoplasms that were present but not diagnosed at the time of prosthetic insertion. Prosthesis-related neoplasms have the same biologic behavior as their de novo counterparts.

SARCOMAS ARISING IN CHRONIC OSTEOMYELITIS

Chronic osteomyelitis with draining sinus tracts is occasionally associated with the development of squamous cell carcinoma (0.5 percent), most of which are well-differentiated neoplasms. Distinction from pseudoepitheliomatous hyperplasia, invariably present around sinus tracts, can be difficult (13,23). Intraosseous sarcomas also arise in this setting, though rarely. Sporadic reports have described myeloma, lymphoma, osteosarcoma, hemangioendothelioma, and "fibrosarcoma" arising in longstanding osteomyelitis (3,7,17,23,24). An associated prosthesis may make it impossible to determine whether either or both factors contributed to the development of the subsequent sarcoma. There is no evidence to suggest that the biologic behavior of these sarcomas differs from that of their de novo counterparts.

REFERENCES

1. Arlen M, Higinbotham NL, Huvos AG, Marcove RC, Miller T, Shah IC. Radiation-induced sarcoma of bone. Cancer 1971;28:1087–99.
2. Bagó-Granell J, Aguirre-Canyadell M, Nardi J, Tallada N. Malignant fibrous histiocytoma of bone at the site of a total hip arthroplasty. A case report. J Bone Joint Surg [Br] 1984;66:38–40.
3. Baitz T, Kyle RA. Solitary myeloma in chronic osteomyelitis. Arch Intern Med 1964;113:872–6.
4. Barwick KW, Huvos AG, Smith J. Primary osteogenic sarcoma of the vertebral column: a clinicopathologic study of ten patients. Cancer 1980;46:595–604.
5. Brien WW, Salvati EA, Healey JH, Bansal M, Ghelman B, Betts F. Osteogenic sarcoma arising in the area of a total hip replacement. A case report. J Bone Joint Surg [Am] 1990;72:1097–9.
6. Cahan WG, Woodard HQ, Higinbotham NL, Stewart FW, Coley BL. Sarcoma arising in irradiated bone: report of eleven cases. Cancer 1948;1:3–29.
7. Campanacci M, Boriani S, Giunti A. Hemangioendothelioma of bone: a study of 29 cases. Cancer 1980;46:804–14.
8. Dube VE, Fisher DE. Haemangioendothelioma of the leg following metallic fixation of the tibia. Cancer 1972;30:1260–6.
9. Frierson HF Jr, Fechner RE, Stallings RG, Wang GJ. Malignant fibrous histiocytoma in bone infarct. Association with sickle cell trait and alcohol abuse. Cancer 1987;59:496–500.
10. Gaucher AA, Regent DM, Gillet PM, Pere PG, Aymard BM, Clement V. Case report 656. Malignant fibrous histiocytoma in a previous bone infarct. Skeletal Radiol 1991;20:137–40.
11. Huvos AG, Butler A, Bretsky SS. Osteogenic sarcoma associated with Paget's disease of bone. A clinicopathologic study of 65 patients. Cancer 1983;52:1489–95.
12. _____, Woodard HQ, Heilweil M. Postradiation malignant fibrous histiocytoma of bone. A clinicopathologic study of 20 patients. Am J Surg Pathol 1986;10:9–18.
13. Johnson LL, Kempson RL. Epidermoid carcinoma in chronic osteomyelitis: diagnostic problems and management. J Bone Joint Surg [Am] 1965;47:133–45.
14. Lee YS, Pho RW, Nather A. Malignant fibrous histiocytoma at site of metal implant. Cancer 1984;54:2286–9.
15. McDonald I. Malignant lymphoma associated with internal fixation of a fractured tibia. Cancer 1981;48:1009–11.
16. Mirra JM. Bone tumors: clinical, radiologic, and pathologic correlations. Philadelphia: Lea & Febiger, 1989:780–94.
17. Morris JM, Lucas DB. Fibrosarcoma within a sinus tract of chronic draining osteomyelitis. Case report and review of literature. J Bone Joint Surg [Am] 1964;46:853–7.
18. Penman HG, Ring PA. Osteosarcoma in association with total hip replacement. J Bone Joint Surg [Br] 1984;66:632–4.
19. Tayton KJ. Ewing's sarcoma at the site of a metal plate. Cancer 1980;45:413–5.

20. Tillotson C, Rosenberg A, Gebhardt M, Rosenthal DI. Postradiation multicentric osteosarcoma. Cancer 1988; 62:67–71.

21. Tountas AA, Fornasier VL, Harwood AR, Leung PM. Postradiation sarcoma of bone: a perspective. Cancer 1979;43:182–7.

22. Tucker MA, D'Angio GJ, Boice JD Jr, et al. Bone sarcomas linked to radiotherapy and chemotherapy in children. N Engl J Med 1987;317:588–93.

23. Unni KK, Dahlin DC. Premalignant tumors and conditions of bone. Am J Surg Pathol 1979;3:47–60.

24. van der List JJ, van Horn JR, Sloof TJ, ten Cate LN. Malignant epithelioid hemangioendothelioma at the site of a hip prosthesis. Acta Orthop Scand 1988; 59:328–30.

25. Weatherby RP, Dahlin DC, Ivins JC. Postradiation sarcoma of bone: review of 78 Mayo Clinic cases. Mayo Clin Proc 1981;56:294–306.

26. Wick MR, Siegal GP, Unni KK, McLeod RA, Greditzer HG 3rd. Sarcomas of bone complicating osteitis deformans (Paget's disease): fifty years' experience. Am J Surg Pathol 1981;5:47–59.

27. Wiklund TA, Blomqvist CP, Räty J, Elomaa I, Rissanen P, Miettinen M. Postirradiation sarcoma. Analysis of a nationwide cancer registry material. Cancer 1991; 68:524–31.

OSSEOUS LESIONS

ENOSTOSIS (BONE ISLAND)

Enostoses are round, usually small (2 to 20 mm) intramedullary nodules of lamellar cortical bone. Most are encountered as incidental, asymptomatic findings in adults. They are not commonly seen by surgical pathologists but are diagnosed radiographically, preventing unnecessary biopsy. Virtually any bone may be involved. Occasionally, however, enostoses may be mistaken for metastases, osteoid osteoma, sclerotic osteosarcoma, calcified enchondroma, bone infarct, or other lesions (3).

Radiographically, enostoses are round or oval, sclerotic lesions (fig. 9). There is no evidence of bony destruction or periosteal reaction. There is a subtle blending into the surrounding medullary bone at the periphery of the mass. Bone scans do not typically detect these relatively inert lesions, although they occasionally can be quite active on bone scan, particularly the larger ones (2,3,6).

There are reports of enostoses slowly enlarging over several years or completely disappearing (1,4). Smith (7) described two giant enostoses that measured 4 cm in greatest dimension, and Gold et al. (2) described one of 5 cm. Lesions of this size may be radiographically confused with a sclerotic osteosarcoma, particularly of the intraosseous well-differentiated type, prompting biopsy. The occasional giant enostosis that exhibits increased radiolabel uptake has even greater potential for confusion with osteosarcoma (3). A lack of symptoms and the radiographic presence of thorny or feather-like radiating spicules of bone merging with the periphery of the lesion and creating a "brush border" are helpful features for recognizing enostoses (3).

Serial radiographs of larger, apparent enostoses may be performed. Mirra (5) suggested repeat radiographs at 1, 3, 6, and 12 months. Enlargement by 25 percent in 6 months or less, or by 50 percent in 1 year or less should prompt biopsy.

Grossly, enostoses are sharply defined hard masses (fig. 10). Microscopically, they usually consist entirely of lamellar cortical bone with a well-developed haversian system (fig. 11). The

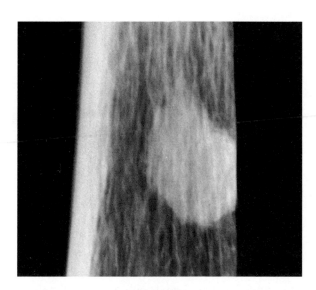

Figure 9
ENOSTOSIS
Specimen radiograph of enostosis that was an incidental finding in an amputation performed for an unrelated reason. A dense, circumscribed island of bone is evident. (Fig. 1D from Greenspan A, Steiner G, Knutzon R. Bone island (enostosis): clinical significance and radiologic and pathologic correlations. Skeletal Radiol 1991;20:85–90.) (Figures 9–11 are from the same patient.)

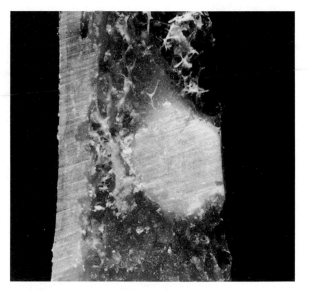

Figure 10
ENOSTOSIS
Cut surface of the enostosis reveals the bone island to be located in the medullary part of the bone. (Fig. 1C from Greenspan A, Steiner G, Knutzon R. Bone island (enostosis): clinical significance and radiologic and pathologic correlations. Skeletal Radiol 1991;20:85–90.)

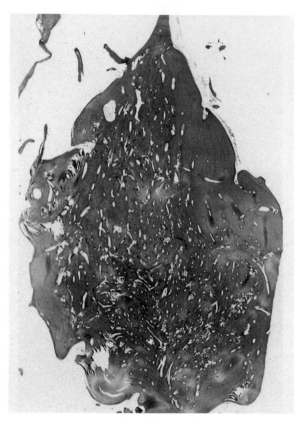

Figure 11
ENOSTOSIS
The entire lesion is seen as compact bone with only a few tiny vascular spaces. (Fig. 1E from Greenspan A, Steiner G, Knutzon R. Bone island (enostosis): clinical significance and radiologic and pathologic correlations. Skeletal Radiol 1991;20:85–90.)

spicules of cortical bone blend into the surrounding medullary bone without peripheral sclerosis. Occasionally there may be a compact mixture of lamellar and woven bone. The latter, usually minor component, is unlikely to cause diagnostic problems and may go unrecognized unless the section is examined under polarized light (2). Giant enostoses are microscopically identical to their smaller counterparts. These "islands" of lamellar cortical bone are easily distinguished from the compact woven osteoid and fibroblastic stroma of a well-differentiated osteosarcoma.

Osteopoikilosis or spotted bone disease is a rare, autosomal dominant condition characterized by multiple small, radiologically and histologically typical enostoses.

OSTEOMA

Definition. A tumor-like mass of abnormally dense, microscopically normal bone occurring almost exclusively in the skull, paranasal sinuses, and facial bones.

General Features. The actual frequency of osteoma is highly debatable due to the potential inclusion of reactive, posttraumatic or postinfectious changes, osseous overgrowth in response to a neoplasm, and old osteochondromas with involuted cartilaginous caps (10). Childrey (9) found radiographic evidence of osteomas in 15 of 3,510 (0.42 percent) paranasal sinus films.

Clinical Features. Osteomas have been reported in patients from 10 to 79 years of age, with most in the fourth or fifth decades of life (15). Sinus osteomas show a male predominance of 2 to 1, whereas lesions of the maxilla and mandible show a 3 to 1 female predominance. The presence of multiple osteomas or osteomas involving the long bones should suggest the possibility of Gardner syndrome (osteomas, cutaneous epidermal cysts, fibromatoses, adenomatous colonic polyposis). Osteomas may be asymptomatic, or, in the head and neck region, present with signs and symptoms of nasal and paranasal sinus obstruction. The symptoms have usually been present for several years. Rarely, there may be extension into the cranial cavity (11). Extracranial osteomas may cause symptomatic nerve compression (13).

Sites. Osteomas are most common in the frontal sinuses, followed by the ethmoids, antrum, and sphenoid sinuses in decreasing order of frequency. They may also involve the maxilla and mandible. Rarely, osteomas may arise from the external surface of long bones and are termed *parosteal osteomas*.

Radiographic Appearance. Radiographs are typically diagnostic and show a sharply circumscribed, radiopaque mass protruding from the bone surface. The surrounding bone typically lacks destructive changes. Osteomas within the sinus generally conform to the sinus contour (fig. 12). Patients with osteomas due to Gardner syndrome may have wavy, irregular cortical thickening of their long bones (8).

Gross and Microscopic Findings. There are two grossly and microscopically distinct patterns. Most lesions are of the "compact" or "ivory" type, grossly resembling dense, cortical bone.

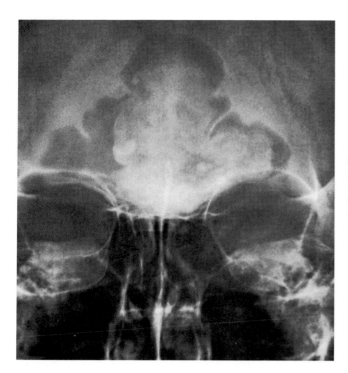

Figure 12
OSTEOMA
A 32-year-old woman complained of a feeling of full-
ness and a sensation of "jostling" in her forehead. The
radiograph disclosed a dense lobular mass in the frontal
sinus that conforms to the sinus contour. It was excised.
(Fig. 111 from Fascicle 5, 2nd Series.) (Figures 12 and 13
are from the same patient.)

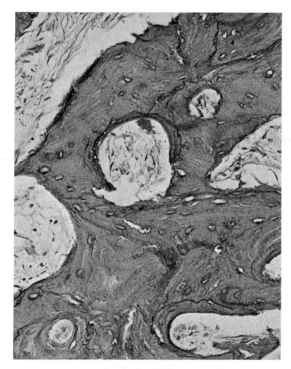

Figure 13
OSTEOMA
The mass consists of thick trabeculae of bone with focally
prominent cement lines. The patient is asymptomatic 7
years later. (Fig. 112 from Fascicle 5, 2nd Series.)

Microscopically, there is dense, lamellar bone
with no medullary component. Less frequently,
osteomas grossly contain both cortical and medullary bone. Microscopically, these "spongy,"
"trabecular," or "mixed" osteomas consist of
dense lamellar cortical bone and a medullary
component with intervening fibrofatty or hematopoietic marrow elements (fig. 13).

Differential Diagnosis. Although osteomas
involving the skull and facial bones represent a
distinct entity, in other locations the diagnosis may
not be clear. Even in the craniofacial region, osteomas can be confused with reactive new bone
formation, densely ossified fibrous dysplasia, or
solid odontomas (10). "Osteomas" of the long bones
may be osteochondromas with eburnated cartilaginous caps (12) or areas of organized periosteal
callus. The rare parosteal osteoma may produce a
radiographic image identical to that of a parosteal
osteosarcoma (10). Mirra (14) emphasized that the
parosteal "osteoma" is more likely to be a parosteal
osteosarcoma with central maturation to lamellar
bone and marrow elements. He described an oste-
oma-like parosteal osteosarcoma in which the neoplastic cells were confined to a microscopically thin
layer on the surface of the lesion. The tumor recurred several times during 30 years and eventually converted to a grade 2 parosteal osteosarcoma.

Treatment and Prognosis. Asymptomatic lesions require no therapy (11). Symptomatic lesions are usually treated by simple excision. This is often aided by the small base of attachment. Recurrences rarely, if ever, develop and malignant transformation has not been described.

OSTEOID OSTEOMA

Definition. A benign, highly vascular, sharply defined osteoblastic proliferation that is usually less than 1 cm in size.

General Features. Osteoid osteoma accounts for 2 to 3 percent of primary excised bone tumors and, in the Mayo Clinic Series, 12 percent of benign bone tumors (20). The nidus of an osteoid osteoma closely resembles, microscopically, the lesional tissue of an osteoblastoma (21). However, most cases can be clearly distinguished based on radiographic and clinical features. Osteoid osteomas are almost always single lesions, although rare multiple lesions have been described, often within the same bone or region (26).

Clinical Features. Osteoid osteomas show a marked predilection for the second decade of life. Most patients (75 to 80 percent) are 25 years of age or younger, and are rarely over 30 years of age. Overall, there is an approximately 2 to 1 male to female ratio. The classic clinical presentation is one of slowly progressive unremitting pain, worse at night and relieved, often dramatically, by aspirin. Although this mode of presentation, especially the marked response to aspirin, is probably overemphasized (19), the vast majority of patients do present with gradually progressing, often severe pain. In the Mayo Clinic series of over 200 cases, only two lesions were nonpainful (20). Frequently, the pain develops prior to a radiographically detectable lesion. Schulman and Dorfman (33), as well as others, have demonstrated the presence of unmyelinated nerve fibers accompanying the fibrovascular tissue in the nidus of osteoid osteoma. Wold et al. (39) have shown that osteoid osteomas, as well as some osteoblastomas, produce high levels of prostaglandin E_2. The prostaglandin inhibiting properties of aspirin may provide the mechanism for pain relief in susceptible patients. Soft tissue swelling and tenderness overlying an osteoid osteoma are also common findings (24).

Osteoid osteomas occurring in specific sites can produce additional site-related symptoms. Tumors near growing epiphyseal plates may accelerate growth in the affected bone, leading to skeletal asymmetry. Epiphyseal lesions are often associated with joint effusion, and this may result in a clinical misdiagnosis of arthritis (17,29,31). This mistake is often compounded when microscopic examination of the associated synovial tissue shows a chronic villous synovitis (17). Although this pattern is nonspecific, it is frequently mistaken for rheumatoid synovitis, further delaying the correct diagnosis and appropriate therapy. Osteoid osteoma of the extremities may cause atrophy of nearby muscles (34). Vertebral lesions may produce muscular spasm with resulting painful scoliosis or peripheral nerve compression (28). Pain may be referred to other sites, often an adjacent joint.

Sites. Virtually any bone may be involved, although in several large series the skull and sternum were not affected and clavicular lesions were rare. There is a predilection for the legs; about 50 percent of cases involve the femur or tibia. Involvement of the femur favors the proximal metaphysis, but tibial involvement occurs more uniformly throughout the bone. About 10 percent of lesions involve the spinal column, most commonly the arch elements rather than the vertebral bodies. The diaphyses and metaphyses are usually affected, but rare osteoid osteomas occur in the epiphyses. Osteoid osteomas are usually intracortical in origin, but can develop within the medullary canal or in the subperiosteal region, especially in the femoral neck, vertebrae, and small bones of the hands and feet (fig. 14) (23).

Radiographic Appearance. When radiographically detectable, osteoid osteoma has a highly characteristic appearance. There is typically a zone of marked sclerosis surrounding a well-demarcated central area of relative radiolucency. Because of the sclerotic reaction, the central lucency or nidus may be difficult to detect. This difficulty increases as the nidus matures and becomes calcified and more radiopaque. Ossification of the nidus usually occurs from the center outward, producing a central zone of density surrounded by a ring of radiolucency (ring sequestrum). Cortical and subperiosteal osteoid osteomas are typically associated with dense reactive sclerosis. The

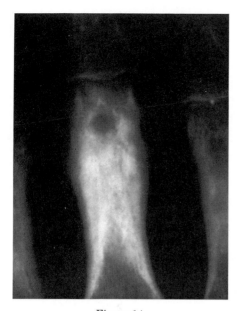

Figure 14
OSTEOID OSTEOMA
Intramedullary sclerosis proximal to a nidus of osteoid osteoma in the phalanx.

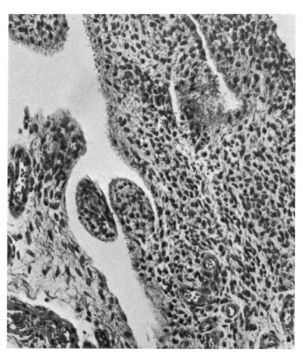

Figure 16
OSTEOID OSTEOMA
Synovitis associated with osteoid osteoma. The synovium from the hip joint contains a chronic inflammatory infiltrate and secondary villous formation. The finding of synovitis and an effusion may obscure or delay the diagnosis of an osteoid osteoma in the nearby bone. (Fig. 114 from Fascicle 5, 2nd Series.)

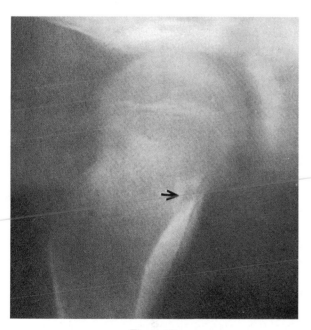

Figure 15
OSTEOID OSTEOMA
This tomogram shows an osteoid osteoma in the femoral neck of a 12-year-old girl treated for arthritis because of a painful effusion. After several months, this radiograph was taken demonstrating sclerosis around the nidus (arrow). There is also periosteal new bone formation that corresponds with the extracapsular reaction to the lesion. Intracapsular reactive bone is lacking. (Fig. 113 from Fascicle 5, 2nd Series.) (Figures 15 and 16 are from the same patient.)

subperiosteal new bone formation typically lacks the "sunburst" or "onionskin" appearance of malignant bone tumors. Intramedullary lesions often evoke a less dense, more diffuse sclerotic reaction (27). Alternately, they may be associated with osteoporosis of the affected bone (35). Intra-articular osteoid osteomas are notoriously difficult to identify because there is no periosteum around the intracapsular bone to produce the periosteal component of the reactive sclerosis (27). If the nidus is not detectable, the patient may be treated for arthritis because of a painful effusion (figs. 15, 16).

When routine radiographs fail to detect the nidus of an osteoid osteoma, standard tomograms, computed tomography, angiography, and magnetic resonance imaging have each been advocated by various authors as the most sensitive technique for nidus localization. Bauer et al. (17) noted that standard tomography detected 9 of 11 intra-articular osteoid osteomas, computed tomography detected 8 of 11 cases, and magnetic resonance imaging detected 3 of 5 cases. In contrast, Bell et al. (18) described a case in which magnetic resonance imaging was the only modality that successfully localized the lesion. Bone scans are of value in documenting increased isotope uptake in the region of a suspected osteoid osteoma, but they usually lack the resolution necessary to localize the nidus and reactive synovitis in an adjacent joint may also stimulate isotope uptake.

Gross Findings. Finding the tiny nidus may pose considerable difficulty for the surgical pathologist, as well as the surgeon. If examination of the submitted fragments does not readily reveal its location, then an overpenetrated specimen X ray may be necessary. Vigorita and Ghelman (37) described a technique of specimen autoradiography following intravenous technitium-99m and excision of the suspected bone fragments. Although quite accurate, this procedure requires up to 8 hours for an image to form on the radiographic film. Alternately, Ayala et al. (16) showed that tetracycline given preoperatively is taken up by the osteoblastic nidus and results in fluorescence of the nidus under ultraviolet light. Others have found this technique to be somewhat insensitive (27).

Once uncovered, the nidus usually appears as a spherical, red to tan mass of gritty, osseous tissue. It is almost always less than 1 cm in greatest dimension and may easily "shell out" from the surrounding reactive bone (fig. 17).

Microscopic Findings. Microscopically, the nidus is sharply demarcated from the surrounding sclerotic bone, often by an intervening fibrovascular zone (fig. 18). It varies in appearance from lesion to lesion but, except for a tendency toward central maturation, is generally uniform in any given case. In poorly ossified osteoid osteomas, the nidus has a highly vascularized stroma and densely packed osteoblasts, producing tangled, thin, lace-like strands of osteoid (fig. 19). Osteoclasts may also be prominent. Intermediate lesions have more abundant osteoid with varying degrees of calcification. Mature nidi consist of well-calcified, compact trabeculae of woven bone and osteoid (fig. 20). The osteoblasts of osteoid osteoma have plump, uniform, active-appearing nuclei, often with mitotic activity. There are no atypical mitotic figures, and the woven bone shows prominent osteoblastic rimming. Cartilage is absent, unless there has been a fracture

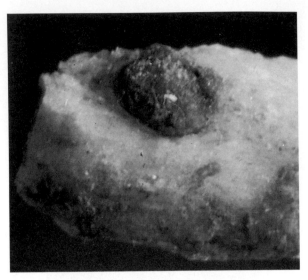

Figure 17
OSTEOID OSTEOMA
Osteoid osteoma from the femur of a 12-year-old girl has a 0.8 cm red nidus, sharply separated from the sclerotic surrounding bone.

through the lesion, previous surgical manipulation, or if it is subarticular. Marrow hematopoietic elements and fat are also absent. Scattered lymphocytes and plasma cells may be seen, but acute inflammation is not present.

Surrounding the central nidus is a variable, 1 to 2 mm zone of less trabeculated fibrovascular tissue. Outside of this fibrovascular zone is a layer of sclerotic, nondiagnostic cortical or medullary bone with a compact, lamellar pattern. The interface between the nidus or fibrovascular zone and the surrounding reactive bone is abrupt, with no evidence of infiltration by the woven bone of the nidus into the surrounding lamellar reactive bone. Occasionally, there is no reactive bone (fig. 21).

Differential Diagnosis. The radiographic differential diagnosis includes intracortical abscess, osteosarcoma, sclerosing osteomyelitis, enostosis, aseptic necrosis, stress fracture, eosinophilic granuloma, and metastasis. Once the nidus is found in the surgical specimen, the diagnosis is usually straightforward.

Confusion with osteosarcoma should seldom if ever occur, given the distinctive clinical setting and small size of this lesion. Rarely, however, small osteosarcomas may be entirely intracortical. These tumors lack the loose, highly vascular

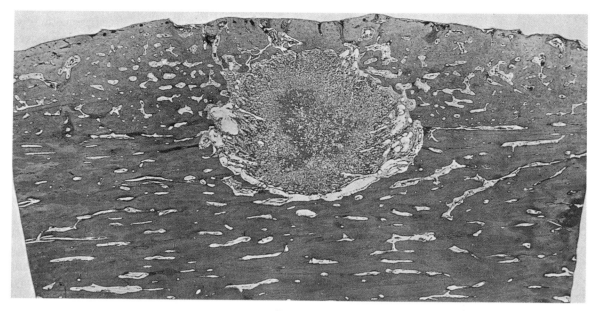

Figure 18
OSTEOID OSTEOMA
This whole mount section from the femur of a 22-year-old man demonstrates densely sclerotic cortical bone surrounding the intact nidus of an osteoid osteoma. (Fig. 116 from Fascicle 5, 2nd Series.)

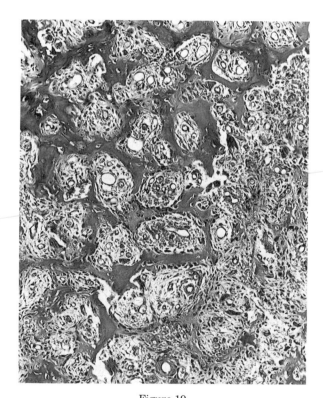

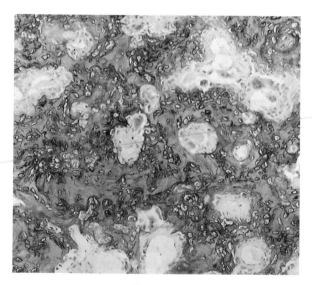

Figure 20
OSTEOID OSTEOMA
Compact bone with minimal stroma can occur in more "mature" osteoid osteomas.

Figure 19
OSTEOID OSTEOMA
The trabeculae of woven bone are lined with osteoblasts and set in a vascular, loosely fibrous stroma.

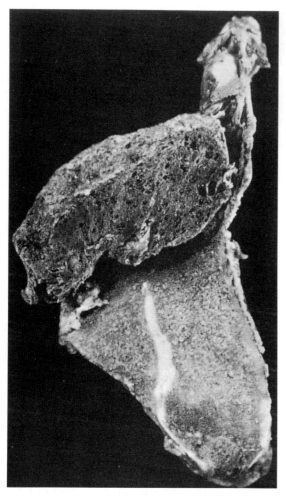

Figure 23
OSTEOBLASTOMA
This osteoblastoma of the ilium is a gritty, well-circumscribed, and highly vascular lesion. The tumor recurred after previous partial removal. (Fig. 139 from Fascicle 5, 2nd Series.)

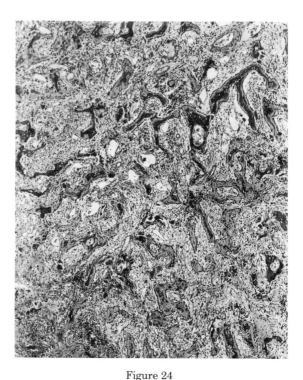

Figure 24
OSTEOBLASTOMA
Osteoblastoma has haphazard proliferation of interlacing trabeculae in a fibrovascular stroma.

the amount of osteoid increases until it accounts for 50 percent or more of the lesional tissue (44). There is also considerable intralesional variation with regard to the thickness of the trabeculae and their degree of calcification. Broad, well-mineralized trabeculae and narrow trabeculae of unmineralized osteoid may exist in close approximation. Some areas of osteoblastoma have rather broad sheets of mineralized osteoid with little intervening stroma. More typically, there is a prominent fibrovascular tissue between the islands and trabeculae that has a loose, areolar configuration with prominent, dilated capillaries (fig. 25) (50). The osteoblasts are plump, active, and have scattered typical-appearing mi-

totic figures. Although osteoblastoma may appear highly cellular, there is little or no cytologic atypia in the conventional form. Prominent osteoblastic rimming of the trabeculae is present, at least focally. Osteoclasts may also be numerous along the trabeculae in areas of resorption. Unless there has been a fracture or a previous curettage, osteoblastoma lacks areas of chondroid differentiation (52,55). Osteoblastoma is one of the many tumors that may undergo secondary aneurysmal bone cyst formation (53,64) and such foci were present in 16 percent of cases in one study (53).

Bizarre Osteoblastoma. A "pseudomalignant" variant of osteoblastoma has been described (54, 57). These lesions contain bizarre multinucleated cells completely devoid of mitotic activity. The authors suggest that the atypical cells are a degenerative change. In the example described in detail by Mirra et al. (57), there was no evidence, microscopically, of cartilage formation. The lesion was well circumscribed, radiographically benign, and the patient is alive and well 8 years later. Bizarre (pseudomalignant) osteoblastoma may

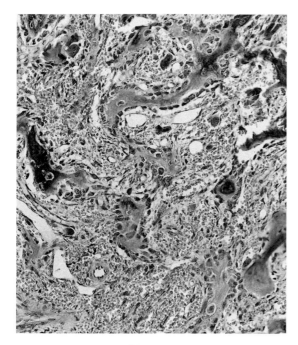

Figure 25
OSTEOBLASTOMA
Trabeculae are lined by large but uniform osteoblasts. Mineralization has taken place focally. The stroma contains many capillaries and much extravasated blood in a loose fibrous background.

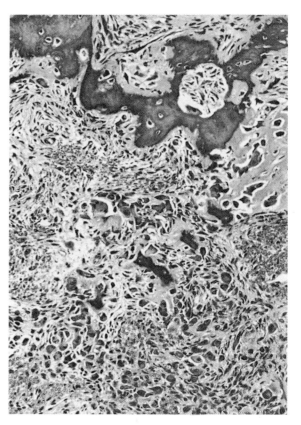

Figure 26
AGGRESSIVE OSTEOBLASTOMA
Orderly mineralized trabeculae of bone characteristic of osteoblastoma are seen on the top adjacent to unorganized osteoid and aggregates of "epithelioid" osteoblasts are at the bottom. (Fig. 506 from Fascicle 5(Suppl), 2nd Series.)

be analogous to other pleomorphic, mitotically inactive mesenchymal lesions such as bizarre leiomyoma of the uterus.

Aggressive Osteoblastoma. Multiple studies have clearly documented a group of osteoblastoma-like neoplasms with a distinctive microscopic appearance and a much more aggressive local behavior than that of conventional osteoblastoma (40,45,46,58,59,61). However, there is considerable dispute regarding the nature of these lesions and their appropriate terminology. The term "aggressive osteoblastoma" was first applied to these lesions by Dorfman in 1973 (45). Schajowicz and Lemos (61) subsequently described eight microscopically similar cases which they chose to label as "malignant osteoblastoma," an arguably confusing term for an apparently nonmetastasizing, albeit locally aggressive variant. In 1984, Dorfman and Weiss (46) reviewed 15 cases of aggressive osteoblastoma and proposed that these lesions were distinct from "innocuous" or low-grade osteosarcoma. Further complicating the issue, Bertoni

and colleagues (40) proposed that aggressive osteoblastomas were, in fact, really osteosarcomas that resembled osteoblastomas.

Although occasional borderline osteoblastic lesions may arise in which the differentiation from osteosarcoma is quite difficult, we believe that aggressive osteoblastoma is a distinct clinicopathologic entity that should not be labeled as a variant of osteosarcoma. Microscopically, these tumors contain a trabecular pattern of osteoid similar to that of typical osteoblastoma, although there is often a tendency toward wider, more irregular trabeculae (fig. 26). As in conventional osteoblastomas, osteoblastic rimming is prominent and scattered osteoclasts are frequent. In 7 of 15 cases reported by Dorfman and Weiss (46), there were small areas of nontrabecular, sheet or "lace-like" osteoid, but these areas were never

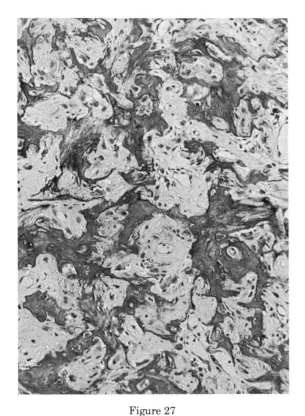

Figure 27
AGGRESSIVE OSTEOBLASTOMA
Calcified osteoid has very few cells. The calcification is dense and irregularly distributed. (Fig. 508 from Fascicle 5(Suppl), 2nd Series.)

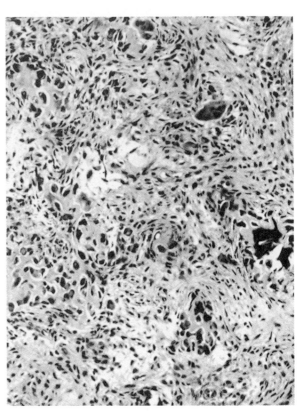

Figure 28
AGGRESSIVE OSTEOBLASTOMA
Minimal osteoid formation is associated with large, "epithelioid" osteoblasts. This poorly organized osteoid set in a moderately cellular fibrous stroma is one of the variable patterns of osseous maturation seen in both typical, as well as aggressive osteoblastomas. (Fig. 507 from Fascicle 5(Suppl), 2nd Series.)

prominent (fig. 27). The stroma separating the trabeculae in aggressive osteoblastoma has the same loose, fibrovascular quality as that seen in more conventional forms (fig. 28). Mitotic rate is variable and may be focally high, but atypical mitotic figures are not present. Cartilage is never present in the absence of fracture or prior surgery.

The most distinctive microscopic feature of aggressive osteoblastoma is the cytologic appearance of many of the osteoblasts. These cells are about twice as large as typical osteoblasts and have a distinctly epithelioid quality with abundant eosinophilic cytoplasm (fig. 29). Nuclei may also be enlarged and often have a vesicular, histiocyte-like appearance (46).

Aggressive osteoblastoma occurs in a broad age range (7 to 80 years), and many patients are over 30 years of age, distinctly older than individuals with typical osteoblastoma. A wide variety of bones may be involved including the femur,

spine, skull, pelvis, bones of the hands and feet, humerus, tibia, and fibula. Radiographically, the tumors tend to be slightly larger than typical osteoblastoma, ranging up to 8.5 cm in greatest dimension. Most have well-defined margins, focal areas of radiographically visible matrix, and variable amounts of perilesional sclerosis. Occasional aggressive osteoblastomas have marginal irregularities or periosteal reactions suggesting possible malignancy and they may invade adjacent bones (fig. 30) (63).

Of 13 patients with follow-up reported by Dorfman and Weiss (46), 7 developed recurrences from 10 months to 2 years after treatment. None had metastases or died of disease. Of the eight cases reported by Schajowicz and Lemos (61), four developed local recurrences, one died of local

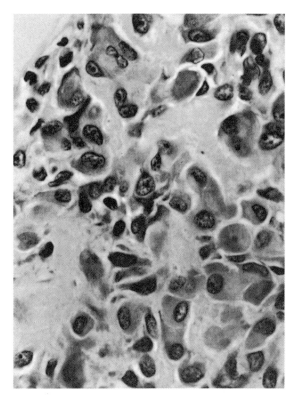

Figure 29
AGGRESSIVE OSTEOBLASTOMA
Large "epithelioid" osteoblasts have abundant, deeply staining cytoplasm. The nuclei are "active" with finely clumped chromatin and small but prominent nucleoli. Osteoid is irregularly intermixed. A field like this could be seen in osteosarcoma, but areas with this appearance must be examined in the context of the entire case. (Fig. 509 from Fascicle 5(Suppl), 2nd Series.)

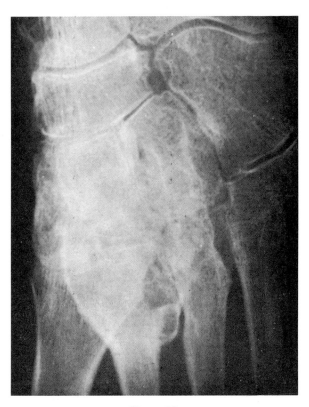

Figure 30
AGGRESSIVE OSTEOBLASTOMA
An expansile lesion of the second metatarsal involves adjacent bones. (Fig. 7 from Steiner GC. Ultrastructure of osteoblastoma. Cancer 1977;39:2127–36.)

disease, and none developed metastases. This locally aggressive but nonmetastasizing behavior strongly suggests that aggressive osteoblastoma should be distinguished from both conventional osteoblastoma and low-grade osteosarcoma. The relationship between aggressive osteoblastoma and deceptively osteoblastoma-like osteosarcoma requires further study. Mitchell and Ackerman (58) described a unique aggressive osteoblastoma which, after radiation therapy, converted to a typical osteosarcoma.

Differential Diagnosis. *Osteosarcoma.* The distinction between typical osteoblastoma and conventional osteosarcoma is almost always straightforward both radiologically and microscopically. However, occasional osteosarcomas have a benign radiographic appearance and, as discussed above, rare osteoblastomas contain cytologically bizarre, but mitotically inactive cells. The differentiating microscopic features for osteoblastoma and osteosarcoma are discussed under the differential diagnosis of conventional osteosarcoma.

Osteoid Osteoma. Osteoid osteoma is rarely confused with osteoblastoma because of the usual clear-cut clinical and radiographic differences. Although the nidus of an osteoid osteoma is quite similar, microscopically, to the lesional tissue of an osteoblastoma, there are minor microscopic differences (60). The periphery of an osteoid osteoma nidus often has a fibrovascular rim, not seen in osteoblastoma. The latter tumor, in contrast, often has a lobulated or multifocal outer margin. The nidus of an osteoid osteoma often shows a distinctly zonal pattern with central maturation to thicker, more highly mineralized woven bone.

Except for this tendency toward central maturation, the osseous tissue in an osteoid osteoma has osteoid and woven bone at a relatively uniform stage of maturation in any given lesion. In contrast, osteoblastomas typically display considerable variation in the thickness and degree of calcification of the woven osteoid trabeculae.

Giant Cell Tumor. As much as 40 percent of giant cell tumors produce woven bone. Distinction from osteoblastoma is important because giant cell tumor is a more aggressive neoplasm. Giant cell tumors of the long bones almost invariably involve the epiphysis, whereas osteoblastomas are rare at this site (53). Giant cell tumors are uncommon in the vertebrae and, when present, almost always arise in the body. Vertebral osteoblastomas favor the arch and processes. In osteoblastoma, the giant cells are smaller, have fewer nuclei, and many represent true osteoclasts that pepper the surfaces of the osteoid and woven bone. Osteoblastoma does not contain the large zones of giant cells and mononuclear stromal cells that are diagnostic of giant cell tumor.

Aneurysmal Bone Cyst. Osteoblastoma and aneurysmal bone cyst have clinical and radiographic similarities (53). Furthermore, as mentioned above, osteoblastomas may have a secondary aneurysmal bone cyst component. Marsh et al. (53) noted such components in 4 of 25 osteoblastomas. Both lesions often involve the spine and, occasionally, may be confused radiographically. Aneurysmal bone cyst is highly unlikely to be misdiagnosed microscopically as osteoblastoma, but all aneurysmal bone cysts must be carefully examined to exclude the presence of an associated primary lesion such as osteoblastoma.

Treatment and Prognosis. In spite of their often alarming histologic appearance, 90 to 95 percent of conventional osteoblastomas are cured by initial therapy. The biologic behavior of the aggressive variant is discussed above. Lesions of the weight-bearing long bones are treated by curettage. Lesions of the small bones of the feet, the fibula, and the rib are more easily removed by complete resection. Partially resected and incompletely curetted osteoblastomas may regress postoperatively, even without radiotherapy, although this is extremely rare. Spinal lesions producing neurologic symptoms may be radiated if unresectable. The efficacy of radiation for osteoblastoma is uncertain and spo-

radic postradiation sarcomas have been reported (53). Recurrences represent regrowth of incompletely resected disease and seldom occur more than 2 years postoperatively. "Osteoblastomas" with rapid, massive local recurrences are likely to be misdiagnosed osteosarcomas and osteoblastomas that recur 5 or more years after initial therapy may represent rare examples of osteoblastoma transforming into osteosarcoma.

CONVENTIONAL INTRAMEDULLARY OSTEOSARCOMA

Definition. A malignant neoplasm of bone that demonstrates at least focal osteoid production by neoplastic cells. In conventional (high-grade) intramedullary osteosarcoma the predominant histologic pattern may be osteoblastic, fibroblastic, chondroblastic, giant cell rich, malignant fibrous histiocytoma-like, or partially telangiectatic. Small cell, pure telangiectatic, well-differentiated, and multifocal variants of intramedullary osteosarcoma have been segregated from the conventional group and are discussed elsewhere, as are intracortical and surface osteosarcoma subtypes.

General Features. Excluding multiple myeloma, osteosarcomas are the most commonly biopsied primary tumors of bone (69). In the Mayo Clinic experience with 8,542 primary osseous neoplasms, osteosarcomas accounted for 16 percent of all such tumors and 19 percent of all malignant tumors of bone (69). More than 90 percent of osteosarcomas are of the "conventional" high-grade intramedullary type.

Osteosarcoma may arise as a de novo lesion or develop secondarily to a known premalignant lesion such as Paget disease, osteogenesis imperfecta, bone infarct, chronic osteomyelitis, fibrous dysplasia, giant cell tumor, osteoblastoma, and others (97), or to a process such as radiation therapy. These secondary osteosarcomas are discussed in a separate chapter and in the sections dealing with the underlying benign neoplasm.

It is well documented that some cases of osteosarcoma appear to be familial (77). In particular, children with familial bilateral retinoblastoma have an incidence of osteosarcoma several hundred times that of an age-matched general population (72). This appears to represent both a genetic predisposition to de novo neoplasia and an increased susceptibility to radiation-induced sarcoma. Retinoblastoma and osteosarcoma, as well as certain other malignancies, share a deletion in chromosome 13 which renders a normally occurring anti-oncogene (termed the retinoblastoma or RB gene) inactive (66). Patients with familial disease inherit one inactive and one active RB gene, requiring only a single "hit" to develop neoplasia, whereas sporadic tumors appear to require the inactivation of the RB gene on both copies of the diploid chromosome 13 before tumorigenesis occurs.

There are various routes to the development of osteosarcomas, since not all such tumors show retinoblastoma gene abnormalities. In vitro, however, osteosarcoma cell lines having retinoblastoma gene deletions lose their neoplastic phenotype when the cells are given a cloned normal RB gene by retrovirus infection (80). Such "gene infusions" do not affect the tumorigenesis of osteosarcomas having normal retinoblastoma genes (80).

Clinical Features. Approximately 85 percent of patients with de novo osteosarcoma present before 30 years of age. More than 60 percent are in their second decade of life. The tubular bones are by far the most frequently involved and the longer the bone grows, both in time and size, the greater the risk for the development of osteosarcoma (89). Thus, the active growth phase appears to be a particularly vulnerable period. Males, perhaps because of greater growth, a longer period of active growth, and a greater volume of actively growing tissue, are affected slightly more often than females by a ratio of about 1.25 to 1 (69).

The most common presenting complaint is pain, usually from 1 to 8 months' duration. Within weeks this is usually accompanied by swelling of the overlying soft tissues. If pain has been present for greater than 1 year, it is highly unlikely that the underlying lesion is a conventional osteosarcoma. Pathologic fractures are uncommon at the time of initial presentation, occurring in less than 5 percent of patients.

Serum alkaline phosphatase levels may be elevated, particularly in patients with heavily osteoblastic tumors. A postexcisional rise in serum alkaline phosphatase generally heralds the development of recurrent or metastatic disease (83). Anaplastic osteosarcomas with little osteoblastic activity may not have elevated serum levels. Conversely, elevated serum alkaline phosphatase may also be seen in benign processes such as osteomyelitis, fracture callus, and osteoblastoma.

Sites. Conventional osteosarcoma shows a marked predilection for the metaphyseal regions of the long bones. Only about 8 percent arise in the diaphysis (69) and rarely in the epiphysis (96). The distal femur accounts for approximately one third of all cases and is the single most common site, followed by the proximal tibia, and the proximal humerus (69). Overall, 75 percent of osteosarcomas arise in the long tubular bones. In patients over 25 years of age, however, almost half occur in the flat bones (99); many of these are secondary lesions associated with premalignant conditions (97).

Osteosarcoma distal to the wrist or ankle does occur (85,86), but is extremely rare, and is most often secondary to a premalignant process such as Paget disease. Florid reactive periostitis of the phalanges (94) should not be confused with an extramedullary osteosarcoma.

Radiographic Appearance. Osteosarcomas may appear either lytic or sclerotic radiographically, but most often they have a mixed lytic and sclerotic appearance. Approximately two thirds have virtually diagnostic radiographs (82). Most of the remainder have a nonspecific but malignant appearance. Osteosarcomas rarely appear benign radiographically (70).

The classic radiographic finding is a large, infiltrating metaphyseal lesion that arises in medullary bone and erodes through the cortex to form a large soft tissue mass. The intramedullary and soft tissue components often contain foci of mineralized tumor osteoid producing fluffy or "cumulus cloud" densities. The soft tissue mass lacks the concentric rim of periosteal bone typically seen surrounding benign, expansile tumors. The overlying periosteal bone is, instead, stimulated to form Codman triangles (fig. 31), sunbursts, and onionskins (fig. 32). These periosteal changes are indicative of a rapidly growing lesion, but are by no means diagnostic of malignancy. A few osteosarcomas are confined to the medullary cavity at the time of presentation. These lesions may be more difficult to diagnose radiographically, and the intramedullary osteoblastic

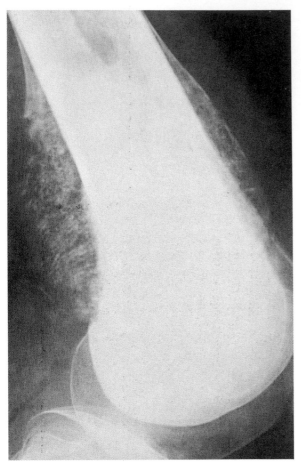

Figure 31
CONVENTIONAL
INTRAMEDULLARY OSTEOSARCOMA

This osteosarcoma from the distal femoral metaphysis arose in a 20-year-old man who had pain for 6 months. There is dense intramedullary bone formation that obscures the cortical markings. A striking periosteal reaction consists of spiculated new bone formation and Codman angles, seen at the upper part of the photograph. (Fig. 143 from Fascicle 5, 2nd Series.)

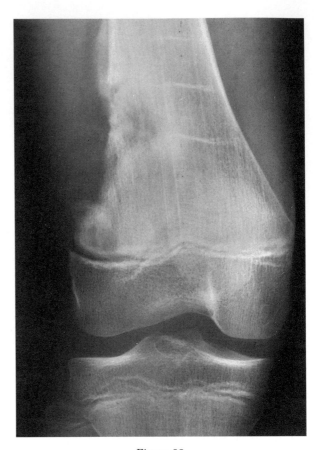

Figure 32
CONVENTIONAL
INTRAMEDULLARY OSTEOSARCOMA

A part of the cortex is destroyed with osteosarcoma. A Codman triangle is seen proximal to the cortical break. The medullary portion of the bone contains irregular calcified matrix.

activity can be confused with benign processes such as stress fractures.

When osteosarcomas lack radiographic evidence of matrix production, their permeative growth is diagnostic of malignancy, but their exact nature can only be suggested. Nonetheless, a radiographically malignant lesion in the metaphysis of a patient under 30 years of age has a very high probability of being an osteosarcoma.

Gross Findings. The great majority of resection specimens demonstrate penetration of the cortex with an often large extraosseous tumor mass (fig. 33). The permeative nature of the intramedullary component is usually obvious, and infiltration of the marrow space may extend for several centimeters from the main tumor mass. Proximal rather than distal extension is favored and occasionally this will be associated with apparent "skip lesions" separated by grossly normal-appearing marrow (73,98). The gross appearance of the neoplastic component is highly variable and reflects the mixture of stromal components present (pl. I). Osteoblastic elements appear as white-tan to yellow, firm, finely gritty tissue; chondroblastic differentiation produces translucent lobules; and fibroblastic or fibrohistiocytic areas appear as tan, soft to firm masses. Foci of hemorrhage and necrosis are common, and large hemorrhagic areas may represent zones of telangiectatic-type change.

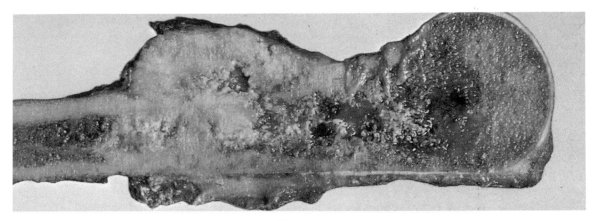

Figure 33
CONVENTIONAL INTRAMEDULLARY OSTEOSARCOMA
This osteosarcoma in the proximal portion of the humerus from a 22-year-old woman shows an intramedullary tumor with cortical destruction and soft tissue extension. The tumor had a hard, gritty consistency indicating a prominent osteoblastic component. (Fig. 147 from Fascicle 5, 2nd Series.)

The periosteal reaction is often grossly visible as spicules or lamellae of new bone at the periphery of the lesion. Metaphyseal osteosarcomas only rarely grossly penetrate an active epiphyseal plate, although one study suggests that microscopic penetration is present in 75 percent of open epiphyses (74). Involvement of the joint space is uncommon and usually develops by cortical penetration and capsular invasion of the soft tissue mass, rather than by extension through the articular cartilage.

Microscopic Findings. Most osteosarcomas are easily recognized, based on their high-grade, obviously anaplastic cells and unequivocal osteoid production (fig. 34). By definition, the sarcomatous component may assume a variety of appearances including osteoblastic, chondroblastic, fibroblastic, malignant fibrous histiocytoma-like, giant cell predominant, small cell, and telangiectatic. The last two variants are discussed in separate sections. Regardless of the predominant microscopic pattern, if focal osteoid production by neoplastic cells is present, the lesion is classified as an osteosarcoma.

The neoplastic cells in most conventional, high-grade osteosarcomas have marked nuclear pleomorphism, conspicuous chromatin abnormalities, prominent nucleoli, and many mitotic figures, some of which are atypical. It is generally easier to identify cytologically malignant

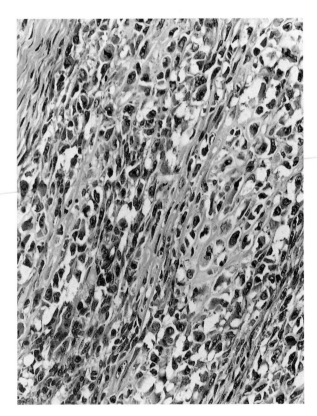

Figure 34
CONVENTIONAL
INTRAMEDULLARY OSTEOSARCOMA
Markedly pleomorphic osteoblasts are separated by delicate, lace-like osteoid or lie in aggregates.

PLATE I

A. TELANGIECTATIC OSTEOSARCOMA

This coronal section through a telangiectatic osteosarcoma is from the upper end of the tibia in a 20-year-old woman. Numerous blood-filled spaces are evident with minimal solid tissue component. In less than a year the patient died with metastases containing similar blood-filled spaces. (Pl. III–D from Fascicle 5, 2nd Series.) (Plates A and B are from the same patient.)

B. TELANGIECTATIC OSTEOSARCOMA

The sparse solid areas of telangiectatic osteosarcoma show pleomorphic cells and irregular deposits of osteoid. (Pl. III–C from Fascicle 5, 2nd Series.)

C. HEMORRHAGIC OSTEOSARCOMA

This hemorrhagic osteosarcoma involves the metaphyseal-diaphyseal regions of the proximal tibia. Cortical destruction and extraosseous extension are obvious. Tumoral osteoid appears yellow-white. (Pl. III–A from Fascicle 5, 2nd Series.)

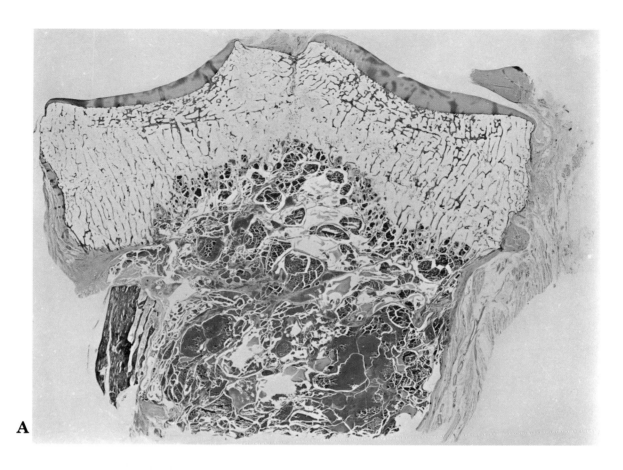

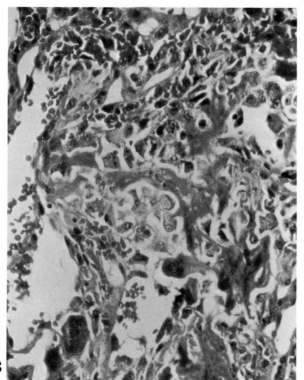

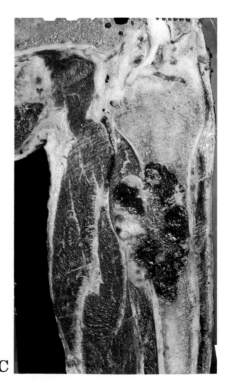

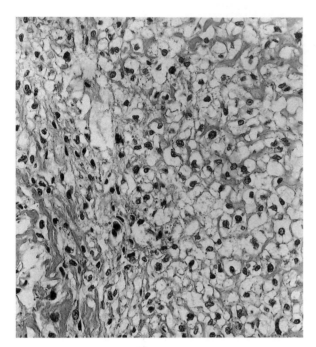

Figure 35
CONVENTIONAL
INTRAMEDULLARY OSTEOSARCOMA
There is focal osteoid formation at the upper right. The malignant osteoblasts have abundant, predominantly clear cytoplasm with minimal pleomorphism.

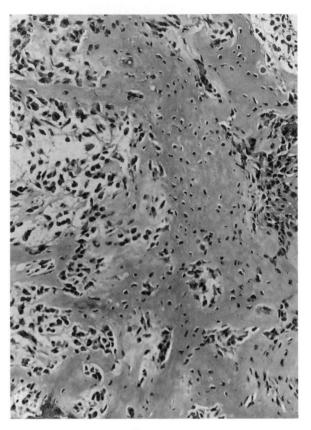

Figure 36
CONVENTIONAL
INTRAMEDULLARY OSTEOSARCOMA
Neoplastic osteoblasts form thin and thick trabeculae of osteoid. The osteosarcoma cells entrapped in the thicker trabeculae have smaller, more uniform nuclei, a phenomenon referred to as "normalization."

cells in more cellular areas, away from prominent osteoid formation. Some osteosarcomas have cells with a low nuclear to cytoplasmic ratio and minimal pleomorphism (fig. 35). There is a tendency for the neoplastic cells to become smaller and less pleomorphic as they become incorporated into the neoplastic osteoid (fig. 36). This well-recognized phenomenon has been referred to as "normalization" of malignant osteoid. Osteosarcoma typically forms closely knit or "streamer" osteoid with little intervening stroma. The neoplastic osteoid lacks the prominent osteoblastic rimming characteristic of osteoblastoma, osteoid osteoma, and reactive proliferations.

Osteoid has variable patterns and degrees of mineralization. Broad islands of osteoid may never mineralize, and conversely, delicate, thin trabeculae of osteoid may become densely mineralized. When narrow, interlacing trabeculae of osteoid are mineralized, the bone stands out with a conspicuously filigreed pattern highly charac-

teristic of osteosarcoma (fig. 37). It is the quantity of mineralization that determines whether the tumor will have a lytic or sclerotic appearance radiographically. The original bone may be focally retained within the neoplasm and serve as a scaffold upon which osteoid is deposited by the neoplastic cells (fig. 38).

Some osteosarcomas consist predominantly or almost exclusively of medium- to high-grade, chondroblastic foci (fig. 39). A careful search should be made between the cartilaginous lobules for areas of unequivocal osteoid production by neoplastic cells. Specimen radiographic and gross correlation may also be necessary to direct the pathologist to areas of apparent osseous matrix production.

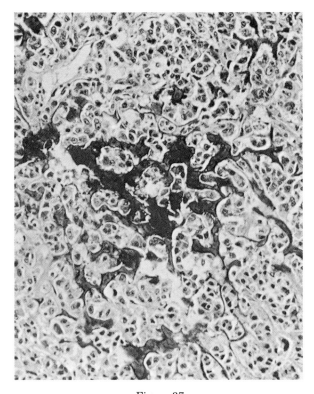

Figure 37
CONVENTIONAL
INTRAMEDULLARY OSTEOSARCOMA
The osteoid in the center of the field is heavily calcified, accentuating its lace-like or filigreed pattern. (Fig. 154 from Fascicle 5, 2nd Series.)

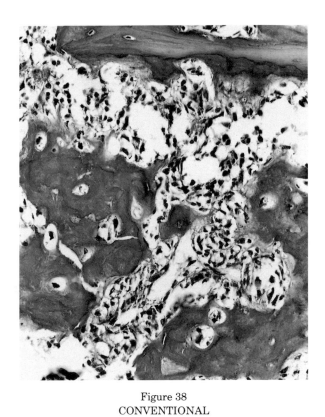

Figure 38
CONVENTIONAL
INTRAMEDULLARY OSTEOSARCOMA
A preexisting, normal trabecula of lamellar bone (top) has formed a "scaffolding" for irregular deposits of "neoplastic" osteoid on its surface. The larger deposits of "neoplastic" osteoid in the bottom two thirds of the figure lack a preexistent scaffolding.

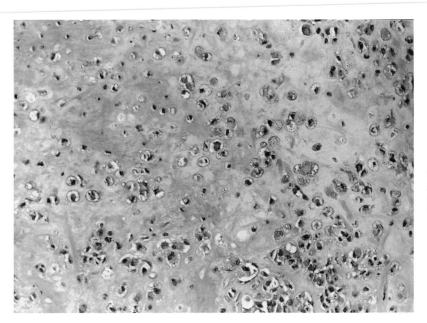

Figure 39
CONVENTIONAL
INTRAMEDULLARY
OSTEOSARCOMA
This predominantly chondroblastic osteosarcoma contained large areas of low-grade cartilaginous differentiation. Clear-cut osteoblastic foci were present elsewhere in the tumor.

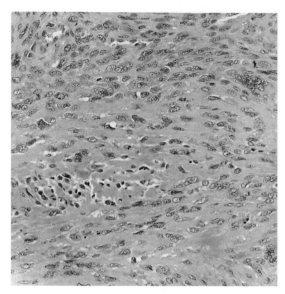

Figure 40
CONVENTIONAL
INTRAMEDULLARY OSTEOSARCOMA
Large areas of some osteosarcomas consist only of spindle cells, often in a "herringbone" pattern, resembling fibrosarcoma.

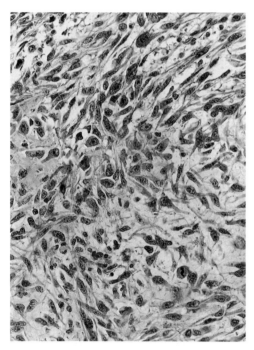

Figure 41
CONVENTIONAL
INTRAMEDULLARY OSTEOSARCOMA
This osteosarcoma contained areas in which spindled, fibroblast-like tumor cells were loosely arranged, often creating centrally radiating or storiform patterns. This appearance overlaps with that of malignant fibrous histiocytoma.

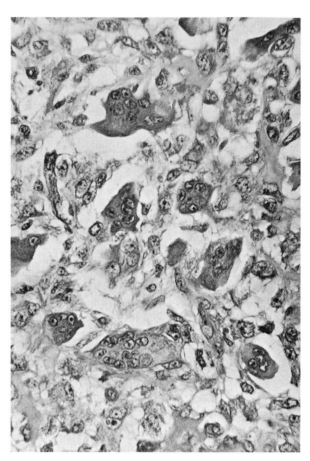

Figure 42
CONVENTIONAL
INTRAMEDULLARY OSTEOSARCOMA
This osteosarcoma shows minimal osteoid deposition and has many non-neoplastic, multinucleated giant cells. The intervening neoplastic mononuclear cells have markedly abnormal nuclei, however. This giant cell–rich pattern of osteosarcoma must not be confused with giant cell tumor. (Fig. 161 from Fascicle 5, 2nd Series.)

In the fibrosarcomatous pattern of osteosarcoma, the stroma is composed of spindle cells (fig. 40) that focally produce a "herringbone" pattern. Osteosarcomas may contain large areas that resemble malignant fibrous histiocytoma (fig. 41), often with a nondiagnostic, storiform pattern. There may be an admixture of pleomorphic spindled cells and enlarged, often bizarre polygonal cells. The presence of focal osteoid production distinguishes this osteosarcoma variant from malignant fibrous histiocytoma of bone.

A particularly treacherous form of conventional osteosarcoma has large numbers of cytologically bland, reactive stromal giant cells (fig. 42) that

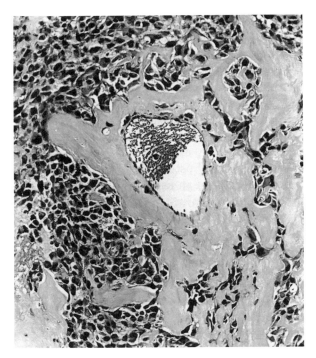

Figure 43
CONVENTIONAL
INTRAMEDULLARY OSTEOSARCOMA
Dense osteoid surrounds a blood vessel. It is associated with closely packed, markedly pleomorphic osteoblasts having dense nuclei.

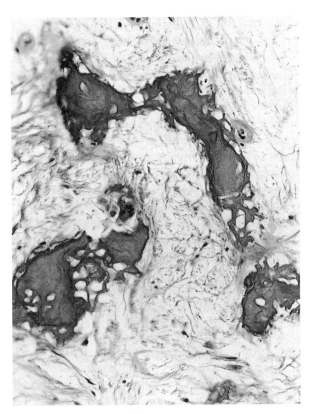

Figure 44
TREATED CONVENTIONAL OSTEOSARCOMA
This osteosarcoma was treated with preoperative chemotherapy and radiation therapy. The remaining calcified trabeculae are almost completely acellular. The intervening tissue is loose, edematous fibrous tissue without recognizable tumor cells.

may obscure the underlying sarcomatous stroma. Osteoid production may be sparse and must be carefully searched for, often with specimen radiographic correlation. Careful study will yield areas of definite stromal anaplasia and osteoid production; the latter may have an unusual, perivascular distribution (fig. 43).

In patients undergoing preoperative chemotherapy, the microscopic appearance of the resultant tumor necrosis varies with the form of preexistent osteosarcoma (91,92). Necrotic osteoblastic foci appear as acellular osteoid matrix (fig. 44). Chondroblastic foci appear similar to acellular chondroid, often with "ghost cells" in lacunae. Areas of fibrous or fibrohistiocytic differentiation are typically replaced by collagen, granulation tissue, and inflammatory cells. Necrotic telangiectatic foci appear as acellular, blood-filled cysts. In all necrotic forms, scattered, single, markedly atypical stromal cells may be present and are of uncertain significance.

Differential Diagnosis. *Osteoblastoma.* The distinction between osteoblastoma and osteosarcoma is typically straightforward, both radiographically and histologically. However, about 10 percent of osteosarcomas may appear radiographically benign and, conversely, up to 25 percent of osteoblastomas may have radiographic features of malignancy (84). Dorfman and Weiss (71) suggested that problems in distinction between osteoblastoma and osteosarcoma can be divided into four categories: osteosarcomas that histologically bear some resemblance to osteoblastomas (68); unusual osteoblastomas that have undergone spontaneous transformation into osteosarcomas; rare clinically and radiographically typical osteoblastomas that show bizarre pseudosarcomatous histologic changes (84,87); and locally aggressive osteoblastomas with distinctive histologic features. For practical purposes, only the first and last

such subtyping does not have prognostic value. The prognostic implications of three specific variants of intramedullary osteosarcoma, telangiectatic, small cell, and intraosseous well-differentiated, are discussed in separate sections.

Clearly, a number of clinical features do affect prognosis. Lesions of flat bones, with the exception of osteosarcoma of the jaw, have a poorer prognosis than extremity lesions. Local extent of tumor, specifically invasion of two or more structures adjacent to the involved bone, has been associated with a significant decrease in disease-free survival (93).

MULTIFOCAL OSTEOSARCOMA

Multifocal osteosarcomas are a distinct and extremely uncommon subgroup of intramedullary osteosarcoma. They should be divided into *synchronous* and *asynchronous types* because of their markedly different biologic behavior. Synchronous lesions appear to develop or are discovered more or less simultaneously. Mirra (103) has suggested that lesions discovered within 6 months of each other be considered as synchronous.

Synchronous multifocal osteosarcomas probably represent multifocal primary lesions and have been divided into childhood-adolescent and adult types. The hypothesis of multiple primaries, rather than osseous metastases, is based on several features including the rapid, simultaneous, and often symmetric appearance of the lesions; their often similar size, without a dominant lesion; rarity of osseous metastases in typical osteosarcoma; and the usual absence of pulmonary metastases early in the clinical course (102). Paget disease or other underlying "premalignant" bone lesions are not seen in these patients. Others have argued, however, in favor of a metastatic origin for the multiple lesions (102). Mahoney et al. (102) have suggested that genetic markers, such as variable expression of X-linked glucose-6-phosphatase dehydrogenase in females, might resolve the issue of separate primaries versus multiple primary tumors.

Patients with the childhood-adolescent form of synchronous multifocal osteosarcoma typically present with symmetric long bone disease. The average patient is 10 years of age; the range is 5 to 17 years (102). The lesions are predominantly osteoblastic (figs. 45–47) and histologi-

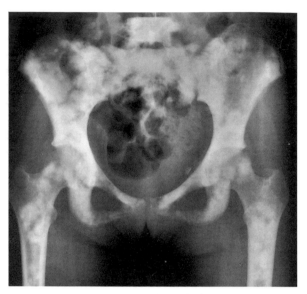

Figure 45
MULTIFOCAL OSTEOSARCOMA
A 15-year-old girl presented with bilateral hip pain of 6 weeks' duration. Multiple osteoblastic lesions are present in both femurs, pelvis, sacrum, and vertebra. (Figs. 45–47 are from the same patient.)

cally high grade. They are often confined to the medullary cavity with little or no extraosseous extension at the time of initial diagnosis. The outcome is invariably fatal, with mean survival of about 6 to 8 months (100).

The adult form of synchronous, multifocal osteosarcoma is less common than the childhood-adolescent form. The patients have varied in age from 23 to 51 (mean, 37) years. In contrast to the childhood-adolescent form, these neoplasms are often better differentiated and resemble intraosseous well-differentiated osteosarcoma. The outcome is again invariably fatal, but the survival ranges from 5 to 70 (mean, 29) months (100,102).

Asynchronous, multifocal osteosarcoma is slightly more common than the synchronous variety. Mahoney et al. (102) suggest that patients developing metachronous lesions less than 24 months after the initial lesion was detected probably have metastases, whereas later lesions may represent delayed metastases or, possibly, new primaries. The literature includes several long-term survivors with metachronous, multifocal osteosarcomas and patients should not be assumed to have the uniformly fatal outcome associated with synchronous disease (101).

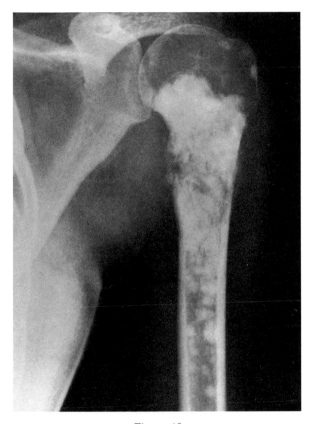

Figure 46
MULTIFOCAL OSTEOSARCOMA
The left humerus has multiple osteoblastic lesions. The distal tumors are separated from one another suggesting multiple sites.

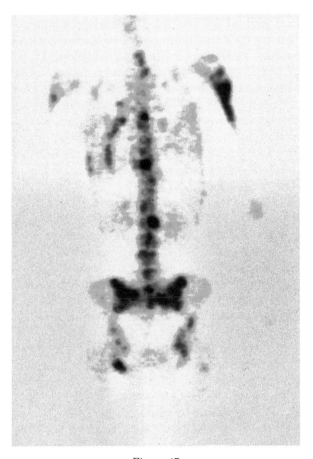

Figure 47
MULTIFOCAL OSTEOSARCOMA
A bone scan shows additional lesions in the vertebra, ribs, and right humerus.

Differential Diagnosis. The possibility of metastatic disease should always be considered in the evaluation of osseous neoplasms, and this is especially true when dealing with multiple lesions. In particular, sarcomatoid renal cell carcinoma may widely involve bones, mimicking a multifocal osteosarcoma. As Mirra (103) has indicated, however, such metastases are quite disseminated and invariably involve the axial skeleton, particularly the skull. Multifocal osteosarcoma is a disease of long bones. Immunohistochemistry may be of value in distinguishing a sarcomatoid carcinoma with exuberant reactive bone from an osteosarcoma. To date, osteosarcomas have not been shown to express epithelial markers such as low molecular weight cytokeratins and epithelial membrane antigens. Such markers are often, but not invariably, present in sarcomatoid carcinomas.

TELANGIECTATIC OSTEOSARCOMA

Definition. A radiographically lytic osteosarcoma variant characterized by cystic vascular spaces separated by thin septa of conventional osteosarcoma.

General Features. This variant has been reported to account for 0.4 to 12 percent of osteosarcomas (108,110,112,116,118). This variation in incidence may be due to the amount of radiographic sclerosis allowed for diagnosis, as well as differences in patient populations. The highest percentages (11 percent and 12 percent) have come from the Memorial Sloan-Kettering Cancer Center (110,116). Several studies indicate that the telangiectatic variant accounts for approximately 4 percent of osteosarcomas (108,113,114,117,118).

Clinical Features. Presenting signs and symptoms are similar to those of conventional osteosarcoma, except that pathologic fractures are present in over 25 percent of patients (118). Pain and swelling of under 1 year's duration involving an extremity is typical. There is a male predilection of about 2 to 1. Patients range in age from 3 to 71 years, but most are in their second decade of life. Older patients and patients with axial skeletal disease often have preexistent Paget disease.

Sites. As with conventional osteosarcoma, there is a predilection for the metaphyseal regions of the long bones. A representative composite series of well-documented cases had the following distribution: distal femur, 48 percent; proximal humerus, 12 percent; proximal tibia, 10 percent; proximal femur, 8 percent; fibula, 5 percent; mid-femur, 2 percent; mid-humerus, 2 percent; rib, 2 percent; with rare cases involving the mid-tibia, distal tibia, pelvis, skull, calcaneus, sternum, distal ulna, and mandible (105). Extraskeletal telangiectatic osteosarcoma has also been reported (110).

Radiographic Appearance. Most radiologists and pathologists have a definitional requirement that telangiectatic osteosarcoma be a purely lytic lesion radiographically (108,113, 114,118). The radiographic appearance is often diagnostic (113). Most are central, metaphyseal defects with permeative margins indicative of aggressive, rapid growth (fig. 48). Occasionally telangiectatic osteosarcomas have better defined margins, but perilesional sclerosis is not seen (118). Cortical destruction, soft tissue extension, and periosteal reaction were each present in 86 percent of cases in one study (118). Codman triangles were documented in 78 percent of cases. The tumors often extend into the epiphysis and up to the articular cartilage in patients with closed growth plates (113). Occasionally this tumor may closely simulate or be radiographically indistinguishable from an aneurysmal bone cyst (111).

Gross Findings. These tumors may assume several appearances grossly. They may appear as a large blood clot, a hemorrhagic and necrotic mass, or a multicystic lesion filled with fluid blood and closely resembling an aneurysmal bone cyst (pl. I–A). By definition, sclerotic or "fleshy" sarcoma-like tissue is not seen.

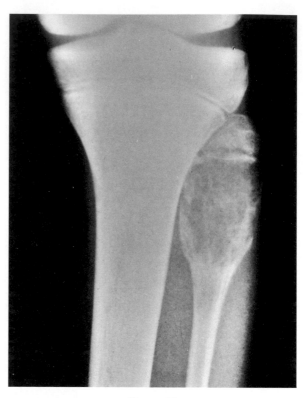

Figure 48
TELANGIECTATIC OSTEOSARCOMA
A 14-year-old girl had pain in the region of her knee. Radiographs showed a destructive, expansile, lytic lesion in the proximal fibula, involving both the metaphysis and epiphysis.

Microscopic Findings. Two microscopic patterns have been identified that correspond to their gross counterparts (108,114). In the hemorrhagic and necrotic variant, recognizably malignant cells are often widely separated in a background of blood and necrotic debris (108,114). It may be necessary to examine several slides before overtly malignant cells are identified (114). Osteoid matrix may be minimal and, in about 20 percent of cases, will not be present in biopsy material (113). Even in the absence of osteoid, the characteristic radiographic and microscopic features should allow diagnosis.

The second variant of telangiectatic osteosarcoma has a low-power appearance identical to that of aneurysmal bone cyst. Curettings from large lesions of this type may yield only sparse fragments of tissue, after exclusion of the cyst contents. Necrosis is typically sparse or absent. At higher magnification, the cyst walls contain overtly malignant cells with enlarged, densely

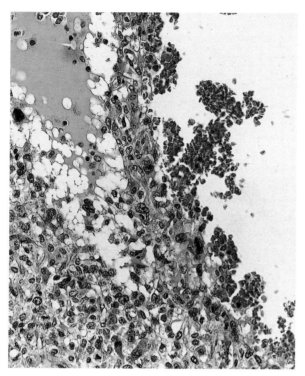

Figure 49
TELANGIECTATIC OSTEOSARCOMA
Cells with markedly abnormal nuclei are present in the septa and line the vascular spaces. An endothelial lining to the vascular spaces is not present. (Courtesy of Dr. M. Kyriakos, St. Louis, MO.)

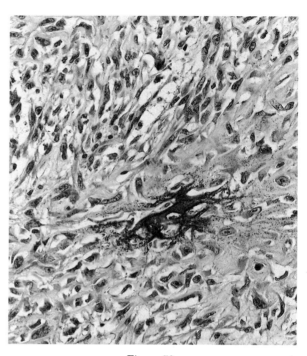

Figure 50
TELANGIECTATIC OSTEOSARCOMA
Delicate, calcified osteoid in a filigree pattern is present within a septum primarily composed of sarcomatous spindle cells. (Courtesy of Dr. M. Kyriakos, St. Louis, MO.)

hyperchromatic nuclei and atypical mitotic figures (pl. II–B). Anaplastic tumor cells often form the actual cyst lining (fig. 49), in combination with benign giant cells. Osteoid production is focal and has a delicate, lace-like appearance in contrast to the denser aggregates of osteoid in the trabeculae of aneurysmal bone cyst (fig. 50).

Ultrastructural study of two cases revealed malignant endothelial cells (angiosarcomatous elements) as well as malignant osteoblasts and malignant fibroblasts (115). Others, however, have been unable to identify malignant endothelial cells (119).

Differential Diagnosis. Typical osteosarcomas may contain areas of telangiectatic change. Such "mixed tumors" should, however, have gross evidence of a solid tumor component, often with radiographic sclerosis. The diagnosis of telangiectatic osteosarcoma should be reserved for pure, lytic lesions. Conventional osteosarcomas may also contain widely dilated, sinusoidal vascular channels. Unlike telangiectatic osteosarcoma, however, the latter are lined by flattened endothelial cells.

The confusion between telangiectatic osteosarcoma and aneurysmal bone cyst represents one of the most treacherous pitfalls in bone pathology (109). Misdiagnoses can be made in both directions. Telangiectatic osteosarcoma is much less common than aneurysmal bone cyst, and the diagnosis should be approached with caution. As discussed above, the radiographic appearance may be nonspecific or misleading. Usually, aneurysmal bone cyst will have more sharply defined radiographic margins, often with peripheral "eggshell" calcification. The distinction must ultimately be made microscopically and rests on finding obviously anaplastic cells in the osteosarcoma. Atypical mitotic figures are frequently present and the osteoid has a delicate "lace-like" pattern. It has been suggested that morphometric studies may be of value in differentiating telangiectatic osteosarcoma from aneurysmal bone cyst (117). Ruiter et al. (117) noted that a computerized analysis allowed discrimination of these lesions with a high degree of certainty. Important discriminants include largest nuclear surface area, mitotic index, and percentage of nuclear cross sections greater than 60 μm^2.

Spread and Metastasis. Telangiectatic osteosarcoma has a metastatic pattern similar to that of conventional osteosarcoma. However, there appears to be an increased tendency for local recurrence following treatment with less than amputation (107,113).

Treatment and Prognosis. Prior to the widespread use of chemotherapy, telangiectatic osteosarcoma, as strictly defined, had an abysmal prognosis (113). Twenty-four of the 25 patients in the original Mayo Clinic study published in 1976 died of disease (113). More recent studies from the postchemotherapeutic era indicate a prognosis at least as good as that of conventional osteosarcoma. Nine of 19 patients diagnosed at the Mayo Clinic after 1976 were alive at last follow-up (108). Rosen et al. (116) reported that 17 of 25 patients with telangiectatic osteosarcoma in their study from Memorial Hospital were free of disease with a mean follow-up interval of 5.5 years. A similar survival was noted in the 33 patients with follow-up from the Istituto Rizzoli (104). Pulmonary metastases have completely regressed with chemotherapy (106).

SMALL CELL OSTEOSARCOMA

Definition. A microscopically and, to a lesser degree, clinically distinct variant of intramedullary high-grade osteosarcoma. The tumor consists of small, malignant cells resembling the cells of Ewing sarcoma or large cell lymphoma. Osteoid production by the neoplastic cells may be focal but, by definition, is always present. Examples of small cell osteosarcoma have been included under older, more general terms such as polyhistioma and primitive multipotential primary sarcoma of bone.

General Features. This unusual variant accounts for 1 to 4 percent of all osteosarcomas, and is considerably less common than Ewing sarcoma. Approximately 75 cases have been reported, most of these in four series from the Mayo Clinic (127), Istituto Rizzoli (121), M.D. Anderson Hospital (120,123), and the National Cancer Institute (128,124). Almost all small cell

osteosarcomas appear to represent de novo lesions, although rare examples have originated in Paget disease (127). The relationship between small cell osteosarcoma and other small cell tumors affecting bone such as Ewing sarcoma and primitive neuroectodermal tumor is unclear. Recent studies indicate that these small cell tumors share a characteristic t(11;22) chromosomal translocation (125). In one tumor, 90 percent of the cells of small cell osteosarcoma were diploid with 13 percent in S-phase, a lower percentage of cells in S-phase than in most conventional osteosarcomas (126). The remaining 10 percent of cells were tetraploid with 23 percent in S-phase, an S-phase fraction comparable to conventional osteosarcomas.

Clinical Features. Patients have findings similar to those associated with conventional high-grade intramedullary osteosarcoma. Pain and swelling are the most common symptoms, seldom present for more than 1 year in the absence of a preexisting lesion (120,121,124,127). There is a slight female predilection of 1.3 to 1. Although patients in their eighties have been reported, about 70 percent are in the first or second decades of life.

Sites. There is a predilection for the metaphyseal regions of the long bones. The 70 patients reported in four series (120,121,127,128) had 71 tumors in the following locations: distal femur, 23; proximal tibia, 8; proximal humerus, 7; proximal femur, 5; mid-femur, 5; pelvis, 5; scapula, 4; distal tibia, 3; fibula, 3; jaw, 2; mid-humerus, 2; mid-tibia, 1; distal humerus, 1; talus, 1; and skull, 1.

Radiographic Appearance. Small cell osteosarcoma almost always has a permeative, "radiographically malignant" appearance. Cortical destruction with extraosseous extension is common. Some lesions may be completely lytic, but over 90 percent have at least focal osteoblastic features. Sometimes the entire lesion, including metastases, is densely osteoblastic (126). Osteoid produced by tumor cells must be distinguished from an osteoblastic reaction in the surrounding, non-neoplastic bone. Irregular, neoplastic osteoid within the soft tissue extension of the tumor may be easier to recognize than its intramedullary counterpart. Edeiken et al. (123) indicate that the diagnosis of small cell osteosarcoma is suggested when osteoblastic foci are seen in the metaphyseal region, associated with a permeative lesion that extends well down into the shaft of the bone. More importantly, the radiographic recognition of tumor osteoid excludes a diagnosis of Ewing tumor when osteoid is missing from a biopsy containing only small blue cells.

Gross Findings. Small cell osteosarcoma cannot be distinguished grossly from conventional high-grade osteosarcoma.

Microscopic Findings. By definition, osteoid production must be present in association with small, round to spindled tumor cells. Typically, the osteoid is sparse and has a delicate, "lace-like" appearance (fig. 51). Rare examples of densely sclerotic small cell osteosarcomas have been described. Foci of cartilaginous differentiation are present in at least one third of cases. Typically, the neoplastic cells grow in sheets and solid nests with densely cellular areas. A focal hemangiopericytoma-like pattern with prominent, branching blood vessels is common. Necrosis is not conspicuous and mitotic figures may be sparse or rare.

Ayala et al. (120) divided small cell osteosarcomas into three histologic patterns. The most common Ewing sarcoma-like pattern, seen in two thirds of their cases, consists of round to polygonal cells with densely hyperchromatic nuclei or coarsely clumped nuclear chromatin. Although the nuclei can be uniform, they often exhibit more variation in size and shape than is typically encountered in Ewing tumors. The second or lymphoma-like pattern consists of cells with slightly larger, more vesicular nuclei and prominent nucleoli (figs. 52, 53). This pattern resembles large cell lymphoma or the large cell variant of Ewing sarcoma. Small cell osteosarcoma may also consist of closely packed, spindle-shaped cells with only scant amounts of indistinct cytoplasm. Mixtures of these patterns may be seen.

Since the cells of small cell osteosarcoma may contain cytoplasmic glycogen, this finding cannot be used for distinction from Ewing sarcoma. Reticulin stains document an abundant, fine reticulin pattern that surrounds individual cells and small cell groups. There are currently no immunohistochemical markers of value to diagnose small cell osteosarcoma, although markers may be used to exclude other possibilities.

Ultrastructural Features. The cells of small cell osteosarcoma generally have scant cytoplasm and few organelles. Free ribosomes are the most consistently prominent organelles

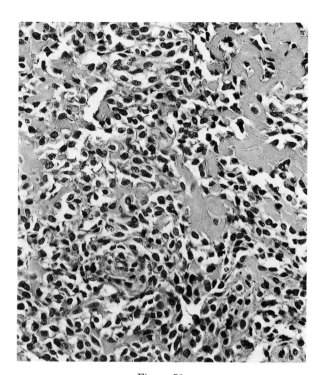

Figure 51
SMALL CELL OSTEOSARCOMA
Small osteoblasts with indistinct cytoplasm are situated within and around delicate deposits of osteoid. (Courtesy of Dr. M. Kyriakos, St. Louis, MO.)

with variable proportions of mitochondria, rough endoplasmic reticulin, golgi apparatus, and filaments (122). Sometimes the nuclei have the finely granular chromatin (eu-chromatin) seen in the cells of Ewing sarcoma (126). The ultrastructural spectrum of these cells overlaps the undifferentiated cells of Ewing sarcoma and mesenchymal chondrosarcoma (122).

Differential Diagnosis. Small cell osteosarcoma should be distinguished from conventional osteosarcoma and from other small cell tumors including Ewing sarcoma, mesenchymal chondrosarcoma, lymphoma, and neuroectodermal tumor. Ewing sarcoma is excluded by the presence of neoplastic osteoid, documented either radiographically or microscopically and abundant reticulin in contrast to the sparse reticulin of Ewing sarcoma. Mesenchymal chondrosarcoma favors the axial skeleton and, although fatal, has a more protracted clinical course. Microscopically, it may contain a small cell population indistinguishable from that of small cell osteosarcoma. However, mesenchymal chondrosarcoma

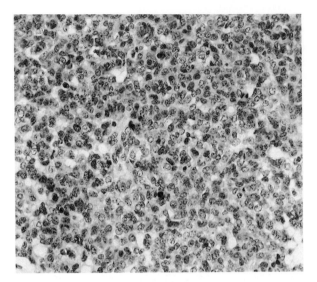

Figure 52
SMALL CELL OSTEOSARCOMA
This small cell osteosarcoma exhibits a lymphoma-like pattern with cells having vesicular nuclei. No osteoid is present in this field. (Courtesy of Dr. M. Kyriakos, St. Louis, MO.) (Figures 52 and 53 are from the same patient.)

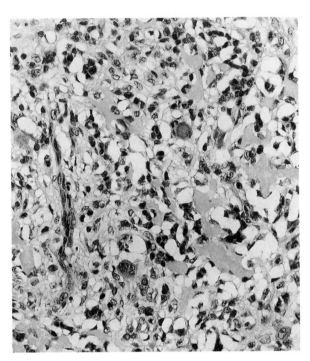

Figure 53
SMALL CELL OSTEOSARCOMA
Small foci of osteoid associated with malignant osteoblasts were present in other areas of the case illustrated in figure 52.

has sharply demarcated nests of low-grade cartilage and not the high-grade chondrosarcoma and osteoid seen in small cell osteosarcoma. The absence of pan-leukocytic markers such as leukocyte common antigen eliminates primary osseous lymphoma from the differential diagnosis. Neuroectodermal tumor of bone should show evidence of neuroendocrine differentiation in the form of positive staining for neuron specific enolase, Leu 7, synaptophysin, chromogranin, or other neural markers and may demonstrate Homer Wright–type rosettes.

Spread and Metastasis. As with conventional osteosarcomas, patients dying with the small cell variant invariably have hematogenously disseminated metastases. The lung is the most common site of metastatic involvement, followed by other bones and the central nervous system.

Treatment and Prognosis. There is no uniform treatment protocol. Local ablation followed by aggressive chemotherapy seems to be used most often. Intra-arterial chemotherapy infusions prior to surgery have also been utilized (120). Ayala et al. (120) noted that, despite aggressive chemotherapy, small cell osteosarcoma had a worse prognosis than conventional osteosarcoma. In their group of 27 patients, 14 died of metastatic disease from 1 to 23 months after initial diagnosis, 1 was living with advanced metastases after 4 months, and 12 were disease free. One patient died of pulmonary and multiple osseous metastases 17 years after diagnosis (126). Only 9 of the disease-free patients had significant follow-ups of 25 to 90 months. Nine of 11 patients in another series died of disease; all but 1 died within the first year (121). In both studies the percent of tumor necrosis following preoperative intra-arterial chemotherapy did not correlate with survival.

The radiation sensitivity of small cell osteosarcoma has been a subject of debate. Sim et al. (127) found that the tumors were less radiation sensitive than Ewing sarcomas. However, another group obtained local tumor control with radiation therapy following only biopsy or limited excision in five of five patients (128); two of these were long-term survivors.

INTRAOSSEOUS WELL-DIFFERENTIATED OSTEOSARCOMA

Definition. A clinically and microscopically distinct intramedullary osteosarcoma variant that is composed mainly of fibrous and osseous tissue with minimal cytologic atypia.

General Features. This variant accounts for about 1 to 2 percent of all skeletal osteosarcomas (131). Approximately 100 cases have been reported, 80 of which were presented in a single review from the Mayo Clinic (131).

Clinical Features. Presenting signs and symptoms are nonspecific and typically consist of pain and swelling. Often, symptoms have been present for more than 1 year (130,131), a rare occurrence for conventional, high-grade osteosarcoma. There is no obvious sexual predilection, although one study suggested a female predominance (130). Patients are distinctly older, on average, than those with conventional osteosarcoma. There is a peak incidence in the third decade of life, but affected individuals are often in their fourth, fifth, sixth, or even seventh decades (131). Although this variant of osteosarcoma affects older adults, it has not been associated with preexisting Paget disease or radiation therapy.

Sites. There is a predilection for the metaphyseal regions of the long bones of the lower extremity. A composite series of cases had the following distribution: distal femur, 43 percent; proximal tibia, 12 percent; distal tibia, 8 percent; fibula, 6 percent; radius, 4 percent; proximal femur, 3 percent; rib, 3 percent; humerus, 3 percent; midfemur, 2 percent; skull, 2 percent; jaw, 2 percent; and hand, 2 percent (130,131). Single cases have also been reported involving the clavicle, vertebra, scapula, ulna, pelvis, and foot.

Radiographic Appearance. About 85 percent of intraosseous well-differentiated osteosarcomas are central medullary lesions (131). The remainder are eccentric with a cortical center. By definition, microscopically similar lesions arising from the periosteum are considered parosteal osteosarcomas. About two thirds are metaphyseal lesions; the remainder are divided equally between the diametaphyseal and diaphyseal regions. In patients with open growth plates, the epiphysis is uninvolved.

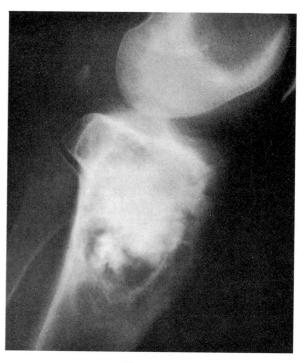

Figure 54
INTRAOSSEOUS
WELL-DIFFERENTIATED OSTEOSARCOMA
This irregularly sclerotic tumor involves the metaphysis and epiphysis of the tibia. The margin is partly sclerotic and sharply defined, suggesting slow growth. (Fig. 511 from Fascicle 5(Suppl), 2nd Series.)

Overall, about 80 percent have a radiographically malignant appearance, and only about 4 percent are interpreted as radiographically benign. Two thirds have poorly defined margins radiographically, about 10 percent have intermediate margins, and 22 percent have sharply defined margins (fig. 54) (130,131). A sclerotic rim surrounded the tumor margins in 12 percent of cases in one study, but no perilesional sclerosis was noted in a smaller series (130). Mineralized matrix is present in 70 percent or more of lesions, but the remainder are entirely radiolucent. Kurt et al. (131) noted that initially lucent lesions ossified with time in serial radiographs. From 55 to 88 percent of these tumors show radiographic evidence of cortical destruction on plain films. CT scans and MRI result in higher levels of detection. About half of intraosseous well-differentiated osteosarcomas have intralesional trabeculations. These may be coarse and quite pronounced; they probably represent incompletely resorbed, nonneoplastic bone.

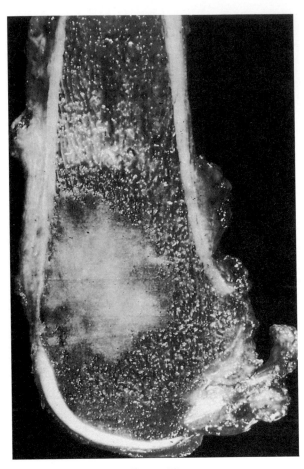

Figure 55
INTRAOSSEOUS
WELL-DIFFERENTIATED OSTEOSARCOMA
An irregularly shaped, sharply circumscribed, and densely sclerotic tumor is present in the medullary cavity. (Courtesy of Dr. L.V. Ackerman, Stony Brook, NY.)

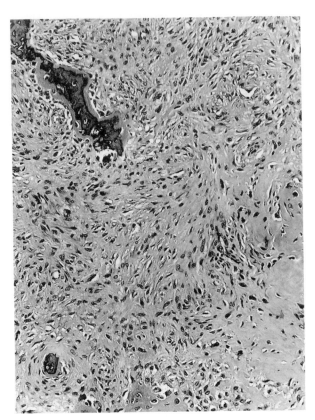

Figure 56
INTRAOSSEOUS
WELL-DIFFERENTIATED OSTEOSARCOMA
The stroma contains amorphous deposits of osteoid, as well as well-formed trabecula of mineralized bone. The stroma is collagenous with fibroblasts having minimal atypia.

Radiographic evidence of soft tissue extension was seen in only 4 of 18 intraosseous well-differentiated osteosarcomas in the original study (136), and in 2 of 7 cases in several subsequent reports (129,132,134,135,137). However, a much larger series from the Mayo Clinic documented soft tissue extension radiographically in 55 percent of cases (131) and Ellis et al. (130) found extraosseous extension radiographically in 75 percent of cases.

Gross Findings. On cut section, the tumors are often well demarcated and yellow to tan (fig. 55). They have a firm, gritty quality due to their mixture of fibrous and osseous elements. Cortical penetration and extraosseous extension are often present, as described above.

Microscopic Findings. Most of these tumors bear a striking resemblance, microscopically, to parosteal osteosarcoma and differ just as strikingly from conventional high-grade osteosarcoma. Fibrous tissue and osteoid form the bulk of the lesion with infrequent cartilaginous foci. The fibroblasts typically have active appearing, but uniform nuclei with only slight atypia (fig. 56). Mitotic figures usually average 1 to 2 per 10 high-power fields, and atypical division figures have not been seen (131).

About 40 percent of well-differentiated osteosarcomas have a heavy osteoid component with sharply demarcated, wide trabeculae of woven to lamellar bone (fig. 57). Sometimes, the neoplastic bone is mature and indistinguishable from normal. About one third have scanty osteoid and a fibroblastic stroma that resembles a desmoid tumor or desmoplastic fibroma. Less often (14 percent),

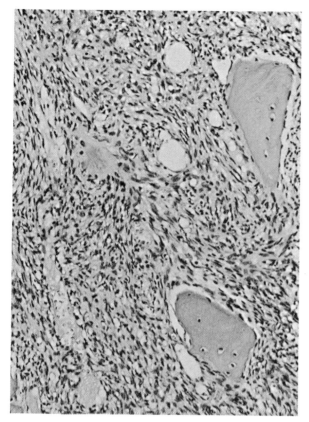

Figure 57
INTRAOSSEOUS
WELL-DIFFERENTIATED OSTEOSARCOMA
Well-differentiated, mature-appearing bone with small central osteocytes lies within a fibroblastic stroma. Despite the normal appearance of the bone, it is judged to be neoplastic, based on its location within the malignant stroma and its association with more immature osteoid. The stromal fibroblasts display minimal cytologic atypia. (Fig. 516 from Fascicle 5(Suppl), 2nd Series.)

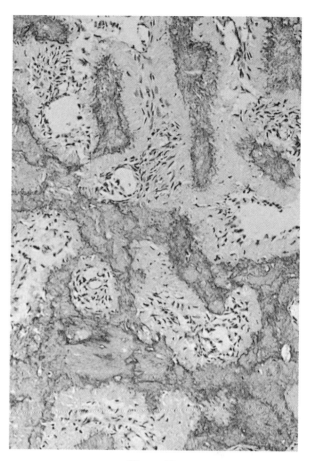

Figure 58
INTRAOSSEOUS
WELL-DIFFERENTIATED OSTEOSARCOMA
Broad trabeculae of bone are heavily mineralized centrally and surrounded by a wide area of unmineralized osteoid. The stroma is sparse, and areas such as this, out of context, are unrecognizable as malignant neoplasm. (Fig. 515 from Fascicle 5, 2nd Series.)

these tumors have osteoid that forms irregular, "Chinese characters" and resembles fibrous dysplasia. About 18 percent have foci of microscopically atypical cartilage. Rare examples have been described that mimic osteoblastoma, chondromyxoid fibroma, and nonossifying fibroma (131,133).

Because well-differentiated intraosseous osteosarcoma lacks the pleomorphism of its more conventional counterpart, it may easily be underdiagnosed as a benign process (fig. 58). Ellis et al. (130) noted that 3 of their 8 cases had initially been interpreted as microscopically benign. These authors noted that all of their cases had a malignant radiographic appearance. As with all osseous lesions, review of the radiographic findings will often prevent such mistakes.

Differential Diagnosis. Conventional, high-grade osteosarcomas may contain densely ossified, sclerotic areas in which the osteoblasts become "normalized" and have an innocuous, deceptively bland appearance. Such densely sclerotic osteosarcomas behave as aggressively as conventional osteosarcoma and are not part of the spectrum of well-differentiated osteosarcoma. Desmoplastic fibromas may infiltrate surrounding trabeculae of bone at their periphery, creating an image similar to that of well-differentiated osteosarcoma. Unlike the latter, however, the central portions of a desmoplastic fibroma will be virtually devoid of osteoid and, perhaps more importantly, the tumor will lack radiographic evidence of matrix production.

Confusion, microscopically, between intraosseous well-differentiated osteosarcoma and fibrous dysplasia is common. Radiographically, fibrous dysplasia has a typical "ground glass" appearance with a sharply demarcated margin, often associated with a rim of reactive sclerosis. Destruction of cortical bone is uncommon. Mirra (133) noted that trabeculations are commonly seen radiographically in well-differentiated osteosarcoma and are less common in fibrous dysplasia. Although well-differentiated osteosarcoma is generally bland, microscopically, it usually contains at least scattered cells with cytologic atypia beyond that seen in fibrous dysplasia. In addition, the bony trabeculae in fibrous dysplasia tend to be short and curled or "C" shaped, whereas in well-differentiated osteosarcoma they are often longer and arranged in roughly parallel arrays.

Well-differentiated osteosarcomas with prominent bony trabeculae could potentially be confused with osteoblastomas. The latter tumors almost invariably have a benign radiographic appearance. Microscopically, osteoblastomas have conspicuous osteoblastic rimming of the bony trabeculae and a characteristic loose, highly vascular stroma, features not found in well-differentiated osteosarcoma.

Spread and Metastasis. Well-differentiated osteosarcoma is fully capable of distant, hematogenous metastasis, usually to the lung, despite its rather bland microscopic appearance. Metastases probably occur in 15 percent or less of all patients, and are related, in large part, to the initial mode of therapy, as discussed below. Metastatic spread usually occurs as a result of anaplastic transformation to a high-grade osteosarcoma following inadequate therapy for the initial low-grade lesion.

Treatment and Prognosis. Curettage is invariably associated with recurrence, often with transformation to a high-grade lesion. In a study of 33 patients seen in consultation at the Mayo Clinic, all 11 patients with intraosseous well-differentiated osteosarcoma who were treated initially with amputation were alive and free of disease (131). Eight of these patients had been followed for more than 6 years. Of 17 patients in

the same study treated by wide excision, 15 were alive and free of disease, although only 5 had been followed for more than 5 years. One patient developed a high-grade (transformed) recurrence with subsequent pulmonary metastasis. The other patient developed a high-grade osteosarcoma at another site. Wide excision or amputation is currently considered appropriate therapy for this lesion. Adjuvant chemotherapy is not currently given, underscoring the need to distinguish this tumor from more aggressively managed forms of osteosarcoma.

INTRACORTICAL OSTEOSARCOMA

Definition. A rare, grossly and radiographically distinct variant of osteosarcoma arising within, and usually confined to, the cortical bone.

General Features. Only seven well-documented cases of intracortical osteosarcoma have been reported (138–140,142,143,145), along with two probable cases (141,144). This is, thus, one of the rarest variants of osteosarcoma, although some cases may have been interpreted as periosteal osteosarcoma.

Clinical Features. Of the seven well-documented cases, there were four male and three female patients who ranged from 10 to 30 (median, 24) years of age. Pain was the most common complaint, and this was occasionally associated with tenderness, swelling, or a palpable lump on the surface of the affected bone. Symptoms ranged from 2 to 12 (median 7) months in duration. A history of trauma to the area was obtained from three of the patients (138).

Sites. All intracortical osteosarcomas have involved the diaphysis of a lower extremity long bone. Of the seven cases, four arose in the tibia and three involved the femur. The two probable cases occurred in the femur and tibia as well.

Radiographic Appearance. Radiographs disclose a zone of intracortical lucency surrounded by sclerosis. The junction of the lucent and sclerotic areas is typically somewhat irregular, but sharply defined (fig. 59). The size of the lesion varies from 1.0 to 4.2 cm in greatest dimension. CT scans may show small foci of cortical permeation. In reported cases, the correct diagnosis was not made preoperatively. Radiographic diagnoses included a variety of benign processes such as nonossifying fibroma, fibrous dysplasia, Brodie abscess,

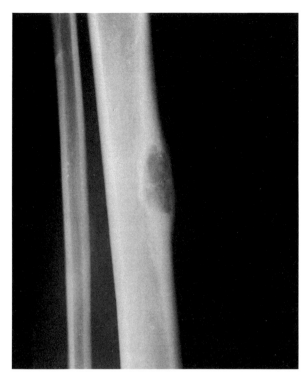

Figure 59
INTRACORTICAL OSTEOSARCOMA
The cortex is expanded by a lytic lesion with focal calcification. The patient, a 24-year-old man, had tenderness over the anterior surface of his leg for 3 months. (Fig. 1 from Kyriakos M. Intracortical osteosarcoma. Cancer 1980;46:2525–33.)

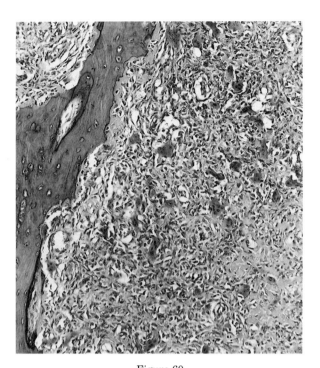

Figure 60
INTRACORTICAL OSTEOSARCOMA
Microscopically conventional osteosarcoma with abundant tumor osteoid at right invades normal bone at left.

osteoid osteoma, and osteoblastoma (138). Adamantinoma was the only malignant preoperative consideration.

Gross Findings. In an en bloc excision or amputation, the surrounding cortical bone is markedly thickened. Sectioning through this reactive bone will yield a dull grey to yellow, gritty central tumor mass with irregular, geographic borders (140). Any extension into the medullary cavity or periosteum should be minimal to avoid confusion with conventional intramedullary or periosteal osteosarcoma.

Microscopic Findings. Virtually all intracortical osteosarcomas have been highly osteoblastic, sclerotic tumors (fig. 60). As in intramedullary osteoblastic osteosarcomas, the neoplastic cells in these osteoid producing areas may become "normalized" with only minimal nuclear pleomorphism. The presence within the lesion of residual cortical bone entrapped by the tumor and serving as a scaffolding for the depo-

sition of tumor osteoid, is a clue to the malignant nature of the lesion (142). Small chondrosarcomatous or fibrosarcomatous foci may be present, but should not predominate.

Differential Diagnosis. Although in tracortical osteosarcoma mimics multiple lesions radiographically, its dominant osteoblastic character considerably narrows the microscopic diagnostic considerations. Intracortical osteosarcoma lacks the loose vascular stroma and osteoblastic rimming typical of osteoid osteoma and osteoblastoma. Conversely, entrapped normal or reactive bone and foci of neoplastic cartilage are virtually never seen within osteoid osteoma or osteoblastoma.

Although some authors consider intracortical osteosarcoma and periosteal osteosarcoma to be essentially the same lesion, Kyriakos (140) has mounted convincing arguments for their distinction. Periosteal osteosarcoma arises from the outer surface of the cortex, and secondarily erodes the underlying cortical bone. It has a predominantly chondroblastic appearance, unlike the sclerotic, osteoblastic appearance, microscopically, of intracortical osteosarcoma.

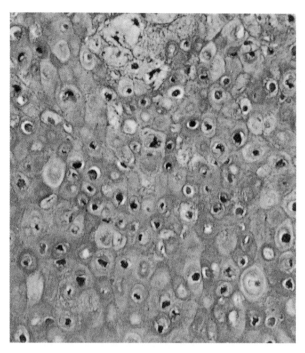

Figure 63
PERIOSTEAL OSTEOSARCOMA
Malignant cartilage in a periosteal osteosarcoma. This often is a major component of the tumor. (Fig. 530 from Fascicle 5(Suppl), 2nd Series.)

Although conventional intramedullary osteosarcomas are typically of somewhat higher histologic grade than most periosteal osteosarcomas, the distinction may not be possible on histologic grounds alone. Because of this potential for confusion, most authors require that periosteal osteosarcomas lack any intramedullary component (see above). The better prognosis of periosteal osteosarcoma justifies its distinction from conventional intramedullary osteosarcoma, although it has been suggested that small foci of intramedullary extension by the former tumors do not adversely affect prognosis (148).

Periosteal osteosarcomas may be confused with high-grade surface osteosarcomas, and Schajowicz et al. (152) suggested that some cases reported as the former would be better classified as the latter. High-grade surface osteosarcomas are highly pleomorphic, predominantly osteoblastic, and lack the cartilaginous lobules seen in periosteal osteosarcoma. Their poorer prognosis warrants distinction from periosteal osteosarcoma.

Periosteal osteosarcoma is easily distinguished from parosteal osteosarcoma on radiographic and histologic grounds. The former tumors

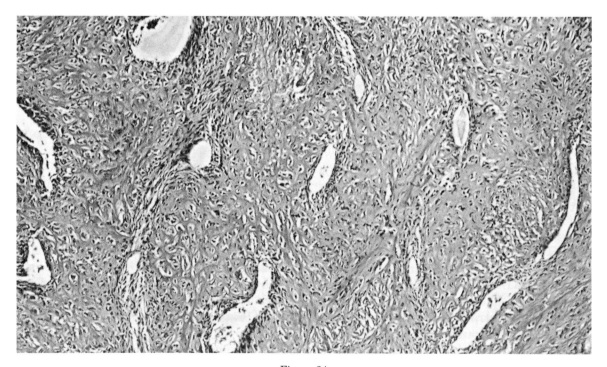

Figure 64
PERIOSTEAL OSTEOSARCOMA
Neoplastic osteoid in a periosteal osteosarcoma confirms the diagnosis. (Fig. 528 from Fascicle 5(Suppl), 2nd Series.)

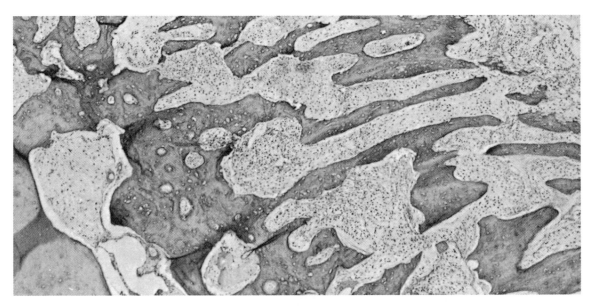

Figure 65
PERIOSTEAL OSTEOSARCOMA
The spiculation of bone seen radiographically in a periosteal osteosarcoma is primarily reactive bone encompassed by tumor. (Fig. 527 from Fascicle 5(Suppl), 2nd Series.)

are radiographically predominantly lytic and spiculated, and involve primarily the diaphysis. The latter tumors are radiographically dense, metaphyseal lesions. Microscopically, parosteal osteosarcomas are very low-grade, fibroblastic lesions; periosteal osteosarcomas are higher grade, predominantly chondroblastic neoplasms. These differences have been reported in detail by deSantos et al. (147).

Spread and Metastasis. When properly defined, and excluding more indolent periosteal chondrosarcomas and more aggressive high-grade surface osteosarcomas, periosteal osteosarcomas have an approximately 15 percent rate of metastasis (146,154). As with other forms of osteosarcoma, metastases primarily involve the lungs.

Treatment and Prognosis. Adequate treatment requires obtaining wide surgical margins around the tumor. Smaller lesions may allow for limb preservation, but larger tumors require amputation. In one series, two of three patients with locally recurrent disease had initially been treated by marginal excisions (150). Recurrent tumors usually develop in less than 1 year and appear to be associated with a higher rate of metastases. Ritts et al. (150) noted an apparently

more aggressive course for periosteal osteosarcomas involving the femur and suggested that these lesions may require more aggressive surgery. Chemotherapy has had no obvious effect on metastatic periosteal osteosarcoma.

PAROSTEAL OSTEOSARCOMA

Definition. A well-differentiated, predominantly fibro-osseous variant of osteosarcoma that arises from the juxtacortical region of the long bones. The term juxtacortical osteosarcoma has been applied to these lesions, but it has also been used for other forms of surface osteosarcoma such as parosteal osteosarcoma, and should probably be abandoned to avoid confusion.

General Features. This variant accounts for up to 5 percent of all osteosarcomas in some series (172). These tumors should be properly defined and distinguished from medullary osteosarcoma with extraosseous extension, periosteal osteosarcoma, and high-grade surface osteosarcoma (159,161,166,168), as well as several reactive processes. Parosteal osteosarcoma shows a strong tendency to undergo "dedifferentiation" to a high-grade sarcoma. One case of postradiation parosteal osteosarcoma has been reported (164).

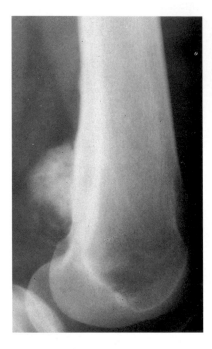 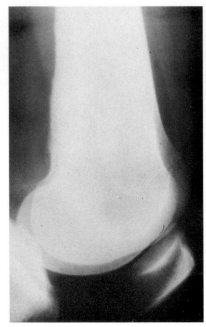 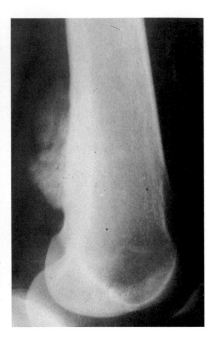

Figure 66
PAROSTEAL OSTEOSARCOMA

A. A 29-year-old woman noticed a painless mass behind her knee. The radiograph showed an irregularly calcified mass in continuity centrally with the cortex. The deeper cortex and medullary part of the bone were uninvolved. Because of a clinical misdiagnosis of osteochondroma, the lesion was locally excised flush with the cortex. B. Two years after local excision, there was no radiographic evidence of recurrent tumor. C. Four years after initial excision, the tumor recurred. An en bloc excision was carried out and the patient remains well 6 years later.

Clinical Features. The most frequent sign is a localized, slowly growing, painless mass in an extremity, usually the leg. Pain may be present and there may be stiffness of the adjacent joint (168). The duration of symptoms is usually for greater than 1 year, and some patients have been symptomatic for more than a decade. Such protracted symptomatology is virtually unheard of for conventional osteosarcoma. Not uncommonly, there will be a history of "recurrent osteochondroma," the lesion having been repeatedly misdiagnosed. Some studies have shown a slight female predilection (168). Patients range in age from childhood to the sixth or seventh decades of life. Although the peak age is in the second decade, many affected individuals are older than patients with conventional intramedullary osteosarcoma.

Sites. Parosteal osteosarcoma shows a striking predilection for the distal femur, particularly its posterior aspect. Between two thirds and three fourths of cases occur in this location. The upper shaft of the tibia is the second most common location, followed by the humerus, radius, ulna, and fibula. Rare cases have involved the skull (160), and the tubular bones of the hands and feet (169). Some lesions in the hands and feet undoubtedly represent the more common reactive processes of florid reactive periostitis or bizarre parosteal osteochondromatous proliferation.

Radiographic Appearance. Parosteal osteosarcoma has a characteristic, frequently diagnostic appearance. It forms a dense, mushroom-shaped mass which is attached to the outer metaphyseal cortex by a broad base (fig. 66). As the tumor grows, it may encircle the involved bone but, except for the base of attachment, it remains separated from the cortex by a narrow lucent zone (fig. 67). The latter feature produces a characteristic radiographic "string sign." Periosteal new bone formation is virtually always absent. Although usually dense, the intralesional sclerosis may be patchy with intralesional lucent zones (157,162). When the lucent areas are located peripherally, they most often consist of

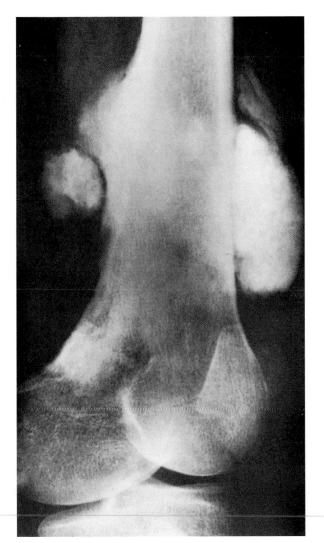 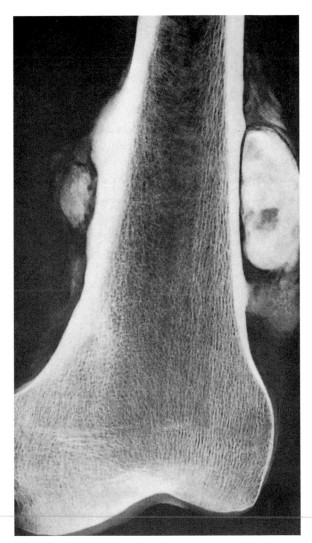

Figure 67
PAROSTEAL OSTEOSARCOMA
A. This oblique-view radiograph shows a recurrent parosteal osteosarcoma involving the femur of a 30-year-old woman. The tumor was locally resected 4 years previously. A lucent line is readily visible on the right between the outer cortex and the tumor. (Fig.180 from Fascicle 5, 2nd Series.) B. This specimen radiograph of a sagittal section from the recurrent parosteal osteosarcoma seen in A clearly demonstrates the cortical component (left) and envelopment of the juxtacortical tissues (right). (Fig. 181 from Fascicle 5, 2nd Series.)

low-grade cartilage, fibrous tissue, or islands of normal fat. Almost half of deep lucencies, in one study, represented areas of dedifferentiation to high-grade sarcoma (157).

Intralesional lucencies are better visualized with CT scans than with conventional radiographs (162). In addition to detecting areas of lucency, CT scans are particularly useful for demonstrating satellite lesions, cortical erosion, and intramedullary extension. Satellite lesions in the surrounding soft tissues most often occur following surgery. Cortical erosion has been reported in 71 percent of cases (162). Intramedullary extension, an important prognostic feature, is rare at the time of initial surgery, but becomes progressively more common with multiple recurrences (165,168). It is unclear whether MRI offers significant advantages over CT scans, although sagittal MRI sections are of some value in detecting intramedullary involvement (162).

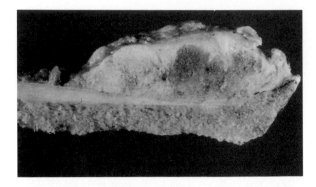

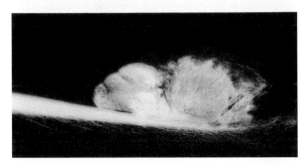

Figure 68
PAROSTEAL OSTEOSARCOMA
An en bloc excision (top) of the posterior distal femur shows the broad attachment of parosteal osteosarcoma to the intact outer cortex. Specimen radiograph (bottom) shows irregular calcification. A radiolucent line between the cortex and tumor is seen at the left. (Figure 16-3 from Fechner RE, Spjut HJ, Haggitt RC. Diseases of bones and joints. Based on the Proceedings of the 51st Annual Anatomic Pathology Slide Seminar of the American Society of Clinical Pathologists. American Society of Clinical Pathologists Press. Chicago, 1985:81.)

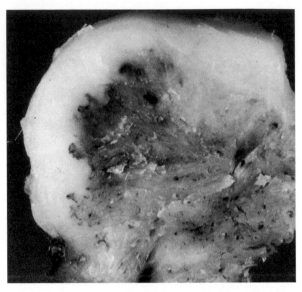

Figure 69
PAROSTEAL OSTEOSARCOMA
This cross section of a parosteal osteosarcoma shows a surface cartilaginous component overlying the osseous tumor. Such lesions may be misinterpreted as osteochondroma.

Gross Findings. A large, ossified, exophytic mass is attached to the involved bone by a broad base (fig. 68). Although much of the lesion may be densely ossified, it is usually possible to find multiple foci of less ossified tissue. These areas should be sectioned. Chondroid areas are commonly recognized, and there may even be a cartilaginous cap, simulating an osteochondroma (fig. 69). If an intramedullary component is present grossly, it should be sampled for microscopic study. By definition, any intramedullary component must have the same well-differentiated appearance typical of parosteal osteosarcoma.

Microscopic Findings. The microscopic appearance of parosteal osteosarcoma is so unlike that of conventional osteosarcoma that features for the diagnosis of the latter lesion do not apply. Typically, there are long, narrow trabeculae or

ill-defined islands of osteoid and woven bone separated by a fibrous stroma (fig. 70). The trabeculae may undergo a maturation that results in the formation of "normalized" lamellar bone. Occasionally, the trabeculae will show osteoblastic rimming (fig. 71).

The spaces between the bony trabeculae are filled with spindled, fibroblastic cells that are often devoid of all but minimal cytologic atypia and contain only scattered, normal-appearing mitotic figures. In about one fourth of cases, the fibrous areas are more cellular, have somewhat more pleomorphism, and an increased mitotic rate (168). These "grade 2" areas still lack the pleomorphism of conventional osteosarcoma (fig. 72).

The islands of cartilage and cartilage "caps" frequently present at the periphery of parosteal osteosarcoma are microscopically low grade, resembling an enchondroma or low-grade chondrosarcoma. The orderly rows of cartilage cell nuclei, as seen in osteochondromas, are not present.

Parosteal osteosarcoma may contain foci of high-grade sarcoma. The term *dedifferentiated parosteal osteosarcoma* has been applied to these lesions (172). In a series of 11 such tumors, only 1 contained dedifferentiated areas at the time of initial presentation; 3 patients had dedifferentiation

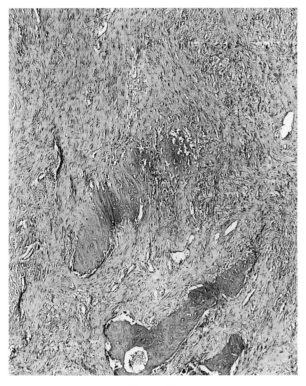

Figure 70
PAROSTEAL OSTEOSARCOMA
An ill-defined island of osteoid is seen in the center, with
a well-formed trabecula of neoplastic bone at the bottom.
Surrounding these areas is a cellular fibrous stroma.

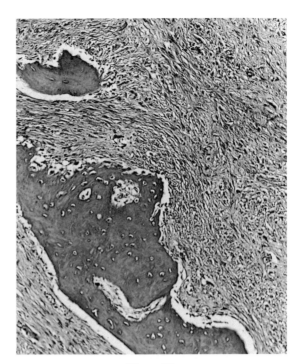

Figure 71
PAROSTEAL OSTEOSARCOMA
Part of the neoplastic bone exhibits osteoblastic rimming. The cells within the neoplastic bone are small and
benign appearing.

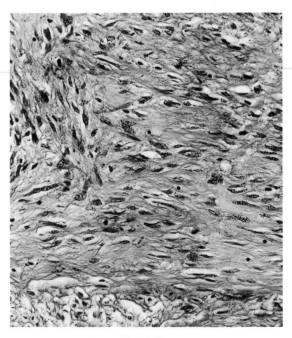

Figure 72
PAROSTEAL OSTEOSARCOMA
Moderately pleomorphic "grade 2" area lacks the marked
pleomorphism of conventional osteosarcoma.

in their first recurrence; 5 patients developed it
in their second recurrence; and 1 developed it in
the third recurrence (172). In one case, the
dedifferentiated component was known to be
aneuploid, and the patient developed pulmonary
metastases 1 year after resection (170).

Differential Diagnosis. Typical parosteal osteosarcoma should be distinguished from high-
grade intramedullary osteosarcoma with a prominent surface component and from high-grade
surface osteosarcoma (171). To avoid confusion
with the former, any intramedullary component of
a parosteal osteosarcoma should have a typical,
well-differentiated fibroblastic appearance (165).
Although otherwise typical parosteal osteosarcomas may contain focal areas of high-grade sarcoma
(dedifferentiation), when surface osteosarcomas
have a uniformly high-grade appearance, they
should be diagnosed as high-grade surface osteosarcoma (161,166,171). Although some studies have
considered such tumors to be "grade 3 parosteal

osteosarcomas," this designation obscures the important clinical and microscopic features of these tumors.

Parosteal osteosarcoma should be distinguished from periosteal osteosarcoma. Although the tumors share a juxtacortical location, they have distinct radiographic, microscopic, and, to a lesser degree, clinical differences, as discussed in a separate section.

Osteochondromas are radiographically and microscopically distinct from parosteal osteosarcomas. However, prior to widespread recognition of the latter tumors in the radiographic and orthopedic literature, it was not uncommon to encounter misdiagnoses. In osteochondromas, the underlying cortex and medullary bone are "drawn into" the lesion, rather than having the appearance of a mass "stuck on" the normal cortex, as is seen in parosteal osteosarcoma, and the maximum lesional sclerosis tends to be located peripherally, with the central portions composed of more lucent normal marrow. In contrast, parosteal osteosarcomas are usually more sclerotic centrally at the site of attachment, with a less mineralized periphery. Microscopically, osteochondromas invariably have normal-appearing hematopoietic or fibrofatty marrow and lack the fibroblastic stroma that is the hallmark of parosteal osteosarcoma.

Reactive soft tissue and periosteal processes produce radiographic images that are indistinguishable at some points in their evolution from parosteal osteosarcoma. A history of trauma may be helpful, but cannot always be elicited. In equivocal cases, serial radiographs over several months will show obvious maturation in reactive processes such as myositis ossificans and reactive periostitis. As these reactive processes mature, areas of lamellar bone and marrow fat develop, imparting a "dotted veil" radiographic appearance. Maturation proceeds from the periphery inward, a pattern opposite to that of parosteal osteosarcoma. The histologic recognition of reactive lesions is based on the finding of zones of maturation showing progression from hypercellular, immature foci to well-formed lamellar bone, often with marrow elements. Paradoxically, the early phases of these reactive processes are far more cellular and active-appearing than typical parosteal osteosarcoma and may be even more likely to be confused with high-grade surface or soft-tissue osteosarcoma.

Frequently in children, the medial posterior portion of the distal femoral metaphysis will show cortical irregularities that may mimic parosteal osteosarcoma (155,156,158,167). This variant of normal has been described in 11.5 percent of boys and 3.6 percent of girls (167). It disappears with closure of the femoral epiphysis and is probably due to the attachment of the adductor magnus muscle to the medial supracondylar ridge (156). It is best seen radiographically in an external rotation. Microscopically, it closely resembles a fibrous cortical defect (158).

Spread and Metastasis. Local recurrence or "satellitosis" is common following inadequate treatment. The frequency of intramedullary extension also increases with the number of recurrences. When metastases develop they disseminate hematogenously, usually to the lungs.

Treatment and Prognosis. Limited forms of excision, such as chiseling the lesion off the underlying bone, invariably result in recurrent disease, although the interval to recurrence may be decades. Small lesions should be treated with en bloc resection with a margin of uninvolved bone (163). Larger lesions may require more complex resections with grafts or amputation. Dedifferentiated parosteal osteosarcoma should be treated as a high-grade, conventional osteosarcoma (172). Recurrences of inappropriately treated lesions carry an increased risk of medullary involvement with associated poorer prognosis (166,168). Whether recurrences are usually of higher microscopic grade is debatable (163,168).

Adequate initial therapy results in cure for most patients and long-term survival is in the range of 80 to 90 percent. Low-grade lesions without intramedullary extension rarely metastasize. Three microscopic factors appear to influence prognosis: grade 2 neoplasms appear to have a somewhat worse prognosis than grade 1 lesions (168); foci of dedifferentiation definitely indicate a poorer prognosis, probably approaching that of conventional osteosarcoma (168,172); and intramedullary extension, a more common finding in recurrences, is also associated with a higher rate of metastatic disease and death (166,168). It should be noted that these factors are interrelated. For example, many parosteal osteosarcomas with intramedullary extension will be higher grade or dedifferentiated tumors.

HIGH-GRADE SURFACE OSTEOSARCOMA

Definition. A lesion that arises from the outer cortex of bone and has a uniformly high-grade microscopic appearance identical to that of conventional intramedullary osteosarcoma. Intramedullary extension is absent or minimal.

General Features. This is the least common variant of surface (juxtacortical) osteosarcoma. The Mayo Clinic experience with over 1,200 osteosarcomas includes 9 high-grade surface osteosarcomas (178). A total of 31 cases have been described in several series under a variety of terms (173–176,178). Additional cases may have been included with lower grade periosteal osteosarcomas (177).

Clinical Features. The following clinical features are summarized from the 31 cases referenced above. Patients ranged from 9 to 62 (median, 20) years of age. There were 22 males and 9 females. Symptoms were nonspecific and typically consisted of a mass or pain. In one series, 7 of 9 patients had been symptomatic for 1 year or more (maximum, 10 years) (174); other studies reported symptoms of 1 year or less in duration (173,176).

Sites. High-grade surface osteosarcoma involves the diaphyseal or, less commonly, the diaphyseal-metaphyseal regions. The distal femur is the most common location, accounting for 11 of the 31 cases (35 percent). Additional sites in order of frequency are: proximal humerus, 8 (26 percent), mid-femur, 3 (10 percent), proximal fibula, 3 (10 percent), proximal ulna, 2 (6 percent), with single cases involving the tibia, proximal femur, interosseous membrane between the tibia and fibula, and the radial shaft.

Radiographic Appearance. Radiographs invariably show a partially mineralized mass attached to the outer cortical surface, with some underlying cortical erosion (fig. 73). The character of the mineralization varies from mature trabeculae to fluffy, "cumulus cloud" calcifications. The amount of mineralization is also highly variable, ranging from dense calcifications to lesions with only small amounts of sclerosis. Mineralization is most frequent and most dense in the region of attachment to the underlying cortex. Periosteal reaction varies from absent to occasional well-formed Codman triangles. The radiographic features may mimic those

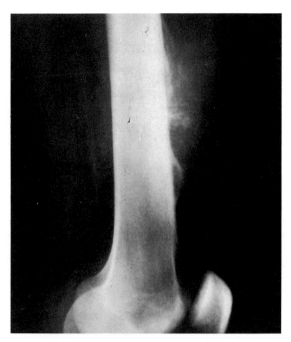

Figure 73
HIGH-GRADE SURFACE OSTEOSARCOMA
The surface osteosarcoma has a broad cortical base with irregular matrix formation. (Fig. 2 from Wold LE, Beabout JW, Unni KK, Pritchard DJ. High-grade surface osteosarcomas. Am J Surg Pathol 1984;8:181–6.)

of periosteal osteosarcoma (176,178) or, less frequently, parosteal osteosarcoma.

Gross Findings. The tumors are bulky, multilobulated masses with firm, soft, and hemorrhagic areas reflecting variation in composition (fig. 74). The characteristic dense sclerosis of parosteal osteosarcoma and the more uniform, chondroid appearance of periosteal osteosarcoma are uncommon. Small, grossly visible foci of intramedullary invasion will be seen in a minority of cases, but larger foci should exclude this diagnosis in favor of conventional intramedullary osteosarcoma.

Microscopic Findings. By definition, these are histologically high-grade neoplasms that are indistinguishable from conventional intramedullary osteosarcoma (fig. 75). To exclude a diagnosis of dedifferentiated parosteal osteosarcoma, a low-grade fibroblastic stroma should be completely absent. Microscopic foci of intramedullary extension will be present in about 60 percent of cases (174,178). The paucity of medullary involvement is the only feature distinguishing these tumors from conventional osteosarcoma (178).

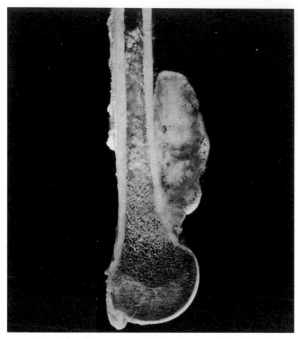

Figure 74
HIGH-GRADE SURFACE OSTEOSARCOMA
Grossly, this high-grade surface osteosarcoma has a multi-lobulated appearance. The medullary canal is not involved. (Fig. 3 from Wold LE, Beabout JW, Unni KK, Pritchard DJ. High-grade surface osteosarcomas. Am J Surg Pathol 1984;8:181–6.)

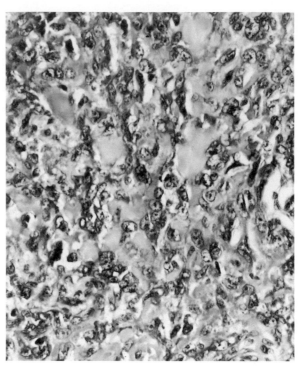

Figure 75
HIGH-GRADE SURFACE OSTEOSARCOMA
This highly anaplastic osteosarcoma is characteristic of surface osteosarcomas. (Fig. 4 from Wold LE, Beabout JW, Unni KK, Pritchard DJ. High-grade surface osteosarcomas. Am J Surg Pathol 1984;8:181-6.)

Differential Diagnosis. High-grade surface osteosarcoma should be distinguished from parosteal osteosarcoma, dedifferentiated parosteal osteosarcoma, periosteal osteosarcoma, and intramedullary osteosarcoma with a prominent surface component. Distinction of high-grade surface osteosarcoma from the variants of parosteal osteosarcoma and from periosteal osteosarcoma are discussed in the sections describing these tumors. These distinctions seem clinically warranted, as high-grade surface osteosarcoma appears to have a worse prognosis than even dedifferentiated parosteal osteosarcoma.

Distinguishing high-grade surface osteosarcoma from intramedullary osteosarcoma with a prominent surface component is of little or no prognostic importance. The definition of high-grade surface osteosarcoma currently allows for "some" intramedullary extension but the limits of this extension remain to be better defined. Certainly, the vast majority of the tumor should be on the cortical surface.

Spread and Metastasis. The biologic behavior of high-grade surface osteosarcoma is virtually identical to that of conventional intramedullary osteosarcoma. Local recurrences develop in a minority of patients and the clinical course is dominated by the development of systemic, usually pulmonary metastases.

Treatment and Prognosis. High-grade surface osteosarcoma requires aggressive therapy identical to that employed for conventional intramedullary osteosarcoma. Although treatment regimens are currently in flux and exhibit considerable inter-institutional variation, most include radical excision and adjuvant chemotherapy (175).

REFERENCES

Enostosis (Bone Island)

1. Blank N, Lieber A. The significance of growing bone islands. Radiology 1965;85:508–11.
2. Gold RH, Mirra JM, Remotti F, Pignatti G. Case report 527. Giant bone island of tibia. Skeletal Radiol 1989;18:129–32.
3. Greenspan A, Steiner G, Knutzon R. Bone island (enostosis): clinical significance and radiologic and pathologic correlations. Skeletal Radiol 1991;20:85–90.
4. Kim SK, Barry WF Jr. Bone islands. Radiology 1968; 90:77–8.
5. Mirra JM. Bone tumors: clinical, radiologic, and pathologic correlations. Philadelphia: Lea & Febiger, 1989: 182–90.
6. Sickles EA, Genant HK, Hoffer PB. Increased localization of 99mTc-pyrophosphate in a bone island: case report. J Nucl Med 1976;17:113–5.
7. Smith J. Giant bone islands. Radiology 1973;107:35–6.

Osteoma

8. Chang CH, Piatt ED, Thomas KE, Watne AL. Bone abnormalities in Gardner's syndrome. Am J Roentgenol Radium Ther Nucl Med 1968;103:645–52.
9. Childrey JH. Osteoma of sinuses, the frontal and the sphenoid bone. Report of fifteen cases. Arch Otolaryngol 1939;30:63–72.
10. Dahlin DC, Unni KK. Bone tumors: general aspects and data on 8,542 cases. 4th ed. Springfield, Ill: Charles C. Thomas, 1986:84–7.
11. Hallberg OE, Begley JW Jr. Origin and treatment of osteomas of the paranasal sinuses. Arch Otolaryngol 1950;51:750–60.
12. Lichtenstein L. Bone tumors. 3rd ed. St. Louis: CV Mosby, 1965:11.
13. Meltzer CC, Scott WW Jr, McCarthy EF. Case report 698. Osteoma of the clavicle. Skeletal Radiol 1991; 20:555–7.
14. Mirra JM. Bone tumors: clinical, radiologic, and pathologic correlations. Philadelphia: Lea & Febiger, 1989: 174–82.
15. Spjut HJ, Dorfman HD, Fechner RE, Ackerman LV. Tumors of bone and cartilage. Atlas of Tumor Pathology, 2nd series, Fascicle 5. Washington, D.C.: Armed Forces Institute of Pathology, 1971:117–9.

Osteoid Osteoma

16. Ayala AG, Murray JA, Erling MA, Raymond AK. Osteoid osteoma: intraoperative tetracycline-fluorescence demonstration of the nidus. J Bone Joint Surg [Am] 1986;68:747–51.
17. Bauer TW, Zehr RJ, Belhobek GH, Marks KE. Juxta-articular osteoid osteoma. Am J Surg Pathol 1991;15:381–7.
18. Bell RS, O'Connor GD, Waddell JP. Importance of magnetic resonance imaging in osteoid osteoma: a case report. Can J Surg 1989;32:276–8.
19. Byers PD. Solitary benign osteoblastic lesions of bone. Osteoid osteoma and benign osteoblastoma. Cancer 1968;22:43–57.
20. Dahlin DC, Unni KK. Bone tumors: general aspects and data on 8,542 cases. 4th ed. Springfield, Ill: Charles C. Thomas, 1986:88–91.
21. De Souza Dias L, Frost HM. Osteoid osteoma-osteoblastoma. Cancer 1974;33:1075–81.
22. Doyle T, King K. Percutaneous removal of osteoid osteomas under CT control. Clin Radiol 1989;40:514–7.
23. Edeiken J, Hodes PJ. Roentgen diagnosis of diseases of bone. Baltimore: Williams and Wilkins, 1967:496–504.
24. Freiberger RH, Loitman BS, Helpern M, Thompson TC. Osteoid osteoma. A report on 80 cases. AJR Am J Roentgenol 1959;82:194–205.
25. Golding JS. The natural history of osteoid osteoma: with a report of twenty cases. J Bone Joint Surg [Br] 1954;36:218–29.
26. Larsen LJ, Mall JC, Ichtertz DF. Metachronous osteoid-osteomas. Report of a case. J Bone Joint Surg [Am] 1991;73:612–4.
27. Klein MH, Shankman S. Osteoid osteoma: radiologic and pathologic correlation. Skeletal Radiol 1992;21:23–31.
28. MacLellan DI, Wilson FC Jr. Osteoid osteoma of the spine. A review of the literature and report of six new cases. J Bone Joint Surg [Am] 1967;49:111–21.
29. Marcove RC, Freiberger RH. Osteoid osteoma of the elbow—a diagnostic problem. Report of four cases. J Bone Joint Surg [Am] 1966;48:1185–90.
30. Moberg E. The natural course of osteoid osteoma. J Bone Joint Surg [Am] 1951;33:166–70.
31. Morton KS, Bartlett LH. Benign osteoblastic change resembling osteoid osteoma. Three cases with unusual radiological features. J Bone Joint Surg [Br] 1966;48:478–84.
32. Regan MW, Galey JP, Oakeshott RD. Recurrent osteoid osteoma. Case report with a ten-year asymptomatic interval. Clin Orthop 1990;253:221–4.
33. Schulman L, Dorfman HD. Nerve fibers in osteoid osteoma. J Bone Joint Surg [Am] 1970;52:1351–6.
34. Sim FH, Dahlin DC, Beabout JW. Osteoid-osteoma: diagnostic problems. J Bone Joint Surg [Am] 1975;57:154–9.
35. Spence AJ, Lloyd-Roberts GC. Regional osteoporosis in osteoid osteoma. J Bone Joint Surg [Br] 1961;43:501–7.
36. Vickers CW, Pugh DC, Ivins JC. Osteoid osteoma. A 15 year follow-up of an untreated patient. J Bone Joint Surg [Am] 1959;41:357–8.
37. Vigorita VJ, Ghelman B. Localization of osteoid osteomas—use of radionuclide scanning and autoimaging in identifying the nidus. Am J Clin Pathol 1983;79:223–5.
38. Voto SJ, Cook AJ, Weiner DS, Ewing JW, Arrington LE. Treatment of osteoid osteoma by computed tomography guided excision in the pediatric patient. J Pediatr Orthop 1990;10:510–3.
39. Wold LE, Pritchard DJ, Bergert J, Wilson DM. Prostaglandin synthesis by osteoid osteoma and osteoblastoma. Mod Pathol 1988;1:129–31.

Osteoblastoma

40. Bertoni F, Unni KK, McLeod RA, Dahlin DC. Osteosarcoma resembling osteoblastoma. Cancer 1985;55:416–26.

41. Bettelli G, Tigani D, Picci P. Recurring osteoblastoma initially presenting as a typical osteoid osteoma. Report of two cases. Skeletal Radiol 1991;20:1–4.

42. Byers PD. Solitary benign osteoblastic lesions of bone. Osteoid osteoma and benign osteoblastoma. Cancer 1968;22:43–57.

43. Dahlin DC, Johnson EW Jr. Giant osteoid osteoma. J Bone Joint Surg [Am] 1954;36:559–72.

44. _____, Unni KK. Bone tumors: general aspects and data on 8,542 cases. 4th ed. Springfield, Ill: Charles C. Thomas, 1986:102–18.

45. Dorfman HD. Malignant transformation of benign bone lesions. 7th National Cancer Conference Proceedings, 1973:901–13.

46. _____, Weiss SW. Borderline osteoblastic tumors: problems in the differential diagnosis of aggressive osteoblastoma and low-grade osteosarcoma. Semin Diagn Pathol 1984;1:215–34.

47. Healey JH, Ghelman B. Osteoid osteoma and osteoblastoma. Current concepts and recent advances. Clin Orthop 1986;204:76–85.

48. Gentry JF, Schechter JJ, Mirra JM. Case report 574. Periosteal osteoblastoma of rib. Skeletal Radiol 1989;18:551–5.

49. Gitelis S, Schajowicz F. Osteoid osteoma and osteoblastoma. Orthop Clin North Am 1989;20:313–25.

50. Lichtenstein L. Benign osteoblastoma. A category of osteoid- and bone-forming tumors other than classical osteoid osteoma, which may be mistaken for giant-cell tumor or osteogenic sarcoma. Cancer 1956;9:1044–52.

51. _____, Sawyer WR. Benign osteoblastoma. Further observations and report of twenty additional cases. J Bone Joint Surg [Am] 1964;46:755–65.

52. Marcove RC, Alpert M. A pathologic study of benign osteoblastoma. Clin Orthop 1963;30:175–80.

53. Marsh BW, Bonfiglio M, Brady LP, Enneking WF. Benign osteoblastoma: range of manifestations. J Bone Joint Surg [Am] 1975;57:1–9.

54. McLeod RA, Dahlin DC, Beabout JW. The spectrum of osteoblastoma. AJR Am J Roentgenol 1976;126:321-5.

55. Mirra JM. Bone tumors: diagnosis and treatment. Philadelphia: JB Lippincott, 1980:108–22.

56. _____, Cove K, Theros E, Paladuga R, Smasson J. A case of osteoblastoma associated with severe systemic toxicity. Am J Surg Pathol 1979;3:463–71.

57. _____, Kendrick RA, Kendrick RE. Pseudomalignant osteoblastoma versus arrested osteosarcoma: a case report. Cancer 1976;37:2005–14.

58. Mitchell ML, Ackerman LV. Metastatic and pseudomalignant osteoblastoma: a report of two unusual cases. Skeletal Radiol 1986;15:213–8.

59. Morton KS, Quenville NF, Beauchamp CP. Aggressive osteoblastoma. A case previously reported as a recurrent osteoid osteoma. J Bone Joint Surg [Br] 1989; 71:428–31.

60. Picci P, Companacci M, Mirra JM. Osteoid osteoma. Differential clinicopathologic diagnosis. In: Mirra JM. Bone tumors. Clinical, radiologic, and pathologic correlations. Philadelphia: Lea & Febiger, 1989:411–4.

61. Schajowicz F, Lemos C. Malignant osteoblastoma. J Bone Joint Surg [Br] 1976;58:202–11.

62. _____, Lemos C. Osteoid osteoma and osteoblastoma. Closely related entities of osteoblastic derivation. Acta Orthop Scand 1970;41:272–91.

63. Steiner GC. Ultrastructure of osteoblastoma. Cancer 1977;39:2127–36.

64. Vade A, Wilbur A, Pudlowski R, Ghosh L. Case report 566. Osteoblastoma of sacrum with secondary aneurysmal bone cyst. Skeletal Radiol 1989;18:475–80.

Conventional Intramedullary Osteosarcoma

65. Belli L, Scholl S, Livartowski A, et al. Resection of pulmonary metastases in osteosarcoma. A retrospective analysis of 44 patients. Cancer 1989;63:2546–50.

66. Benedict WF, Fung YK, Murphree AL. The gene responsible for the development of retinoblastoma and osteosarcoma. Cancer 1988;62:1691–4.

67. Benjamin RS. Chemotherapy for osteosarcoma. In: Unni KK, ed. Bone tumors. New York: Churchill Livingstone, 1988:149–56.

68. Bertoni F, Unni KK, McLeod RA, Dahlin DC. Osteosarcoma resembling osteoblastoma. Cancer 1985;55:416–26.

69. Dahlin DC, Unni KK: Bone tumors: general aspects and data on 8,542 cases. 4th ed. Springfield, Ill: Charles C. Thomas, 1986:269–307.

70. deSantos LA, Edeiken B. Purely lytic osteosarcoma. Skeletal Radiol 1982;9:1–7.

71. Dorfman HD, Weiss SW. Borderline osteoblastic tumors: problems in the differential diagnosis of aggressive osteoblastoma and low-grade osteosarcoma. Semin Diagn Pathol 1984;1:215–34.

72. Draper GJ, Sanders BM, Kingston JE. Second primary neoplasms in patients with retinoblastoma. Br J Cancer 1986;53:661–71.

73. Enneking WF, Kagan A. "Skip" metastases in osteosarcoma. Cancer 1975;36:2192–205.

74. _____, Kagan A II. Transepiphyseal extension of osteosarcoma: incidence, mechanism, and implications. Cancer 1978;41:1526–37.

75. Fechner RE, Huvos HG, Mirra JM, Spjut HJ, Unni KK. A symposium on the pathology of bone tumors. Pathol Annu 1984;19(Pt 1):125–94.

76. Giuliano AE, Feig S, Eilber FR. Changing metastatic patterns of osteosarcoma. Cancer 1984;54:2160–4.

77. Glass AG, Fraumeni JF Jr. Epidemiology of bone cancer in children. JNCI 1970;44:187–99.

78. Glasser DB, Lane JM, Huvos AG, Marcove RC, Rosen G. Survival, prognosis, and therapeutic response in osteogenic sarcoma. The Memorial Hospital experience. Cancer 1992;69:698–708.

79. Goorin AM, Abelson HT, Frei E III. Osteosarcoma: fifteen years later. N Eng J Med 1985;313:1637–43.

80. Huang HJ, Yee JK, Shew JY, et al. Suppression of the neoplastic phenotype by replacement of the RB gene in human cancer cells. Science 1988;242:1563–6.

81. Huvos AG, Heilweil M, Bretsky SS. The pathology of malignant fibrous histiocytoma of bone. A study of 130 patients. Am J Surg Pathol 1985;9:853–71.
82. Lindbom Å, Söderberg G, Spjut HJ. Osteosarcoma. A review of 96 cases. Acta Radiol 1961;56:1–19.
83. McKenna RJ, Schwinn CP, Soong KY, Higinbotham NL. Sarcomata of the osteogenic series (osteosarcoma, fibrosarcoma, chondrosarcoma, parosteal osteogenic sarcoma, and sarcomata arising in abnormal bone). An analysis of 552 cases. J Bone Joint Surg [Am] 1966;48:1–26.
84. McLeod RA, Dahlin DC, Beabout JW. The spectrum of osteoblastoma. AJR Am J Roentgenol 1976;126:321–5.
85. Mirra JM. Bone tumors: diagnosis and treatment. Philadelphia: JB Lippincott, 1980:111–22.
86. _____, Kameda N, Rosen G, Eckardt J. Primary osteosarcoma of toe phalanx: first documented case. Review of osteosarcoma of short tubular bones. Am J Surg Pathol 1988;12:300–7.
87. _____, Kendrick RA, Kendrick RE. Pseudomalignant osteoblastoma versus arrested osteosarcoma: a case report. Cancer 1976;37:2005–14.
88. Picci P, Manfrini M, Zucchi V, et al. Giant-cell tumor of bone in skeletally immature patients. J Bone Joint Surg [Am] 1983;65:486–90.
89. Price CH. Primary bone-forming tumours and their relationship to skeletal growth. J Bone Joint Surg [Br] 1958;40:574–93.
90. Pritchard DJ. Surgical management of osteosarcoma. In: Unni KK, ed. Bone tumors. New York: Churchill Livingstone, 1988:135–48.
91. Raymond AK, Ayala AG. Specimen management after osteosarcoma chemotherapy. In: Unni KK, ed. Bone tumors. New York: Churchill Livingstone, 1988:157–81.
92. _____, Chawla SP, Carrasco CH, et al. Osteosarcoma chemotherapy effect. A prognostic factor. Semin Diagn Pathol 1987;4:212–36.
93. Spanier SS, Shuster JJ, Vander Griend RA. The effect of local extent of the tumor on prognosis in osteosarcoma. J Bone Joint Surg [Am] 1990;72:643–53.
94. Spjut HJ, Dorfman HD. Florid reactive periostitis of the tubular bones of the hands and feet. A benign lesion which may simulate osteosarcoma. Am J Surg Pathol 1981;5:424–33.
95. Taylor WF, Ivins JC, Pritchard DJ, Dahlin DC, Gilchrist GS, Edmonson JH. Trends and variability in survival among patients with osteosarcoma: a 7-year update. Mayo Clin Proc 1985;60:91–104.
96. Tsuneyoshi M, Dorfman HD. Epiphyseal osteosarcoma: distinguishing features from clear cell chondrosarcoma, chondroblastoma, and epiphyseal enchondroma. Hum Pathol 1987;18:644–51.
97. Unni KK, Dahlin DC. Premalignant tumors and conditions of bone. Am J Surg Pathol 1979;3:47–60.
98. Weatherby RP, Unni KK. Practical aspects of handling orthopedic specimens in the surgical pathology laboratory. Pathol Annu 1982;17(Pt 2):1–31.
99. Weinfeld MS, Dudley HR Jr. Osteogenic sarcoma. A follow-up study of the ninety-four cases observed at the Massachusetts General Hospital from 1920 to 1960. J Bone Joint Surg [Am] 1962;44:269–76.

Multifocal Osteosarcoma

100. Amstutz HC. Multiple osteogenic sarcomata—metastatic or multicentric? Report of two cases and review of literature. Cancer 1969;24:923–31.
101. Fitzgerald RH Jr, Dahlin DC, Sim FH. Multiple metachronous osteogenic sarcoma. Report of twelve cases with two long-term survivors. J Bone Joint Surg [Am] 1973;55:595–605.
102. Mahoney JP, Spanier SS, Morris JL. Multifocal osteosarcoma: a case report with review of the literature. Cancer 1979;44:1897–907.
103. Mirra JM. Bone tumors: clinical, radiologic, and pathologic correlations. Philadelphia: Lea & Febiger, 1989: 344–50.

Telangiectatic Osteosarcoma

104. Bertoni F, Bacchini P, Pignatti G, Picci P. Telangiectatic osteosarcoma. Survival compared to that of "conventional" osteosarcoma [Abstract]. Mod Pathol 1988;1:10A.
105. Chan CW, Kung TM, Ma L. Telangiectatic osteosarcoma of the mandible. Cancer 1986;58:2110–5.
106. Chawla SP, Benjamin RS. Effectiveness of chemotherapy in the management of metastatic telangiectatic osteosarcoma. Am J Clin Oncol 1988;11:177–80.
107. Chowdhury K, Bachynski B, Alport EC. Telangiectatic osteosarcoma: unusual behavior. Can J Surg 1986;29: 29–31.
108. Dahlin DC, Unni KK. Bone tumors: general aspects and data on 8,542 cases. 4th ed. Springfield, Ill: Charles C. Thomas, 1986:290–2.
109. Gomes H, Menanteau B, Gaillard D, Behar C. Telangiectatic osteosarcoma. Pediatr Radiol 1986;16:140–3.
110. Huvos AG, Rosen G, Bretsky SS, Butler A. Telangiectatic osteogenic sarcoma: a clinicopathologic study of 124 patients. Cancer 1982;49:1679–89.
111. Kaufman RA, Towbin RB. Telangiectatic osteosarcoma simulating the appearance of an aneurysmal bone cyst. Pediatr Radiol 1981;11:102–4.
112. Larsson SE, Lorentzon R, Boquist L. Telangiectatic osteosarcoma. Acta Orthop Scand 1978;49:589–94.
113. Matsuno T, Unni KK, McLeod RA, Dahlin DC. Telangiectatic osteogenic sarcoma. Cancer 1976;38:2538–47.
114. Mirra JM. Bone tumors: clinical, radiologic, and pathologic correlations. Philadelphia: Lea & Febiger, 1989: 316–25.
115. Roessner A, Hobik HP, Immenkamp M, Grundmann E. Ultrastructure of telangiectatic osteosarcoma. J Cancer Res Clin Oncol 1979;95:197–207.
116. Rosen G, Huvos AG, Marcove R, Nirenberg A. Telangiectatic osteosarcoma. Improved survival with combination chemotherapy. Clin Orthop 1986;207:164–73.
117. Ruiter DJ, Cornelisse CJ, van Rijssel TG, van der Velde EA. Aneurysmal bone cyst and telangiectatic osteosarcoma. A histopathological and morphometric study. Virchows Arch [A] 1977;373:311–25.

118. Vanel D, Tcheng S, Contesso G, et al. The radiological appearances of telangiectatic osteosarcoma. A study of 14 cases. Skeletal Radiol 1987;16:196–200.

119. Yoshida H, Adachi H, Naniwa S, Yumoto T, Morimoto K, Furuse K. High alkaline phosphatase activity of telangiectatic osteosarcoma (TOS) and its diagnostic significance. Acta Pathol Jpn 1987;37:305–13.

Small Cell Osteosarcoma

120. Ayala AG, Ro JY, Raymond AK, et al. Small cell osteosarcoma. A clinicopathologic study of 27 cases. Cancer 1989;64:2162–73.

121. Bertoni F, Present D, Bacchini P, Pignatti G, Picci P, Campanacci M. The Istituto Rizzoli experience with small cell osteosarcoma. Cancer 1989;64:2591–9.

122. Dickersin GR, Rosenberg AE. The ultrastructure of small-cell osteosarcoma, with a review of the light microscopy and differential diagnosis. Hum Pathol 1991;22:267–75.

123. Edeiken J, Raymond AK, Ayala AG, Benjamin RS, Murray JA, Carrasco HC. Small-cell osteosarcoma. Skeletal Radiol 1987;16:621–8.

124. Martin SE, Dwyer A, Kissane JM, Costa J. Small-cell osteosarcoma. Cancer 1982;50:990–6.

125. Noguera R, Navarro S, Triche TJ. Translocation (11;22) in small cell osteosarcoma. Cancer Genet Cytogenet 1990;45:121–4.

126. Roessner A, Immenkamp M, Hiddemann W, Althoff J, Miebs T, Grundmann E. Case report 331: small cell osteosarcoma of the tibia with diffuse metastatic disease. Skeletal Radiol 1985;14:216–25.

127. Sim FH, Unni KK, Beabout JW, Dahlin DC. Osteosarcoma with small cells simulating Ewing's tumor. J Bone Joint Surg [Am] 1979;61:207–15.

128. Stea B, Cavazzana A, Kinsella TJ. Small-cell osteosarcoma: correlation of in vitro and clinical radiation response. Int J Radiat Oncol Biol Phys 1988;15:1233–8.

Intraosseous Well-Differentiated Osteosarcoma

129. Campanacci M, Bertoni F, Capanna R, Cervellati C. Central osteosarcoma of low grade malignancy. Ital J Orthop Traumatol 1981;7:71–8.

130. Ellis JH, Siegel CL, Martel W, Weatherbee L, Dorfman HD. Radiologic features of well-differentiated osteosarcoma. AJR Am J Roentgenol 1988;151:739–42.

131. Kurt AM, Unni KK, McLeod RA, Pritchard DJ. Low-grade intraosseous osteosarcoma. Cancer 1990;65:1418–28.

132. Lodwick GS. Case report 169: low-grade osteosarcoma of the tibia. Skeletal Radiol 1981;7:139–41.

133. Mirra JM. Bone tumors: clinical, radiologic, and pathologic correlations. Philadelphia: Lea & Febiger, 1989: 359–83.

134. Sundaram M, Herbold DR, McGuire MH. Case report 370: low-grade (well-differentiated) intramedullary osteosarcoma. Skeletal Radiol 1986;15:338–42.

135. Unni KK. Case report 136. Central low-grade osteosarcoma of tibia. Skeletal Radiol 1981;6:65–7.

136. _____, Dahlin DC, McLeod RA, Pritchard DJ. Intraosseous well-differentiated osteosarcoma. Cancer 1977;40:1337–47.

137. Xipell JM, Rush J. Case report 340. Well-differentiated intraosseous of the left femur. Skeletal Radiol 1985;14:312–6.

Intracortical Osteosarcoma

138. Anderson RB, McAlister JA Jr, Wrenn RN. Case report 585: intracortical osteosarcoma of tibia. Skeletal Radiol 1989;18:627–30.

139. Jaffe HL. Intracortical osteogenic sarcoma. Bull Hosp Joint Dis 1960;21:189–97.

140. Kyriakos M. Intracortical osteosarcoma. Cancer 1980:46:2525–33.

141. Lichtenstein L. Bone tumors. 5th ed. St. Louis: CV Mosby, 1977:225.

142. Mirra JM. Bone tumors: clinical, radiologic, and pathologic correlations. Philadelphia: Lea & Febiger, 1989:384–9.

143. Picci P, Gherlinzoni F, Guerra A. Intracortical osteosarcoma: rare entity or early manifestation of classical osteosarcoma? Skeletal Radiol 1983;9:255–8.

144. Scranton PE Jr, DeCicco FA, Totten RS, Yunis EJ. Prognostic factors in osteosarcoma. A review of 20 years' experience at the University of Pittsburgh Health Center Hospitals. Cancer 1975;36:2179–91.

145. Vigorita VJ, Jones JK, Ghelman B, Marcove RC. Intracortical osteosarcoma. Am J Surg Pathol 1984;8:65–71.

Periosteal Osteosarcoma

146. Bertoni F, Boriani S, Laus M, Campanacci M. Periosteal chondrosarcoma and periosteal osteosarcoma. Two distinct entities. J Bone Joint Surg [Br] 1982;64:370–6.

147. deSantos LA, Murray JA, Finklestein JB, Spjut HJ, Ayala AG. The radiographic spectrum of periosteal osteosarcoma. Radiology 1978;127:123–9.

148. Hall RB, Robinson LH, Malawar MM, Dunham WK. Periosteal osteosarcoma. Cancer 1985;55:165–71.

149. Levine E, De Smet AA, Huntrakoon M. Juxtacortical osteosarcoma: a radiologic and histologic spectrum. Skeletal Radiol 1985;14:38–46.

150. Ritts GD, Pritchard DJ, Unni KK, Beabout JW, Eckhardt JJ. Periosteal osteosarcoma. Clin Orthop 1987;219:299–307.

151. Schajowicz F. Juxtacortical chondrosarcoma. J Bone Joint Surg [Br] 1977;59:473–80.

152. _____, McGuire MH, Santini Araujo E, Muscolo DL, Gitelis S. Osteosarcomas arising on the surfaces of long bones. J Bone Joint Surg [Am] 1988;70:555–64.
153. Spjut HJ, Ayala AG, deSantos LA, Murray JA. Periosteal osteosarcoma. In: Clinical Conference on Cancer. Management of primary bone and soft tissue tumors: a collection of papers presented at the twenty-first annual Clinical Conference on Cancer. Chicago: Year Book Medical Publishers, 1977:79–95.
154. Unni KK, Dahlin DC, Beabout JW. Periosteal osteogenic sarcoma. Cancer 1976;37:2476–85.

Parosteal Osteosarcoma

155. Allen DH. A variation of diaphyseal development which simulates the roentgen appearance of primary neoplasms of bone. AJR Am J Roentgenol 1953;69:940–3.
156. Barnes GR Jr, Gwinn JL. Distal irregularities of the femur simulating malignancy. Am J Roentgenol Radium Ther Nucl Med 1974;122:180–5.
157. Bertoni F, Present D, Hudson T, Enneking WF. The meaning of radiolucencies in parosteal osteosarcoma. J Bone Joint Surg [Am] 1985;67:901–10.
158. Brower AC, Culver JE Jr, Keats TE. Histological nature of the cortical irregularity of the medial posterior distal femoral metaphysis in children. Radiology 1971;99:389–92.
159. Campanacci M, Picci P, Gherlinzoni F, Guerra A, Bertoni F, Neff JR. Parosteal osteosarcoma. J Bone Joint Surg [Br] 1984;66:313–21.
160. Hinton CE, Turnbull AE, O'Donnell HD, Harvey L. Parosteal osteosarcoma of the skull. Histopathology 1989;14:322–3.
161. Levine E, De Smet AA, Huntrakoon M. Juxtacortical osteosarcoma: a radiologic and histologic spectrum. Skeletal Radiol 1985;14:38–46.
162. Lindell MM Jr, Shirkhoda A, Raymond AK, Murray JA, Harle TS. Parosteal osteosarcoma: radiologic-pathologic correlation with emphasis on CT. AJR Am J Roentgenol 1987;148:323–8.
163. Luck JV Jr, Luck JV, Schwinn CP. Parosteal osteosarcoma: a treatment-oriented study. Clin Orthop 1980;153:92–105.
164. Masuda S, Murakawa Y. Postirradiation parosteal osteosarcoma. A case report. Clin Orthop 1984;184:204–7.
165. Picci P, Campanacci M, Bacci G, Capanna R, Ayala A. Medullary involvement in parosteal osteosarcoma. A case report. J Bone Joint Surg [Am] 1987;69:131–6.
166. Schajowicz F, McGuire MH, Santini Araujo E, Muscolo DL, Gitelis S. Osteosarcomas arising on the surfaces of long bones. J Bone Joint Surg [Am] 1988;70:555–64.
167. Simon H. Medial distal metaphyseal femoral irregularity in children. Radiology 1968;90:258–60.
168. Unni KK, Dahlin DC, Beabout JW, Ivins JC. Parosteal osteogenic sarcoma. Cancer 1976;37:2466–75.
169. van der Walt JD, Ryan JF. Parosteal osteogenic sarcoma of the hand. Histopathology 1990;16:75–8.
170. van Oven MW, Molenaar WM, Freling NJ, et al. Dedifferentiated parosteal osteosarcoma of the femur with aneuploidy and lung metastases. Cancer 1989;63:807–11.
171. Wold LE, Unni KK, Beabout JW, Pritchard DJ. High-grade surface osteosarcomas. Am J Surg Pathol 1984;8:181–6.
172. _____, Unni KK, Beabout JW, Sim FH, Dahlin DC. Dedifferentiated parosteal osteosarcoma. J Bone Joint Surg [Am] 1984;66:53–9.

High-Grade Surface Osteosarcoma

173. Ahuja SC, Villacin AB, Smith J, Bullough PG, Huvos AG, Marcove RC. Juxtacortical (parosteal) osteogenic sarcoma: histologic grading and prognosis. J Bone Joint Surg [Am] 1977;59:632–47.
174. Campanacci M, Picci P, Gherlinzoni F, Guerra A, Bertoni F, Neff JR. Parosteal osteosarcoma. J Bone Joint Surg [Br] 1984;66:313–21.
175. Levine E, De Smet AA, Huntrakoon M. Juxtacortical osteosarcoma: a radiologic and histologic spectrum. Skeletal Radiol 1985;14:38–46.
176. Schajowicz F, McGuire MH, Santini Araujo E, Muscolo DL, Gitelis S. Osteosarcomas arising on the surfaces of long bones. J Bone Joint Surg [Am] 1988;70:555–64.
177. Spjut HJ, Ayala AG, De Santos LA, Murray JA. Periosteal osteosarcoma. In: Clinical Conference on Cancer. Management of primary bone and soft tissue tumors: a collection of papers presented at the twenty-first annual Clinical Conference on Cancer. Chicago: Year Book Medical Publishers, 1977:79–95.
178. Wold LE, Unni KK, Beabout JW, Pritchard DJ. High-grade surface osteosarcomas. Am J Surg Pathol 1984;8:181–6.

❖❖❖

CARTILAGINOUS LESIONS

OSTEOCHONDROMA

Definition. An outgrowth of medullary and cortical bone, covered with a cartilaginous cap, which projects from the cortical surface of the involved bone.

The term *exostosis* is sometimes used for osteochondroma. This is a generic term referring to any outgrowth of bone that is capped with cartilage. The marginal osteophytes near the joints of patients with degenerative joint disease (osteoarthritis) fulfill the definition of an exostosis, however, the pathogenesis is completely different for osteophytes and osteochondromas. Therefore, the term exostosis should not be applied interchangeably with osteochondroma.

General Features. The prevalence of osteochondroma is unknown because many are asymptomatic and found incidentally on radiographs taken for other reasons. Symptomatic lesions usually present during the first 20 years of life. Most osteochondromas probably result from displaced epiphyseal cartilage that herniates through a periosteal defect (12), and then proceeds to grow at 90 degrees to the normal growth plane. Osteochondromas ultimately are covered completely with periosteum. In a sense, osteochondromas are not true neoplasms but rather a malformation that grows synchronously with the epiphyseal plate during the first two decades of life. Epiphyseal cartilage of rabbits transplanted beneath the periosteum results in a lesion similar to an osteochondroma (5).

Osteochondromas develop in approximately 12 percent of patients receiving therapeutic radiation during childhood for such conditions as osseous eosinophilic granuloma and a variety of nonosseous malignant neoplasms. Radiation doses have ranged from less than 1,000 to 6,000 rads. Any open epiphysis is susceptible, including those of the pelvis and the vertebra (9). The lesions can appear from 17 months to 16 years later and may be multiple (10). Multiple osteochondromas have the same gross and microscopic features as solitary ones. One case of chondrosarcoma has been reported in a radiation-induced osteochondroma 10 years after radiation therapy for metastatic neuroblastoma (14).

Clinical Features. In some series, males are reported to be affected approximately twice as often as females (4). In other series, there is no predilection. Patients usually complain of a mass, often of long duration. Occasionally, there is pain if the osteochondroma impinges on nerves. Rarely, there is fracture through the stalk (4), or painful spontaneous infarction (15). Some lesions have an overlying bursa that may accentuate the mass and be painful (6). Rarely, the bursa contains cartilaginous loose bodies (1). Enlargement of the bursa may mimic malignant transformation (8). Popliteal vein thrombosis and popliteal artery pseudoaneurysm are rare complications (11).

Sites. Just over 50 percent of osteochondromas involve the lower end of the femur, the upper end of the humerus, and the upper end of the tibia. Except for the craniofacial bones, any bone may be involved, although lesions in the hands, feet, and vertebrae are extremely uncommon.

Radiographic Appearance. Osteochondromas have highly characteristic, although widely variable appearances. The osteochondroma projects from the involved bone with a narrow to broad stalk. Its medullary bone is continuous with that of the affected bone. Osteochondromas point toward the mid-shaft and away from the nearest epiphysis (fig. 76). Flocculent densities may be seen within the medullary bone that represent calcified lobules of cartilage (see below). The surface of the osteochondroma may be smooth or irregular. The cartilaginous cap is not detectable on ordinary films because it is not calcified, however magnetic resonance imaging is quite sensitive in accurately measuring its thickness (3).

Gross Findings. Externally, a resected osteochondroma consists of normal cortical bone, usually with a cartilaginous cap. The cap may be round and smooth or knobby (fig. 77). A thin, fibrous periosteal layer covers the entire lesion. On cut surface, the cartilage may cover the majority of the lesion or only its central, most peripheral part. Generally, the younger the patient the greater the proportion of the surface is cartilage covered. The thickness of the cartilage is not uniform. In younger patients, it may measure 0.1 to 3 cm in thickness. Usually, however, it is less than 0.5 cm in depth. The cartilage ceases to grow in adults, and

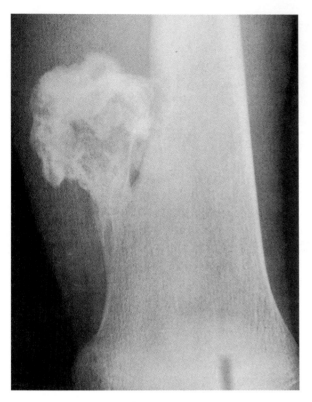

Figure 76
OSTEOCHONDROMA
An osteochondroma involving the distal portion of the femur in a 13-year-old boy has a well-circumscribed, knobby surface. The lesion forms an acute angle with the cortex of the femur, and the cartilaginous cap is pointed away from the adjacent epiphysis. (Fig. 42 from Fascicle 5, 2nd Series.)

usually involutes so that it is only a few millimeters in thickness. It is often missing altogether, with a thin plate of eburnated bone forming the surface.

The central portion of an osteochondroma consists of normal medullary bone. One or more irregular, yellow, gritty foci may be present within the bone, representing densely calcified mosaics of cartilage, osteoid, and amorphous debris.

A bursa is occasionally present, and is generally attached around the base of the osteochondroma. The wall of the bursa is usually thin, but may be up to 1 cm in thickness. The bursa infrequently contains deposits of fibrin, rice bodies, or calcified cartilaginous bodies.

Microscopic Findings. The cap of an osteochondroma is covered by an outermost layer of thin fibrous periosteum that is often almost imperceptible and blends into the underlying cartilage (fig. 78). The hyaline cartilage cap has fairly evenly distributed chondrocytes that usually appear normal. There may, however, be nuclei up to five times the normal diameter, with mild to moderate nuclear atypia (fig. 79). Such foci may form poorly circumscribed aggregates of chondrocytes lying in an otherwise sparse matrix. These areas are not of importance, as long as the cartilaginous cap is less than 3 cm in thickness, there are no cartilaginous masses beyond the periosteum, and there is no radiographic evidence of destruction of the underlying bone.

The junction of the cartilage cap and the underlying bone sometimes resembles an epiphyseal plate, with linear columns of closely approximated chondrocytes (fig. 80). Bone is deposited along these columns (enchondral ossification), resulting in irregularly shaped cartilaginous islands encased in bone. The medullary bone usually contains fatty marrow, but hematopoietic elements also may be seen.

In addition to the minute foci of cartilage surrounded by bone in the deeper portion of the stalk, there may be large disorganized aggregates of cartilage, bone, and amorphous calcified debris. The cartilage is often necrotic in these foci. These calcified areas correspond to the flocculent densities seen on radiographs as described above.

Differential Diagnosis. Chondrosarcoma arising in osteochondroma is the only tumor that enters into the microscopic differential diagnosis. The radiograph is usually diagnostic in such cases, showing a focally calcified mass that is larger than 2 cm. In some instances, however, the only clue is a fuzzy or indistinct surface to an otherwise typical osteochondroma. The interior of the osteochondroma may have radiographically lucent areas that represent resorbed bone invaded by nonmineralized cartilage. The persisting stalk may be discernible, or have been completely destroyed by the sarcoma. In the latter instance, the cartilaginous mass appears to lie directly on the cortical surface.

Grossly, chondrosarcomas arising in osteochondromas have bosselated cartilaginous caps that range in thickness from 2 to 12 cm when accurately measured on perpendicular sections. Separate lobules of cartilage may be in the adjacent soft tissue. Most chondrosarcomas are grade 1 and the criteria described in the section on chondrosarcoma apply to chondrosarcomas arising in osteochondromas as well.

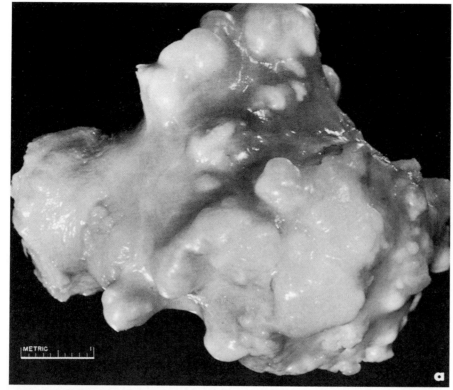

Figure 77
OSTEOCHONDROMA

A. The outer surface of this resected osteochondroma has knobby gray cartilaginous areas.

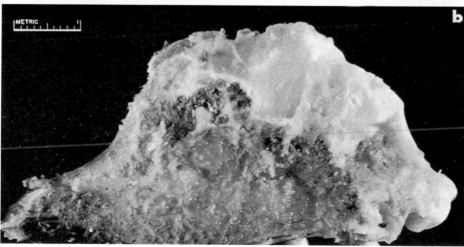

B. On cut surface, the central portion of the osteochondroma is cancellous bone covered with hyaline cartilage. (Fig. 43 from Fascicle 5, 2nd Series.)

Distinction of osteochondroma from parosteal osteosarcoma is typically straightforward both radiographically and microscopically. Distinguishing features are discussed in the chapter dealing with the latter lesion.

Treatment and Prognosis. Osteochondromas almost always cease to grow when the epiphyses close and are removed only when symptomatic or causing cosmetic distress. There does not appear to be a correlation between size and the risk for chondrosarcoma. Osteochondromas up to 14 cm in greatest dimension have been left untreated for as long as 40 years without further growth or malignant transformation (2). Dahlin and Unni (4) reported that approximately 2 percent of osteochondromas recurred from 1 to 26 years later. The second operation was curative. Recurrence was presumably due to failure to remove the entire cartilaginous cap or, possibly, incomplete removal of the overlying periosteum.

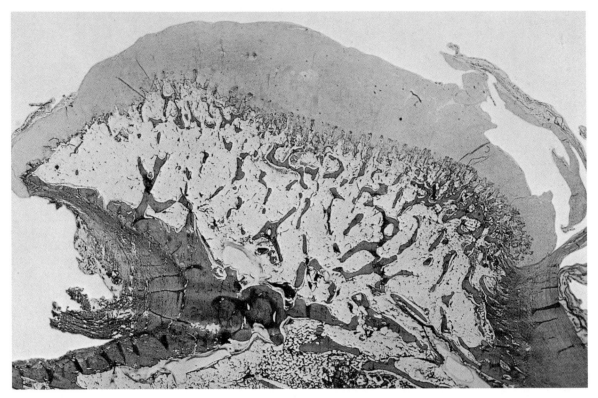

Figure 78
OSTEOCHONDROMA
A whole mount section of an osteochondroma has periosteum covering the cartilage (right). The cartilaginous cap has a zone of enchondral ossification. The stalk is fatty marrow and normal trabeculae of bone. (Fig. 44 from Fascicle 5, 2nd Series.)

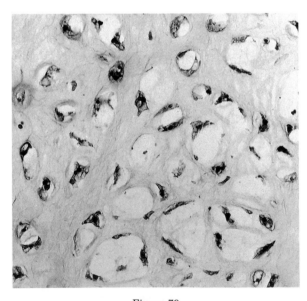

Figure 79
OSTEOCHONDROMA
Some osteochondromas have cellular cartilaginous foci with chondrocytes having moderately atypical nuclei.

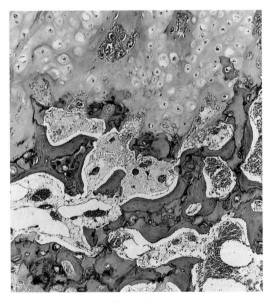

Figure 80
OSTEOCHONDROMA
Junction of cartilage cap and underlying bone resembles an epiphyseal plate with enchondral bone formation.

There is one report of a spontaneously disappearing osteochondroma (13). It ceased to grow prior to skeletal maturation and was incorporated into the growing metaphysis.

Rarely, osteochondromas give rise to chondrosarcomas (7). The risk has been estimated at 1 to 2 percent of solitary osteochondromas, but since the prevalence of asymptomatic lesions is unknown, this is almost certainly an artificially high estimate. The chondrosarcomas occur in patients between the ages of 10 and 75 years, but most show a rather even distribution between the ages of 15 and 50 years. Symptoms consist of pain, a mass, or enlargement of a previously palpable but quiescent osteochondroma. The radiographic, gross, and microscopic features are discussed above under differential diagnosis.

OSTEOCHONDROMATOSIS (MULTIPLE OSTEOCHONDROMAS)

Definition. A familial disorder manifested by multiple osteochondromas, defective metaphyseal remodeling, and asymmetric retardation of longitudinal bone growth. A few patients have only two or three osteochondromas, but most have many tumors involving several bones. In the most severe cases, virtually every bone (except the craniofacial bones) is involved. Other terms for this condition include *multiple hereditary exostoses*, *diaphysial aclasis*, and *hereditary deforming chondrodysplasia*.

General Features. Osteochondromatosis is inherited as an autosomal-dominant gene with incomplete penetrance in females. Thus, males are affected more often in a ratio of about 7 to 3 (17). Whether the pathogenesis of multiple lesions is the same as for solitary lesions is unknown. Clearly, osteochondromatosis is manifested by a much greater derangement of the epiphyseal cartilage than occurs in patients with solitary osteochondromas. Patients with multiple osteochondromas usually have deformities of the forearm, wrist, knee, and ankle because of discrepancies in the growth rate of the radius and ulna, or tibia and fibula. Phalanges may be shortened, and long tubular bones are frequently shortened and broadened with an abnormally wide flaring of the metaphysis. Shapiro et al. (22) found that 60 percent of patients had moderate to severe deformities of the forearms with shortening of the ulna.

Clinical Features. The disease is rarely diagnosed in infancy, but palpable osteochondromas and deformities are noticeable after the age of two. Additional lesions become clinically apparent throughout adolescence, and cease to appear in adulthood. There may be spinal cord compression by vertebral lesions (18).

Radiographic Appearance. Individual osteochondromas are not qualitatively different from solitary lesions. The deformities of the forearm and leg, however, are an intrinsic part of osteochondromatosis, and are not seen in patients with solitary osteochondromas.

Gross and Microscopic Findings. The lesions have the same gross and microscopic appearances as described under solitary osteochondroma.

Treatment and Prognosis. The deformities with resultant discrepancies in arm and leg length often require corrective surgery (19). The osteochondromas themselves are dealt with singly, if they are symptomatic, using the same management criteria as for solitary lesions.

Reports in the literature repeatedly state that the frequency of developing malignancy is 5 to 25 percent. This is, however, a highly biased figure introduced by the referral nature of the reporting institutions. Peterson (21) summarized reports of three pedigrees spanning several generations and found that only 1 of 134 affected patients developed a malignancy. A similar figure (1.3 percent) was determined by Voutsinas and Wynne-Davies (23). Most of the malignancies have been chondrosarcomas. A few osteosarcomas and a malignant fibrous histiocytoma have also been reported (20).

Interestingly, Garrison et al. (16) found that chondrosarcomas arising from solitary osteochondromas were distributed about equally between flat and long bones, whereas 80 percent of those associated with osteochondromatosis arose from flat bones. The same criteria for a diagnosis of secondary chondrosarcoma apply to patients with multiple osteochondromas as is described for patients with solitary lesions. High-grade neoplasia is far more common in association with osteochondromatosis than in patients with solitary lesions who develop secondary chondrosarcoma. Ten of eleven grade 3 secondary chondrosarcomas were in patients with osteochondromatosis (16).

ENCHONDROMA

Definition. A benign, intramedullary neoplasm of hyaline cartilage. It is sometimes called a *central chondroma* or, less specifically, a *chondroma*. The latter term also includes extramedullary lesions.

General Features. Enchondroma is a relatively common lesion, accounting for about 10 percent of benign osseous tumors. It has been postulated that these neoplasms arise from cartilaginous cell nests that are displaced from the growth plate during development. Although unproven, this theory would explain the exclusive occurrence of enchondromas in bones that form by enchondral ossification. It would also account for the development of multiple enchondromas in association with the growth plate abnormalities of Ollier disease and Maffucci syndrome.

Clinical Features. Patients range from 5 to 79 years of age. However, about 60 percent are between the ages of 15 and 40 years. In some series, males are reported to be affected slightly more often than females, but most studies show no sexual predilection.

Some enchondromas are asymptomatic and are detected as incidental radiographic abnormalities, sometimes as "hot" spots in patients having a skeletal scan for other reasons. Symptomatic lesions may present as painless swellings. Most enchondromas of the phalanges present with pain due to small stress fractures.

Sites. Enchondromas occur almost exclusively in the appendicular skeleton. About half involve the hands and feet, chiefly the phalanges of the hand. The proximal humerus and the proximal or distal femur are other affected sites. Increased and improved radiographic surveillance may lead to detection of a higher percentage of asymptomatic, quiescent enchondromas involving the long bones. Enchondromas of the pelvis, vertebrae, or ribs are uncommon.

Radiographic Findings. The lesions are predominantly lucent with some mineralization. The calcified foci vary from powder-like to dense aggregates. The tumors may be located centrally, eccentrically, or are occasionally multicentric (32). The bone may be eccentrically or concentrically expanded, especially in the phalanges (fig. 84). The expanded cortex is thinned but intact. In large tubular bones, enchondromas produce

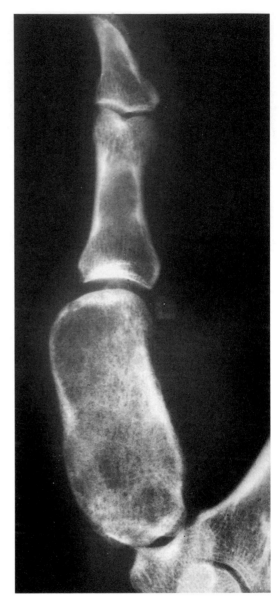

Figure 84
ENCHONDROMA
A 33-year-old woman noted discomfort and slight swelling in her finger for 2 months. An enchondroma expands the proximal phalanx and focally thins, but does not penetrate the cortex.

little if any endosteal cortical erosion and do not expand the involved bone (fig. 85). Rarely, enchondromas result in eccentric, exophytic masses termed *enchondroma protuberans* (29).

Gross Findings. Most enchondromas are satisfactorily treated by curettage and resected specimens are rare. The fragments consist of blue-white, glistening hyaline cartilage, sometimes mixed with yellow, calcified foci. Resected

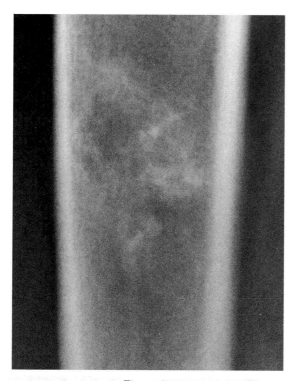

Figure 85
ENCHONDROMA
An enchondroma of the distal femur was an incidental finding in a 56-year-old man who had a radiograph taken because of trauma to the knee. The inner part of the cortex is not eroded, and curettings disclosed sparsely cellular, benign-appearing hyaline cartilage.

tumors have discrete, focal lobules of mature hyaline cartilage ranging from a few millimeters to up to a centimeter in diameter (fig. 86).

Microscopic Findings. A lobular arrangement of the neoplastic cartilage is often apparent microscopically (fig. 87). The lobules are frequently rimmed by a narrow band of reactive bone directly apposed to the cartilage and blending imperceptibly with it. The lobules may also be surrounded by bone marrow, between trabeculae of normal bone. This should not be interpreted as an infiltrative or permeative growth pattern. In fact, it has been suggested that the presence of many such islands located within the marrow indicate an enchondroma, and that this feature can be used as a microscopic criterion for distinction from chondrosarcoma (33).

Most enchondromas consist of normal-appearing chondrocytes in lacunar spaces separated by abundant hyaline chondroid matrix (fig.

88). However, the cellularity in enchondromas varies greatly. Several chondrocytes may lie within a single lacuna, and lacunae can be closely approximated, so that the tumor is very cellular (fig. 89). Binucleated or trinucleated chondrocytes are occasionally evident, as are chondrocytes with large nuclei. The cartilage may be necrotic and, occasionally, the stroma is myxoid, especially in enchondromas of the small bones.

Differential Diagnosis. The differential diagnosis lies exclusively with chondrosarcoma. Histologic features alone are often inadequate to differentiate a hypercellular enchondroma from a chondrosarcoma. Mirra (33) found that careful counts of cellularity, mitotic activity, and other cytologic features showed an overlap between enchondromas and grade 1 chondrosarcomas in 25 percent of cartilaginous neoplasms. The radiograph and clinical history are critical for distinction. The presence of pain in the absence of a fracture is highly suspicious for a chondrosarcoma. Radiographically, destruction of the cortex is evidence of malignancy. In chondrosarcomas of the hands and feet, cortical destruction was present in all but one case, and, often, there was extraosseous extension (31). When most or all of the lesion has the hypercellularity and nuclear abnormalities of a grade 2 or grade 3 chondrosarcoma, a diagnosis of malignancy is straightforward. A radiograph showing aggressiveness will invariably support the diagnosis of chondrosarcoma in these higher grade tumors.

The differential diagnosis is further complicated by chondrosarcomas that appear to arise in preexisting enchondromas, sometimes as long as 40 years after the radiographic diagnosis of the precursor lesion (38). Thus, one may have sparsely cellular, essentially normal-appearing cartilage (enchondroma) plus hypercellular, cytologically atypical cartilage (secondary chondrosarcoma). Recognition of this coexistence is important when interpreting small biopsies. Nevertheless, from a practical standpoint, the radiograph in this situation will nearly always show evidence of destruction by the sarcomatous component. It may also provide convincing evidence of the previous enchondroma (30). Rarely, osteosarcomas, fibrosarcomas, or malignant fibrous histiocytomas have arisen adjacent to preexisting enchondromas (35,36). This phenomenon is discussed further under Dedifferentiated Chondrosarcoma.

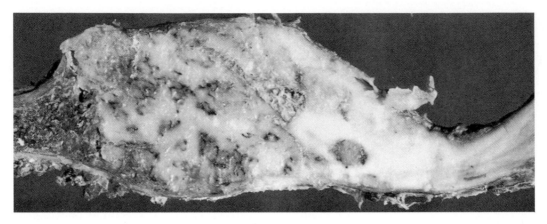

Figure 86
ENCHONDROMA
An enchondroma expands the rib but does not transgress its cortex. Most of the tumor consists of confluent cartilage, but a nodular pattern is seen at the left. (Fig. 61 from Fascicle 5, 2nd Series.)

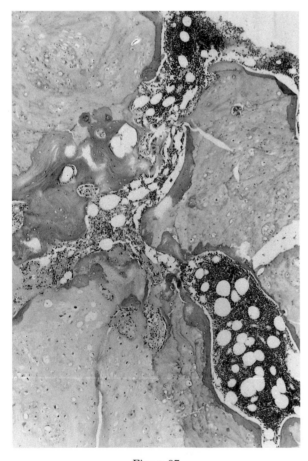

Figure 87
ENCHONDROMA
Islands of cartilage, partly cuffed by thin layers of bone, are separated by normal bone marrow.

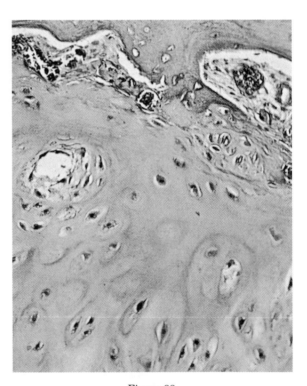

Figure 88
ENCHONDROMA
Sparsely cellular cartilage with minimal nuclear variation abuts surrounding normal bone (top). (Fig. 62 from Fascicle 5, 2nd Series.)

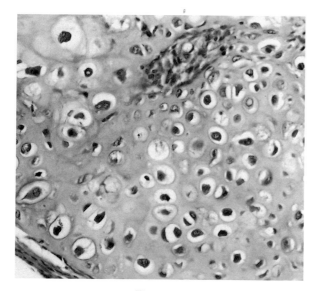

Figure 89
ENCHONDROMA
Enchondromas may have cellular areas with moderate nuclear pleomorphism indistinguishable from grade 1 chondrosarcoma.

Treatment and Prognosis. Most enchondromas are treated by curettage, with or without bone grafting. The recurrence rate for curetted enchondromas is less than 5 percent (37). Patients treated only with splinting may have long-term resolution of symptoms (34), occasionally associated with improvement in the radiograph, indicating that the lesion has not only ceased to grow but may be resolving (37).

ENCHONDROMATOSIS (OLLIER DISEASE)

Enchondromatosis is a rare, nonhereditary disorder characterized by multiple cartilaginous tumors. The extremities are usually affected and the extent of the disease is variable. Enchondromatosis is usually confined to all or a portion of one extremity. The affected limb is often shortened and deformed (fig. 90). Enchondromatosis rarely progresses after puberty.

The enchondromas involve the metaphysis, diaphysis, epiphyseal plates, and articular cartilage. Whole mount sections of involved bones show intracortical, as well as periosteal lesions that are not in continuity (42).

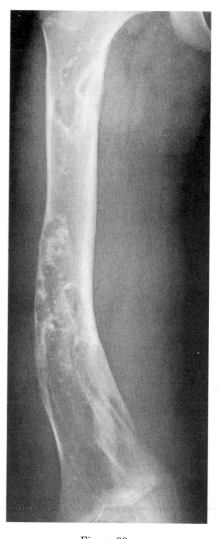

Figure 90
ENCHONDROMATOSIS (OLLIER DISEASE)
This radiograph shows typical features of enchondromatosis in the right femur of a 13-year-old boy. Spotty calcifications in multiple foci reflect multiple tumors. There is a bowing deformity as well. (Fig. 65 from Fascicle 5, 2nd Series.)

Microscopically, the enchondromas in this disease are often very cellular with large numbers of binucleated chondrocytes. The degree of cellularity and cytologic atypia is greater than for solitary enchondromas. The microscopic distinction between the benign cartilage of enchondromatosis and low-grade chondrosarcoma is especially difficult. Necrosis and myxoid stroma strongly favor the diagnosis of chondrosarcoma (40).

Approximately 30 to 50 percent of patients with enchondromatosis develop an associated sarcoma.

This is usually manifest by pain or an enlarging mass. Radiographs show intralesional lucencies or cortical destruction. Most sarcomas in this setting are low-grade chondrosarcomas, but dedifferentiated chondrosarcomas and, rarely, osteosarcomas also occur. In one series of 16 sarcomatous transformations, the patients ranged from 13 to 69 years of age (41). Most were in their fifth decade of life, and the average age was 40 years. Some patients with enchondromatosis develop multiple sarcomas (39). Multiple malignancies in varying stages of evolution may be found in a single amputation specimen (40).

The survival rate for patients with sarcomas arising in enchondromatosis is the same as that associated with their de novo microscopic counterparts. As expected, patients with grade 1 chondrosarcomas (the most common sarcoma) do well, whereas those with dedifferentiated chondrosarcoma have a very high mortality rate.

MAFFUCCI SYNDROME

Maffucci syndrome is a rare, nonhereditary, congenital disorder consisting of enchondromatosis in association with hemangiomas. The latter may occur anywhere in the skin and subcutaneous tissues of the body, including the extremity with the enchondromas. The hemangiomas usually are cavernous and may be unilateral or bilateral, localized or extensive. Phleboliths are commonly seen radiographically (fig. 91). A total of 129 cases had been reported by 1985 (44).

Patients with Maffucci syndrome are susceptible to the development of malignant tumors (figs. 92, 93). Lewis and Ketcham (43) reviewed 105 cases of the syndrome and found that 15 percent developed chondrosarcoma, 3 percent had a vascular sarcoma or fibrosarcoma, and 5 percent had malignancies unrelated to bone or soft tissue. The lower rate of chondrosarcoma in Maffucci syndrome, as opposed to enchondromatosis, may relate to a greater mortality from complications of hemangiomatosis and extraskeletal malignancies, thereby reducing the patient population at risk for malignant transformation of osseous lesions in middle age.

In the series reported by Sun et al. (44), chondrosarcomas developed only in patients with widespread involvement and not in those with disease confined to an extremity. Four out of the

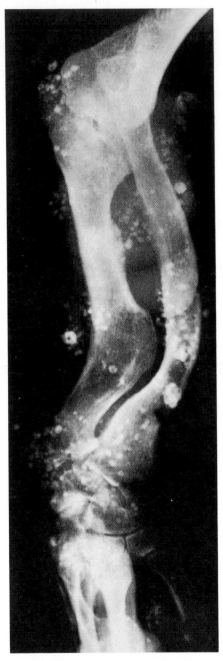

Figure 91
MAFFUCCI SYNDROME
The radius and ulna are deformed by enchondromas. Numerous phleboliths are present. (Fig. 72 from Fascicle 5, 2nd Series.) (Figs. 91–93 are from the same patient.)

five patients were at least 40 years old and presented with pain. Long bones, small bones of the hands or feet, or flat bones were involved. Most patients died of their disease.

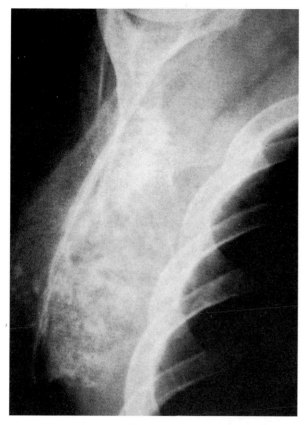

Figure 92
MAFFUCCI SYNDROME WITH CHONDROSARCOMA
A large, but fairly well-demarcated mass involves the scapula and contains flocculent and ring-like calcifications suggestive of chondrosarcoma. (Fig. 73 from Fascicle 5, 2nd Series.)

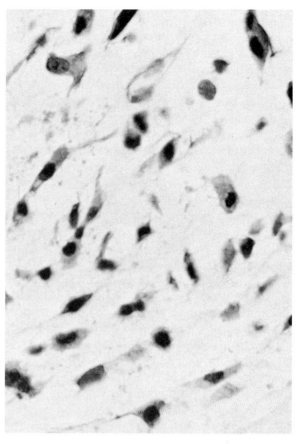

Figure 93
MAFFUCCI SYNDROME WITH CHONDROSARCOMA
This biopsy of the scapular lesion shows a poorly differentiated chondrosarcoma with immature cells in a myxoid matrix. (Fig. 74 from Fascicle 5, 2nd Series.)

CHONDROBLASTOMA

Definition. An almost invariably benign neoplasm showing a marked predilection for the epiphysis and comprised predominantly of ovoid, round, and spindled cells, some of which resemble immature chondrocytes (chondroblasts). Mature hyaline cartilage is present only focally in some tumors.

General Features. Chondroblastoma accounts for fewer than 1 percent of osseous neoplasms, and is thus about one fifth as common as giant cell tumor, a lesion with which it has often been confused (48). In fact, chondroblastomas were initially lumped with giant cell tumors, then considered a variant of giant cell tumor and, finally, identified as a distinct entity. As discussed below, ultrastructural and immunohistochemical studies have clearly documented the chondroid nature of the neoplastic cells.

Clinical Features. Patients range from 3 to 72 years of age. However, 95 percent of tumors occur in patients between the ages of 5 and 25 years, and the majority occur in teenagers, especially in the latter part of that decade (47). Males are affected about twice as often as females. The most common symptom is pain. It is often mild and may have been present for several months or even several years. About one third of patients have joint effusion (59), and swelling or limitation of motion may also occur.

Sites. About 98 percent of chondroblastomas are located in the epiphysis with a predilection for the distal femur, proximal tibia, and proximal humerus. Lesions confined to the metaphysis are well documented but infrequent, with 13 cases reported by 1986 (62). Rarely, two entirely separate bones may be involved (58). About 20 percent of chondroblastomas affect flat bones or tubular bones of the hands and feet, with an affinity for the calcaneus and talus (46). Chondroblastomas may occur in the craniofacial bones, especially the temporal bone, which is formed in part by enchondral ossification (45).

Radiographic Appearance. These are typically sharply delimited, lytic lesions with a thin margin of increased bone density. The tumor may be confined to the epiphysis, but a majority extend across the growth plate to involve the metaphysis. In about 70 percent the epiphyses are still open. Most tumors fill less than half the diameter of the epiphysis. Occasionally, a lesion may be initially confined to the epiphysis followed by growth into the metaphysis (fig. 94) (46). Scattered, stippled calcifications or a sparsely trabecular pattern is sometimes evident. Chondroblastomas are nearly always confined within the involved bone, but on rare occasions they can penetrate the cortex or enter the joint space. In one series, 15 percent of chondroblastomas had a secondary aneurysmal bone cyst component. This secondary change was not recognizable radiographically (46).

A few chondroblastomas, especially recurrent ones, are quite large and appear radiographically aggressive, with "blowout" destruction of the cortex. These "aggressive chondroblastomas" are discussed below.

Gross Findings. Chondroblastomas have a grossly variable appearance (fig. 95). They are usually finely granular and grey, yellow, or brown with interspersed irregular red areas that represent foci of hemorrhagic necrosis or an aneurysmal bone cyst component. There may be blue-grey areas that correspond to chondroid matrix. Punctate yellow, gritty foci, when present, represent calcified tumor, or less commonly, reactive bone within the lesion. In completely resected specimens, a rim of sclerotic bone is often visible.

Microscopic Findings. There is a broad histologic spectrum that varies with the amount of matrix produced by the tumor, the extent of necrosis, and the presence of microscopic foci of aneurysmal bone cyst in about 40 percent of cases (53). The cytologic spectrum is large as well. The most typical cell has a sharply defined cytoplas-

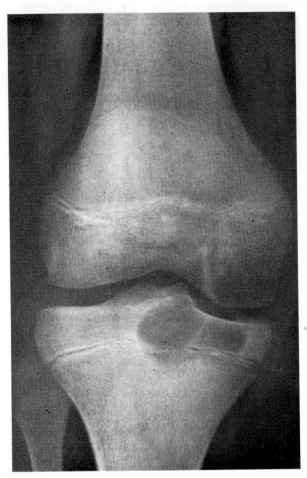

Figure 94
CHONDROBLASTOMA
This radiograph of the tibia of a 12-year-old girl shows a sharply demarcated, radiolucent area located mainly in the epiphysis and extending for a short distance into the metaphysis. (Fig. 15 from Fascicle 5, 2nd Series.)

mic border, lightly staining or focally clear cytoplasm, and an ovoid or round nucleus (fig. 96). Nuclear clefts, grooves, or invaginations are commonly seen. These features permit diagnosis on fine-needle aspiration (49). The chromatin may be evenly dispersed or irregularly clumped. Mitotic figures are present in approximately 75 percent of cases, but usually only a few are seen in all of the sections. Rarely, there may be more than 4 mitotic figures per 10 high-power fields (53). Atypical forms are not seen. Approximately 20 to 30 percent of chondroblastomas have atypical cells with enlarged, irregularly shaped, hyperchromatic nuclei. These do not appear to indicate an adverse prognosis (59,63).

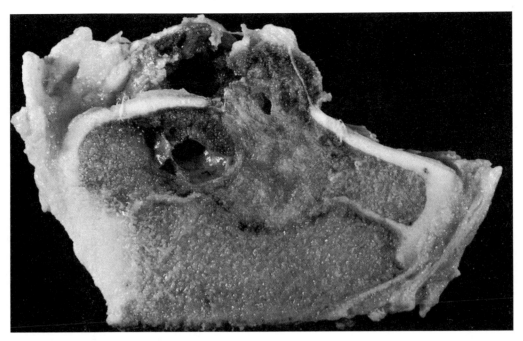

Figure 95
CHONDROBLASTOMA
A hemisection of a chondroblastoma from the proximal tibial epiphysis shows a well-demarcated lesion which is partially cystic. There is focal extension through the growth plate into the metaphysis, and the articular cartilage is also partially disrupted. (Fig. 26 from Fascicle 5, 2nd Series.)

Although most chondroblastoma cells have sharply defined borders, many lack well-defined cellular margins, creating a syncytial appearance to the cytoplasm. Spindle cells are commonly seen, either as nests or interspersed among the more typical chondroblasts (fig. 97). Multinucleated cells with nuclei identical to those of the mononuclear chondroblasts are common. In addition, huge osteoclast-like giant cells may be present, either in large aggregates or as single cells.

Almost all chondroblastomas have areas of chondroid differentiation, but these may be minimal and widely scattered. The chondroid matrix typically is eosinophilic rather than basophilic (53). The cells within the matrix maintain their chondroblastic appearance; mature chondrocytes with small, dense nuclei are rare (fig. 98). Occasionally there are areas of myxoid stroma with spindle cells having a stellate cytoplasmic configuration. The latter are identical to the myxoid stromal cells seen in chondromyxoid fibroma.

Calcifications are found either within the matrix or, more commonly, surrounding individual

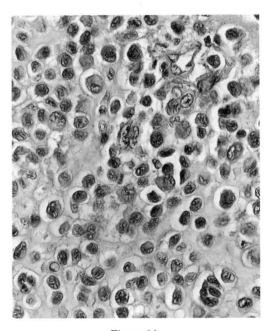

Figure 96
CHONDROBLASTOMA
Chondroblasts have cell borders ranging from well demarcated to ill defined. Nuclei vary in size and configuration, with numerous multilobed forms. Some nuclei have vesicular chromatin and others are quite dense. Multinucleated cells are also present.

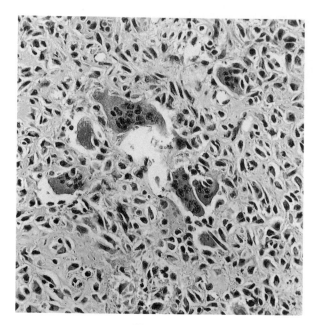

Figure 97
CHONDROBLASTOMA
The neoplastic cells in this field have ovoid to spindled nuclei. There is a moderate amount of matrix. Several osteoclastic-like, multinucleated giant cells are also present.

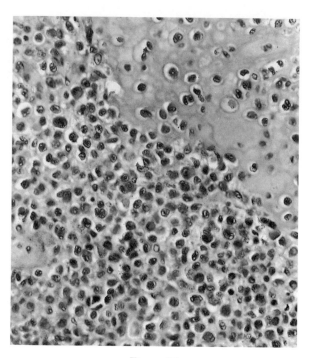

Figure 98
CHONDROBLASTOMA
The cells embedded in well-formed chondroid matrix (top right) are cytologically identical to the chondroblasts in sheets, unassociated with matrix.

cells. The latter pattern is especially frequent in partly or totally necrotic areas (fig. 99). The deposition of calcium around individual cells results in a "chicken-wire" appearance that is highly characteristic of chondroblastoma, although it is seen in only about two thirds of cases.

Ultrastructurally, the cells have numerous, long cytoplasmic processes, prominent Golgi complexes, and abundant rough endoplasmic reticulum. These features are typical of both fetal chondroblasts and adult chondrocytes. The cells of chondroblastoma differ only by having extremely irregular nuclear shapes (64).

Chondroblastomas have been the subject of multiple immunohistochemical studies (52,55, 60,65), which have clearly demonstrated the presence of S-100 protein in the neoplastic cells, supporting their chondroid differentiation and providing a potential diagnostic tool. The tumor cells are also strongly positive for neuron specific enolase and vimentin (52,60). Positivity for epithelial markers including cytokeratin and epithelial membrane antigen has been reported in some studies (60), but others have noted an absence of epithelial markers in these tumors.

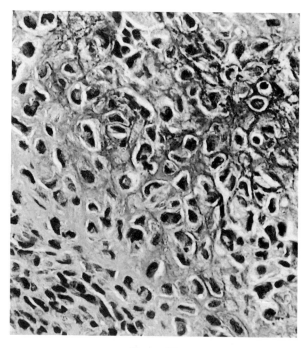

Figure 99
CHONDROBLASTOMA
The deposition of a thin layer of calcium around individual, often degenerating cells produces a "chicken-wire" appearance.

Differential Diagnosis. Because of its epiphyseal location and lytic radiographic appearance, chondroblastoma may be confused with giant cell tumor. There are significant clinical and radiographic differences, however. The majority of chondroblastomas occur when the epiphyses are still open, and most involve less than half the epiphyseal diameter. In contrast, giant cell tumors tend to be larger lesions occurring in skeletally mature individuals. Microscopically, chondroblastoma often has large numbers of giant cells, many of which are identical to cells seen in giant cell tumor. The distinguishing feature is the background mononuclear cells, which, in giant cell tumors, resemble histiocytes with folded nuclei and lack the irregularly vacuolated and indented nuclei of chondroblasts. In addition, the matrix of chondroblastoma is missing, as is the calcification around necrotic cells. In rare cases, S-100 positivity in the neoplastic cells may be helpful in establishing a diagnosis of chondroblastoma.

Clear cell chondrosarcoma enters into the differential diagnosis because it frequently involves the epiphysis and may contain large numbers of giant cells. However, it has broad sheets of cells that have voluminous clear or nearly clear cytoplasm. Although cells indistinguishable from chondroblasts are found focally in clear cell chondrosarcoma, they account for only a small part of the tumor. S-100 staining is of no value in this distinction, as clear cell chondrosarcoma has been demonstrated to be S-100 positive (55,65).

Treatment and Prognosis. About 90 percent of chondroblastomas are successfully treated by curettage and bone chip grafting. Virtually all recurrences develop within 3 years, and 99 percent of these are cured by a second curettage or by resection. Huvos and Marcove (50) noted greater recurrence when the chondroblastoma had an aneurysmal bone cyst component, but others have not found this association (46).

Approximately 1 percent of reported chondroblastomas are associated with aggressive local invasion, with or without pulmonary metastasis. The actual frequency of this phenomenon is undoubtedly far less because of the tendency to preferentially report tumors behaving in an unusual manner. Some locally aggressive or metastasizing chondroblastomas may be microscopically indistinguishable from conventional tumors (fig. 100) (51,66). Metastases may not appear until more than 30 years after the initial diagnosis. In other aggressive or metastasizing tumors, recurrence or metastasis ceases to resemble chondroblastoma and assumes the appearance of an unclassifiable pleomorphic sarcoma (54,56,61).

There is no consistent correlation between tumors with aggressive local behavior and pulmonary metastases. Some chondroblastomas have invaded soft tissues, including neurovascular bundles, necessitating an amputation or hemipelvectomy, but have not developed metastases. Conversely, one patient with pulmonary metastases had no difficulty with local recurrence (54).

Pulmonary metastases of chondroblastoma are often satisfactorily treated by surgical removal. In one instance, a nodule of metastatic chondroblastoma was removed, but three other presumed metastases left in place remained unchanged over a 5-year period (57). One patient with persistent local disease for 34 years had small pulmonary metastases discovered at autopsy when the patient was 71 years old (66). There are, however, cases in which the metastases continued to grow and contributed to the patient's death. There is only one case in which pulmonary metastases were detected at the time of initial presentation (54). Other metastases have followed surgical intervention and may represent the "transport" or "implant" phenomenon seen in giant cell tumors.

Some irradiated chondroblastomas have been followed several years later by a fibrosarcoma or osteosarcoma at the prior treatment site. These are viewed as postradiation sarcomas rather than spontaneous malignant transformation of chondroblastoma.

CHONDROMYXOID FIBROMA

Definition. A benign tumor characterized by lobules of spindle shaped or stellate cells in an abundant myxoid to chondroid stroma. The lobules are separated by a more cellular stroma rich in spindle shaped to rounded cells and containing varying numbers of pleomorphic cells or multinucleated giant cells.

Clinical Features. Patients range from 3 to 70 years of age; about 60 percent are between 10 and 30 years of age. A male predominance of approximately 2 to 1 has been reported in many series (69), whereas others have found an equal predilection (77).

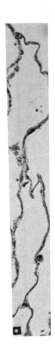

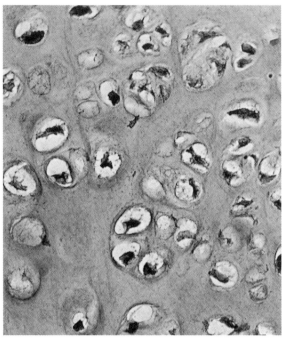

Figure 120
CHONDROSARCOMA
Well-differentiated chondrosarcoma retains cellular groupings in the hyaline cartilage matrix. Nuclei are moderately enlarged, elongated, and irregular in shape. (Fig. 95 from Fascicle 5, 2nd Series.)

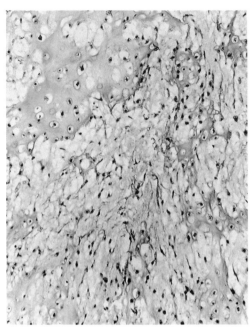

Figure 121
CHONDROSARCOMA
Well-formed chondroid matrix at the upper left of the figure is in continuity with myxoid stroma. Nuclei are fairly uniform and small in this grade 1 chondrosarcoma.

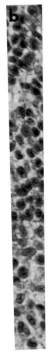

encase small lobules of cartilage (fig. 123). Similar foci or reactive bone may be present deep within the tumor, but not closely apposed to the cartilaginous lobules (fig. 124). Sections taken at the edge of intramedullary chondrosarcomas show cartilage invading the marrow between trabeculae of bone (fig. 125). Most of the host bone is resorbed, but partially replaced trabeculae may become completely surrounded by proliferating cartilage, remaining as islands of usually necrotic bone within the neoplasm (fig. 126). Invasion and resorption of the cortex occurs as the first step in extraosseous extension (fig. 127). Microscopically, fingers of tumor infiltrate the adjacent soft tissue. This process may not be grossly discernible (fig. 128). Such foci are obvious sources for local recurrence, however. Many peripheral chondrosarcomas have a pushing margin that is more amenable to en bloc excision (fig. 129).

Microscopic Grading. The broad microscopic spectrum of chondrosarcomas lends itself to grading, and this has been shown to have prognostic value. A three-grade system is commonly used.

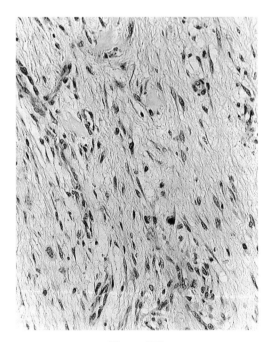

Figure 122
CHONDROSARCOMA
Spindle cells are occasionally seen in chondrosarcomas, especially high-grade lesions. When they lack pleomorphism or nuclear atypia, such as in this field, they should not be interpreted as areas of dedifferentiation.

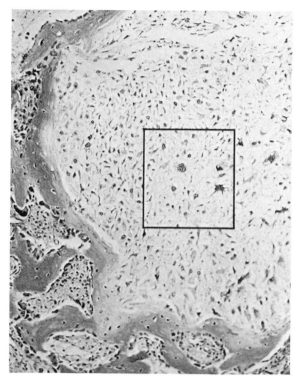

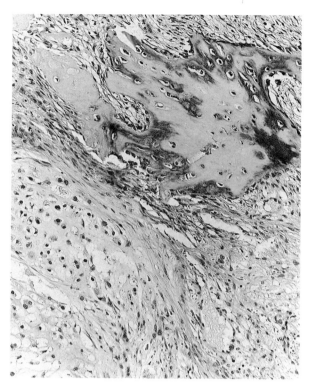

Figure 123
CHONDROSARCOMA

A lobule of grade 2 chondrosarcoma with myxoid stroma is encased in a thin rim of reactive bone. Osteoblasts are prominent on the side of the trabeculae away from the lobule. The bone and neoplasm imperceptibly meld together on the inside of the trabeculae. The area outlined is seen at higher magnification in figure 132. (Fig. 96 from Fascicle 5, 2nd Series.) (Figures 123 and 132 are from the same patient.)

Figure 124
CHONDROSARCOMA

Reactive new bone, partially lined by osteoblasts is adjacent to neoplastic cartilage, but it does not rim the cartilaginous lobule. The fibrous stroma may be the spindle cell component of chondrosarcoma or it may be reactive. Such fibro-osseous foci must not be misinterpreted as osteosarcoma or dedifferentiated chondrosarcoma.

Figure 125
CHONDROSARCOMA

The edge of a chondrosarcoma infiltrates the bone marrow. One trabecula of normal host bone has been engulfed by the tumor (upper left).

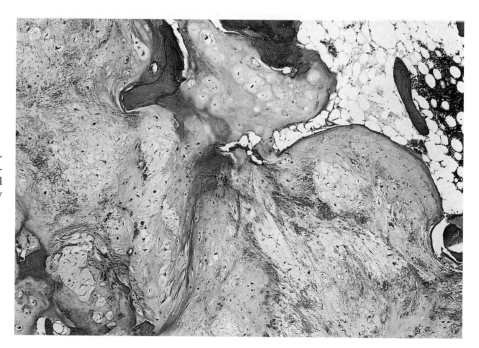

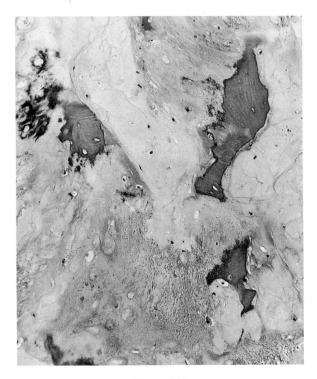

Figure 126
CHONDROSARCOMA
Necrotic, partly resorbed fragments of host bone are situated deeply within this grade 1 chondrosarcoma.

Grade 1 lesions have chondrocytes with small, dense nuclei, although some slightly enlarged nuclei (i.e., >8 μm) and a few multinucleated cells, usually binucleated, are present. The stroma is mainly chondroid, and myxoid areas are sparse or absent. Occasionally, there are isolated areas of widely spaced, large, pleomorphic nuclei, but this does not indicate a higher grade, as long as there is not increased cellularity or mitotic activity (fig. 130) (85).

Grade 2 chondrosarcomas have less matrix and are correspondingly more cellular (see figs 117, 123). The increased cellularity is especially prominent at the periphery of tumor lobules where matrix may be completely absent. Rarely, mitotic figures are found in this zone. The chondrocyte nuclei in the center of the lobules are enlarged and either vesicular or hyper chromatic. Often there is more than one cell in a lacuna. Necrosis ranges from small, microscopic foci to completely necrotic lobules. The stroma is frequently myxoid.

Grade 3 chondrosarcomas exhibit even greater cellularity and nuclear pleomorphism than the grade 2 tumors (fig. 131). Chondroid matrix is

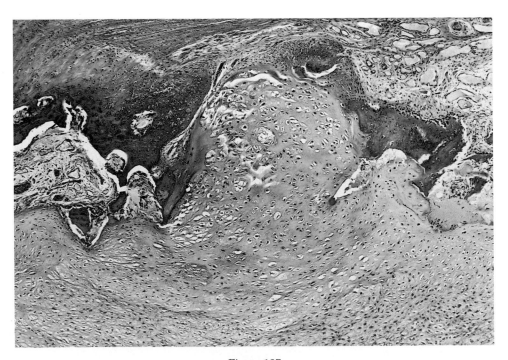

Figure 127
CHONDROSARCOMA
This chondrosarcoma penetrates the cortex and abuts connective tissue near a tendon.

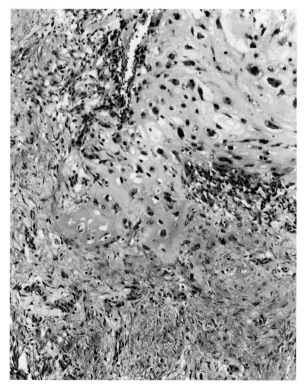

Figure 128
CHONDROSARCOMA
Soft tissue extension by grade 2 chondrosarcoma has an irregular margin infiltrating the surrounding fibrovascular tissue.

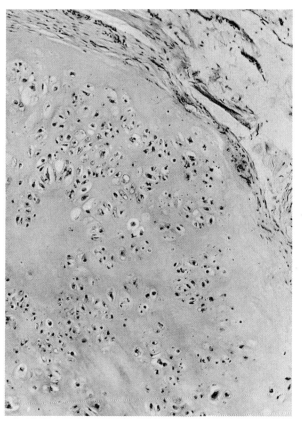

Figure 129
CHONDROSARCOMA
The outermost margin of this grade 1 peripheral chondrosarcoma is well demarcated, readily allowing for complete en bloc excision. (Fig. 93 from Fascicle 5, 2nd Series.)

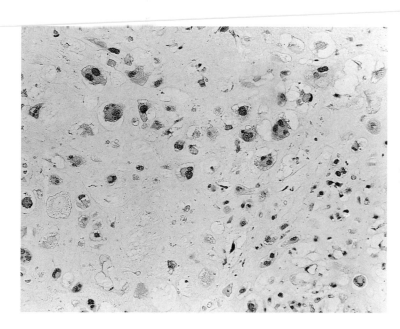

Figure 130
CHONDROSARCOMA
Widely spaced, markedly atypical, multinucleated chondrocytes are present in this otherwise typical, grade 1 chondrosarcoma.

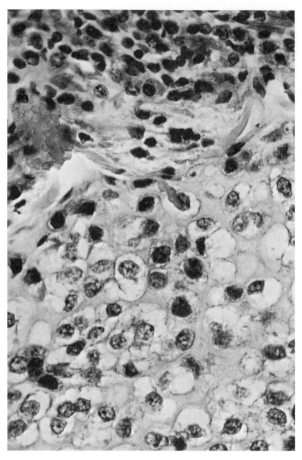

Figure 131
CHONDROSARCOMA
Grade 3 chondrosarcoma has sparse matrix and chondrocytes with large vesicular to dense nuclei. This rare lymph node metastasis has normal lymphocytes at the top for comparison of nuclear size with the neoplastic chondrocytes. (Fig. 103 from Fascicle 5, 2nd Series.)

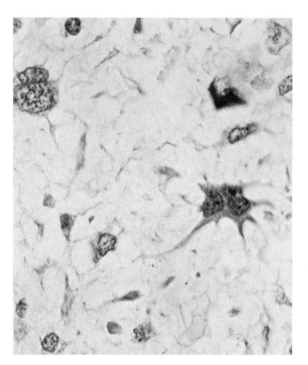

Figure 132
CHONDROSARCOMA
This higher magnification of the tumor seen in figure 123 shows a multinucleated stellate cell. Nuclei of other cells are markedly abnormal, due to enlargement and coarse chromatin. (Fig. 97 from Fascicle 5, 2nd Series.)

sparse or absent, and the small amount of intercellular material present tends to be myxoid. The neoplastic chondrocytes are often arranged in cords and clumps. The individual cells frequently have stellate or grotesquely irregular shapes (fig. 132). Foci of necrosis are almost invariably seen and are frequently extensive. Nuclei are typically vesicular, are often spindle shaped, and may be 5 to 10 times larger than normal. Evans et al. (85) use mitotic figures as a criterion for grade 3 lesions, but others classify tumors as grade 3 even in the absence of mitotic figures, when the cellularity and pleomorphism are extreme.

Although most chondrosarcomas have a dominant microscopic grade, many have small microscopic foci that range from grade 1 to grade 3. Whether such tumors should be graded based on their highest grade or their predominant grade is not currently clear. We believe that the presence of small, high-grade foci should be indicated in the pathology report, at least as an accompanying note. Wide sampling is important to avoid missing small high-grade foci, since these heterogenous areas can be overlooked in small biopsies. Large biopsies should be completely sectioned, and resected specimens should be liberally sampled to identify possible high-grade areas. Soft, tan, myxoid or hemorrhagic foci are especially likely to be high grade.

The proportion of chondrosarcomas having a given grade varies from series to series. This is a reflection, in part, of the difficulty inherent in categorizing the diverse images presented by cartilaginous tumors, as well as differing emphasis on various features such as cellularity, mitotic count, and nuclear pleomorphism. The greatest variation is in the proportion of cases that are grade 1 or grade 2. In three large series, grade 1 chondrosarcoma varied from 26 to 50 percent of cases, grade 2 ranged from 30 to 60 percent of cases, and grade 3 varied from 8 to 25 percent of cases (85,86,98).

Differential Diagnosis. Grade 1 chondrosarcomas pose the greatest diagnostic dilemma because their microscopic appearance can be identical to the more cellular and cytologically atypical areas of enchondromas, osteochondromas, and other benign cartilaginous lesions such as synovial chondromatosis (102). Thus, the diagnosis of histologic grade 1 chondrosarcoma often relies exclusively on the radiographic findings of cortical bone destruction or, in the case of a peripheral cartilaginous mass, the lack of features of benign peripheral lesions such as periosteal chondroma or osteochondroma. Occasionally, a tumor that could be either a histologic grade 1 chondrosarcoma or an enchondroma will have radiologic findings such as endosteal scalloping of the cortex that are considered by the radiologist as suggestive, but not unequivocal, evidence of aggressive growth. Since endosteal scalloping can be seen in chondrosarcomas as well as enchondromas, the pathologist may be left with a diagnosis such as "cartilaginous neoplasm of uncertain malignant potential" or "borderline cartilaginous neoplasm."

Enchondroma. A few microscopic findings are helpful in distinguishing grade 1 chondrosarcoma from enchondroma. Sections from the edge of a chondrosarcoma may show growth of cartilage between trabeculae of bone (see fig. 125), a pattern lacking in enchondromas. Chondrosarcomas can also contain, within the neoplasm, islands of viable or necrotic preexisting bone (see fig. 126), a feature also absent in enchondroma. As discussed above, enchondromas tend to consist of cartilaginous islands, partly or completely rimmed with lamellar bone with normal bone marrow intervening. There may be osseous rimming of small lobules of cartilage in chondrosarcoma, but the lobules will be completely surrounded by other lobules of tumor rather than intervening marrow. Bands of fibrous tissue seen between lobules of chondrosarcoma do not occur in enchondromas (see fig. 117). Rarely, chondrosarcoma infiltrates the haversian system (97).

Whether chondrosarcomas arise from solitary, preexistent enchondromas has been a subject of debate. Some authors found no evidence of this (86,98), but Mirra et al. (97) believe that approximately 50 percent of chondrosarcomas contain areas fulfilling their criteria for a preexisting enchondroma.

Chondroblastic Osteosarcoma. These tumors contain large quantities of cartilage, and are occasionally confused with chondrosarcoma. The osteoid of osteosarcoma has cytologically atypical osteoblasts and anomalous patterns of deposition. In addition to a rim of reactive osteoid surrounding neoplastic cartilaginous nodules, chondrosarcomas may have foci of osseous metaplasia or reactive osteoid within the tumor. These trabeculae are lined by cytologically uniform osteoblasts. The trabeculae appear mature, and they are evenly spaced in contrast to the irregular, lace-like osteoid of osteosarcoma.

Spread and Metastasis. Chondrosarcoma readily spreads within the medullary cavity. The overlying cortex is often intact, but is frequently eroded, thinned, or expanded. Cortical permeation with extension of tumor into the surrounding soft tissues is also common. Pelvic chondrosarcomas may invade the bladder or colon, and, rarely, there is grossly visible extension into large veins.

Distant metastases are most often to the lungs, followed by skin and soft tissue. Lymph node metastases are uncommon (85). Metastases to brain, liver, and bone are rare.

Treatment and Prognosis. En bloc excision is the preferred therapy (88) because curettage is associated with a greater than 90 percent rate of local recurrence, even for grade 1 or 2 tumors (85). Limb-saving resections are feasible for some peripheral tumors and central lesions that have not broken through the cortex (84). Local recurrences can usually be controlled by subsequent amputation. Tumors of the pelvis pose special problems. Complete excision is often not feasible or, if attempted, is accompanied by a high rate of local recurrence.

The prognosis depends on two major factors: the stage and the histologic grade. If the chondrosarcoma is completely resectable, the prognosis depends mainly on the histologic grade, because this feature correlates with metastatic rate. As many as 70 percent of grade 3 tumors metastasize, including cases with adequate initial local control (85). By contrast, metastasis is uncommon for a grade 1 chondrosarcoma, unless it is a high stage lesion (86). Between 10 and 33 percent of grade 2 chondrosarcomas metastasize (85,86, 98,101). It is likely that some lesions reported as grade 3 chondrosarcomas would be classified by others as so-called dedifferentiated chondrosarcomas: lesions with an extremely high rate of metastasis.

For chondrosarcomas of the rib that are less than 4 cm in diameter, stripping the rib from the adjacent pleura and removal is sufficient. However, lesions larger than 4 cm in diameter require en bloc excision, including adjacent uninvolved ribs, as well as the pleura. Lesser excisions for large tumors are followed by local recurrence and may result in death (95).

The prognosis of grade 1 and grade 2 chondrosarcomas is predominately governed by their resectability which, in turn, is often a function of location. Tumors of the distal extremities have a good prognosis because amputation will totally ablate the lesion, and many tumors of the extremity are amenable to en bloc resection that preserves the limb. Conversely, chondrosarcomas of the pelvis or shoulder girdle often pose formidable problems for resection, especially when they are large. Thus, even if they are grade 2 tumors (which most are) the risk of local recurrence due to incomplete resection or intraoperative implantation of tumor is very high. Repeated recurrences may extend over many years, finally reaching a point where resection is impossible and the patient dies. Interestingly, the local recurrence rate is about the same (27 to 35 percent) regardless of the grade (85).

Local recurrences or metastases usually occur within the first 5 years after diagnosis, although many patients who die of their disease do so after this time period (96). In fact, more than 80 percent of deaths due to peripheral chondrosarcomas are after 5 years, and one third of patients with central chondrosarcomas who die of their disease do so after 5 years. Patients younger than 20 years of age have been reported by some to have a worse prognosis, even when the diagnosis of chondroblastic osteosarcoma has been carefully excluded (95); others find no difference in the prognosis in children (103).

Some authors have noted that recurrences of chondrosarcoma are often of a higher grade than the original tumor (80,91,98,100). It is likely that the higher grade was present in the original lesion but not included in the samples examined microscopically. Evans et al. (85) did not find that recurrences had a higher grade, even when they were multiple and developed over a long period of time. They did note, however, that metastatic tumors often had greater cellularity and an increased mitotic rate, as compared with the primary neoplasms.

Kreicbergs and associates (90), using cytophotometry, found that ploidy complemented grading in identifying tumors with metastatic potential. Seven of eight patients with metastases had hyperploid tumors and only one was diploid. All of the patients were free of local recurrence. Flow cytometry has no value in the separation of enchondroma from low-grade chondrosarcoma (78,94).

DEDIFFERENTIATED CHONDROSARCOMA

Definition. A high-grade, nonchondroid sarcoma such as malignant fibrous histiocytoma, osteosarcoma, fibrosarcoma, rhabdomyosarcoma, or angiosarcoma associated with, and apparently arising from, a low-grade cartilage-forming tumor. The longer, albeit more accurate, term of *chondrosarcoma with additional mesenchymal component* is synonymous.

General Features. Dedifferentiated chondrosarcomas comprise approximately 11 percent of all chondrosarcomas (111). Using the term "dedifferentiation" to reflect a high-grade, noncartilaginous component is probably mechanistically incorrect. It is more likely that the high-grade elements represent a failure of maturation in mitotically active "stem cells," rather than a "dedifferentiation" of mature chondroid cells. The adjective dedifferentiated is, nonetheless, widely established in the literature and is retained in this discussion.

Controversy remains as to whether the dedifferentiated component is derived from cartilage precursors or represents a completely separate line of cells. Ultrastructural and immunohistochemical studies can be interpreted to support both viewpoints and indeed, different pathogenetic pathways may exist in different tumors. Most evidence, however, suggests that the noncartilaginous element is derived from a separate noncartilaginous clone (or clones) of cells (104,117,118).

In their original paper on the topic, Dahlin and Beabout (108) noted that the cartilaginous tumors were often so bland that the diagnosis of chondrosarcoma, as opposed to enchondroma, was difficult. This probably accounts for reports of osteosarcomas arising within enchondromas (115,116).

Clinical Features. Patients range from 19 to 82 years of age, but most are beyond the age of 50 years. Pain, with or without pathologic fracture, swelling, and paresthesias are the most frequent complaints. Symptoms can be present from a few weeks to up to 10 years and average approximately 6 to 10 months in duration (107,108,112).

Sites. The distribution of dedifferentiated chondrosarcoma parallels that of conventional chondrosarcoma. Therefore, the most common sites are the bones of the pelvis, followed by the proximal femur, proximal humerus, distal femur, and ribs (111).

Radiographic Appearance. The distinctive radiographic finding is an ill-defined, lytic intraosseous lesion or an extraosseous soft tissue mass that is devoid of calcifications but is in continuity with a lesion having the features of a cartilaginous tumor (fig. 133). There is frequently cortical perforation, and when extraosseous extension of the tumor occurs, the mass is usually large. Characteristically, there is an abrupt transition between the chondroid tumor and the dedifferentiated, lytic component. The bone may be expanded, which indicates the initial slow growth of the chondrosarcomatous component. CT scans are particularly useful in identifying extraosseous extension that may not be seen on radiographs (109).

It may be difficult to determine whether the original cartilaginous component had radiographic features of enchondroma or chondrosarcoma. This is because the dedifferentiated portion of the tumor destroys the cortex, preventing radiographic evaluation of the cartilaginous tumor-cortical interface. Dedifferentiated chondrosarcoma almost always originates from a central chondrosarcoma. Occasionally, the chondrosarcoma has arisen in turn from a preexistent enchondroma (113). A minority of dedifferentiated chondrosarcomas arise from peripheral chondrosarcomas that, in turn, were superimposed on osteochondromas (105). The osteochondromas may be solitary or occur in patients with multiple hereditary osteochondromatosis.

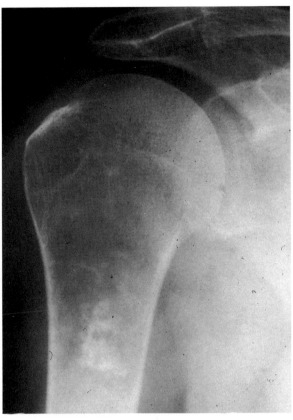

Figure 133
DEDIFFERENTIATED CHONDROSARCOMA
Cartilaginous matrix is seen centrally with lytic areas and destruction of cortex around it. The latter corresponds to the dedifferentiated component in this 72-year-old man.

Gross Findings. The cut surface of a resected specimen has areas with the typical lobular, blue-gray myxoid or overtly cartilaginous appearance of mature hyaline cartilage. In addition, there are zones of brown, tan, or hemorrhagic tissue lacking the consistency of cartilage (fig. 134). The dedifferentiated component may be only a minor portion of the overall tumor, or it may be so extensive that very little residual cartilage is recognizable.

Microscopic Findings. The chondrosarcoma component is often grade 1 (108,112). In one study, however, high-grade chondrosarcomas predominated (107). The junction of cartilaginous and noncartilaginous elements is nearly always sharp (fig. 135).

The predominant noncartilaginous component has varied from series to series. Fibrosarcoma and malignant fibrous histiocytoma have

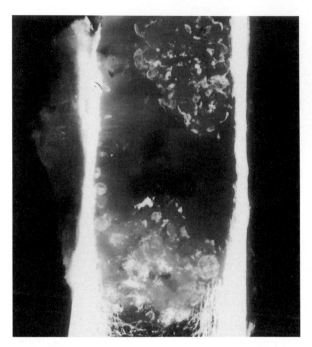 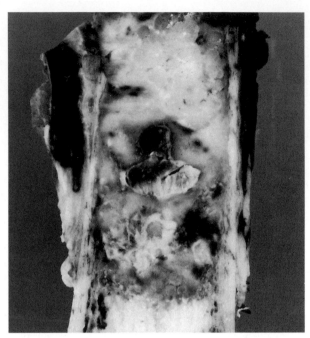

Figure 134
DEDIFFERENTIATED CHONDROSARCOMA
A. Specimen radiograph of dedifferentiated chondrosarcoma in the mid-shaft of the femur in a 62-year-old man. The ring-like calcifications of the preexisting cartilage neoplasm are seen on either side of a central lytic area, representing the dedifferentiated component. B. The gross specimen shows lobules of cartilage above and below a central, variegated area which microscopically resembles malignant fibrous histiocytoma. (Fig. 1 from Wick MR, Siegal GP, Mills SE, Thompson RC, Sawhney D, Fechner RE. Dedifferentiated chondrosarcoma of bone. An immunohistochemical and lectin-histochemical study. Virchows Arch [A] 1987;411:23–32.)

been the most frequently reported (111,112,114), but osteosarcoma, rhabdomyosarcoma, and angiosarcoma also have been described (106,110). In our experience, as well as the series of Johnson et al. (112), malignant fibrous histiocytoma is by far the most frequent dedifferentiated component. High-grade spindle cells are typically arranged in a storiform pattern with intermixed giant cells. The fibrohistiocytic nature of the dedifferentiated component is supported with immunohistochemical studies (112,118). In a few tumors, there is striated muscle differentiation and cytokeratin formation (110).

Differential Diagnosis. Dedifferentiated chondrosarcoma may be confused with high-grade chondrosarcoma having spindle cell areas, mesenchymal chondrosarcoma, chondroblastic osteosarcoma, malignant fibrous histiocytoma, and fibrosarcoma. The latter two diagnoses are eliminated by the presence of cartilage. High-grade chondrosarcomas with spindle cell areas show multiple zones of transition and intermix-

ing of the spindle cell foci with the hyaline cartilage. In dedifferentiated chondrosarcomas, the spindle cell foci and hyaline cartilage are only juxtaposed at the interface of the two tumor components. There is not an intimate mixture throughout the lesion. Similarly, mesenchymal chondrosarcoma has its cartilaginous component speckled throughout the tumor and mixed with the spindle cell or small round cell noncartilaginous component. Chondroblastic osteosarcoma has neoplastic osteoid irregularly mixed with usually high-grade cartilage, and it lacks two grossly separate malignant elements, as is the case in dedifferentiated chondrosarcoma.

When the biopsy contains only high-grade elements such as osteosarcoma, malignant fibrous histiocytoma, or fibrosarcoma, the proper diagnosis rests on finding areas of cartilage. Attention to the calcified areas on the radiograph should facilitate identifying the cartilaginous components in the gross specimen, or in directing biopsies to these areas, in addition to the high-grade component.

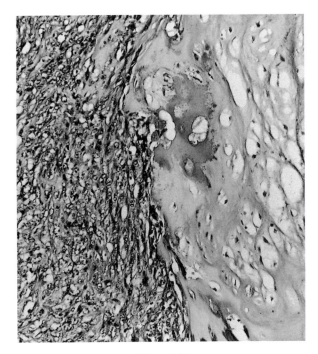

Figure 135
DEDIFFERENTIATED CHONDROSARCOMA
A low-grade cartilaginous neoplasm is seen at the right with a spindle cell component of malignant fibrous histiocytoma at the left.

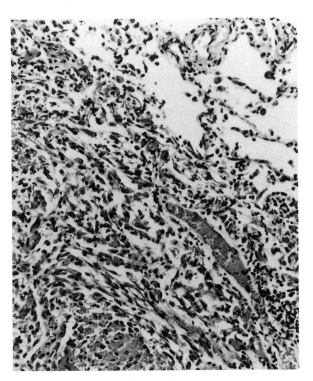

Figure 136
DEDIFFERENTIATED CHONDROSARCOMA
Pulmonary metastasis from a dedifferentiated chondrosarcoma contains only the malignant fibrous histiocytoma-like component.

Treatment and Prognosis. Regardless of the extent of local resection, the prognosis is almost hopeless. Approximately 90 percent of patients are dead with distant metastases within 2 years, and most of these die within 1 year of diagnosis. Metastases consist solely of the high-grade, noncartilaginous component (fig. 136) and predominately involve the lungs. Spread may also occur to other bones and visceral organs.

CLEAR CELL CHONDROSARCOMA

Definition. A malignant tumor comprised of neoplastic chondrocytes having abundant, predominately clear cytoplasm with little intervening matrix. Foci of conventional chondrosarcoma may also be present.

General and Clinical Features. This uncommon variant accounts for about 2 percent of all chondrosarcomas (122,124). The approximately 2 to 1 male predominance in patients with conventional chondrosarcoma is also seen with the clear cell subtype. Patients range from 14 to 84 years of age, with most in their third or fourth decades of life.

The most common symptoms are pain and swelling. Because these tumors tend to involve the epiphyses of long bones, there may be interference with motion in the adjacent joint. Symptoms are often of long duration. Of 38 patients, 17 (45 percent) had symptoms for less than 1 year, 14 (37 percent) were symptomatic for 1 to 5 years, and 7 (18 percent) had symptoms for more than 5 years (120). One patient had swelling for 20 years. Occasional clear cell chondrosarcomas may be detected as incidental findings (123).

Sites. The epiphyses of long bones are characteristically involved. Rarely, lesions are confined to the diaphysis or metaphysis; larger lesions may extensively involve the epiphysis, metaphysis, and diaphysis. The most common sites of involvement are the proximal femur, proximal humerus, distal femur, and proximal tibia. Cases have been reported in the ulna, rib, small bones of the hand, pelvis, vertebrae, and temporal bone. Infrequently, patients may have two clear cell chondrosarcomas (124).

Radiographic Appearance. Clear cell chondrosarcoma is usually an osteolytic, expansile lesion (fig. 137), which may be focally calcified. There is often a sharp interface between tumor and surrounding normal bone, although a sclerotic rim is uncommon. The margin is indistinct in about half of the cases. The overlying cortex is usually thinned but intact. Destructive cortical penetration is rare, but has been reported. In the series of Bjornsson et al. (120), soft tissue masses were present in only three cases: tumors associated with a rib, vertebra, and the calvarium. Pathologic fractures are also rare, and periosteal new bone formation occurs only in the presence of fracture.

Gross Findings. On cut surface, clear cell chondrosarcoma typically lacks the appearance of conventional chondrosarcoma and is, instead, usually red, soft, and granular. There may be multiple cysts. Small areas of gray or white cartilage may be irregularly interspersed.

Microscopic Findings. These lesions can have the same lobular pattern seen in most cartilaginous neoplasms, although it is usually much less conspicuous. Sometimes, the microlobules are separated by a delicate fibrovascular stroma. The dominant cell is a chondrocyte with variably clear cytoplasm and a sharply defined cell border (figs. 138, 139). Many of the clear cells have a condensation of powdery cytoplasm near the cell membrane or clumped near the nucleus (fig. 140). Scattered eosinophilic cells often have a similar powdery cytoplasm irregularly filling much of the cell. The nuclei of both clear and eosinophilic cells are enlarged and, rarely, binuclear. Mitotic figures are extremely rare.

Matrix formation is sparse, with only small deposits of chondroid material between the clear cells. The matrix may be focally calcified. More

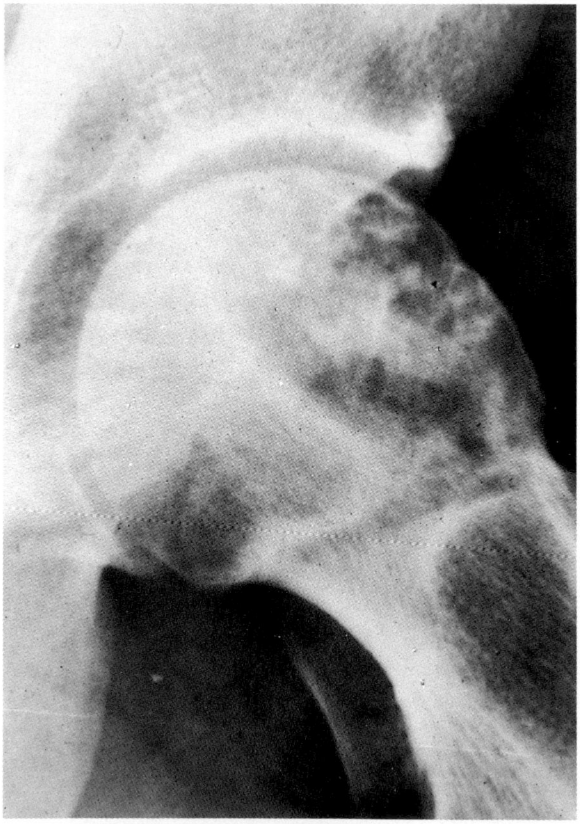

Figure 137
CLEAR CELL CHONDROSARCOMA
The tumor is located in the head of the femur of a 46-year-old man. It is lytic with floccular calcified matrix and involves the epiphysis. (Courtesy of Dr. A. G. Ayala, Houston, TX.)

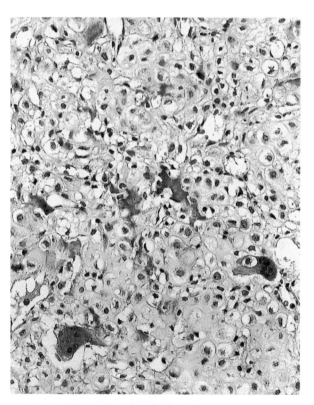

Figure 138
CLEAR CELL CHONDROSARCOMA
The tumor cells have delicate powdery-to-clear cytoplasm. A small area of calcified matrix is present centrally. Multinucleated giant cells are scattered in the tumor.

abundant matrix is present in the areas of conventional chondrosarcoma that are found in approximately half of the clear cell variants (fig. 140). These areas may form small foci or, occasionally, broad zones that blend imperceptibly into the clear cell component. The conventional chondrosarcoma component is usually grade 1.

Small deposits of uncalcified or calcified osteoid may occur in clear cell chondrosarcoma. These trabeculae are indented by the cartilaginous cells. The long trabeculae that intimately encase nodules of cartilage in conventional osteosarcoma do not occur. Rarely, the osteoid has a more disorganized appearance somewhat resembling that of osteosarcoma (120). Multinucleated osteoclast-like giant cells are frequently present, either as individual cells or small clusters. This contrasts with conventional chondrosarcoma, which almost never contains giant cells.

Ultrastructurally, the cells of clear cell chondrosarcoma exhibit the features of chondrocytes,

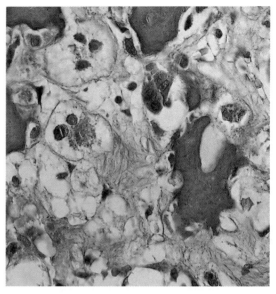

Figure 139
CLEAR CELL CHONDROSARCOMA
Cells have variably clear cytoplasm. Binucleate clear cells are present and calcified matrix is interspersed.

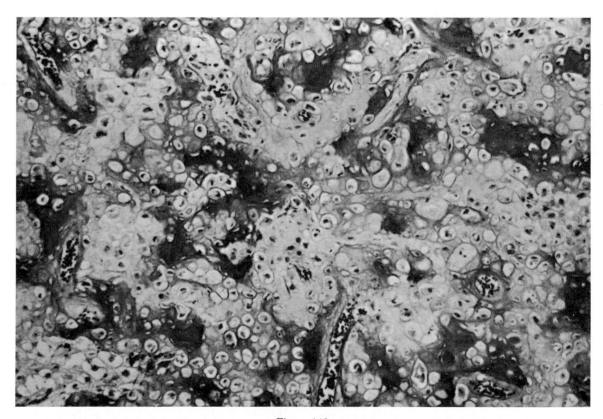

Figure 140
CLEAR CELL CHONDROSARCOMA
An area of well-differentiated chondrosarcoma with conventional pattern coexists in this clear cell chondrosarcoma. (Fig. 522 from Fascicle 5(Suppl), 2nd Series.)

including deeply indented nuclei, large, dilated rough endoplasmic reticulum cisternae, and substantial quantities of glycogen (121). Angervall and Kindblom (119) noted that the clear areas in the cytoplasm corresponded to low density granular material, distinct from glycogen, that was devoid of organelles. Although none of these features is specific, the ultrastructural spectrum is similar to that of normal chondrocytes in varying degrees of differentiation, as well as that of cartilaginous neoplasms such as chondroblastoma or low-grade chondrosarcoma.

Differential Diagnosis. Chondroblastoma is a major consideration, because many clear cell chondrosarcomas occur in the epiphyseal ends of long bones. Although chondroblastomas may have cells with clear cytoplasm and well-defined cell borders, they are not the predominate cell type, as in clear cell chondrosarcoma. Chondroblastoma cells are oval or spindled and have lightly staining eosinophilic cytoplasm, in contrast to the cells of clear cell chondrosarcoma.

Metastatic clear cell carcinomas, such as from the kidney, may cytologically resemble clear cell chondrosarcoma, although the glandular architecture or lumen formation of the former is not seen in clear cell chondrosarcoma. If immunohistochemistry is employed to facilitate the differential diagnosis in suspicious cases, it should be interpreted with caution. Clear cell chondrosarcomas, as well as other cartilaginous neoplasms, express S-100 protein, but this antigen will also be present in about two thirds of metastatic renal cell carcinomas. Renal cell carcinomas express large amounts of epithelial membrane antigen and cytokeratin, and often also contain vimentin. Cartilaginous tumors have been clearly demonstrated to express vimentin, and some authors have reported epithelial antigens, including cytokeratin and epithelial membrane antigen as well.

Treatment and Prognosis. En bloc resection with a wide margin of normal bone and soft tissue is the procedure of choice. Bjornsson et al. (120) reported that simple excision or curettage had an 80 percent risk of local recurrence while only 1 of 13 patients treated with en bloc resection developed local recurrence. That patient underwent amputation and remains well 3 years later. One patient developed metastases 2 years after en bloc resection. The clear cell chondrosarcomas that metastasized did not appear to have distinguishing

microscopic or clinical differences. Seven of their 47 (15 percent) patients died with metastases between 2 and 12 years after the initial procedure. Four of the 7 patients who died had been treated initially with local excision, usually curettage. However, metastases also occurred in 2 patients treated initially with amputation.

MESENCHYMAL CHONDROSARCOMA

Definition. A malignant, cartilage-forming tumor comprised predominantly of noncartilaginous small, round, oval, or spindle shaped cells. Osteoid is often present as well, and the tumor frequently has a hemangiopericytoma-like appearance.

General Features. This variant accounts for about 2 percent of all chondrosarcomas (125). Some of the tumors reported as polyhistioma and primitive multipotential primary sarcoma of bone appear to be mesenchymal chondrosarcomas (127,129).

Clinical Features. Patients with mesenchymal chondrosarcoma range from 5 to 74 years of age. However, 80 percent are between the ages of 10 and 40 years. There is no sexual predilection. Presenting complaints typically consist of pain and, occasionally, swelling. Approximately one third of patients are symptomatic for more than 1 year.

Sites. Mesenchymal chondrosarcoma favors the maxilla, mandible, ribs, and vertebrae. The pelvis and femur are additional common sites of involvement. Other long tubular bones and, rarely, the phalanges, may also be affected. A few patients have presented with multiple sites of bone involvement (132).

Radiographic Appearance. A lytic defect that often contains stippled densities corresponding to small islands of mineralized cartilage is seen radiographically (fig. 141). Calcified tumors are indistinguishable, radiographically, from conventional chondrosarcoma. Most mesenchymal chondrosarcomas have an indistinct border. Some, however, have sharply defined or, rarely, sclerotic margins (132). The cortex is destroyed in approximately half of the cases, with associated extension of tumor into the adjacent soft tissues. A subperiosteal mesenchymal chondrosarcoma has been reported (133).

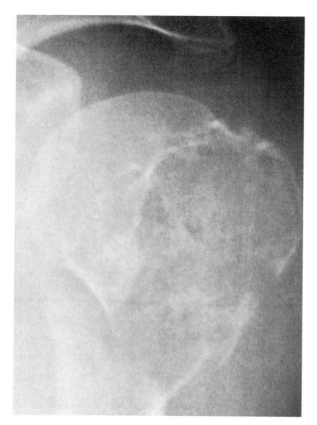

Figure 141
MESENCHYMAL CHONDROSARCOMA
Radiograph demonstrates an expansile, predominately lytic lesion with irregular, fine calcifications and extension into soft tissue. This 31-year-old man had discomfort for 3 years with onset of sudden pain due to pathologic fracture. (Fig. 104 from Fascicle 5, 2nd Series.)

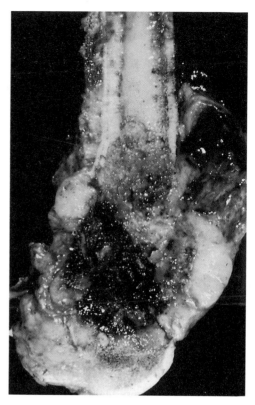

Figure 142
MESENCHYMAL CHONDROSARCOMA
This amputation specimen demonstrates a hemorrhagic mesenchymal chondrosarcoma involving the distal femur and extending into the surrounding soft tissue. Foci of cartilaginous differentiation are recognizable proximally. (Courtesy of Dr. K.W. Barwick, Jacksonville, FL.)

Gross Findings. The gross appearance is quite variable, ranging from soft to firm, gray to pink, and, occasionally, having a faintly lobulated pattern (fig. 142). Grossly obvious cartilage is rarely discernible.

Microscopic Findings. The microscopic appearance is highly variable, both from lesion to lesion and within any given example. The neoplastic cells may be small, round, oval, or spindle shaped with scant cytoplasm (fig. 143). The nuclei usually have irregular clumping of the chromatin and small nucleoli. Regardless of the shape of the cells, they tend to be only modestly pleomorphic. Mitotic figures are usually sparse, but occasionally may be numerous.

The cartilaginous component of mesenchymal chondrosarcoma is usually only a small part of

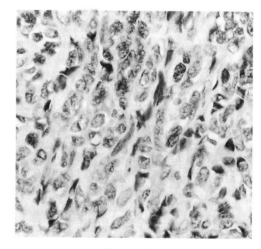

Figure 143
MESENCHYMAL CHONDROSARCOMA
Neoplastic cells are moderately pleomorphic with nuclei that are round, ovoid, or spindle shaped. There is variation in nuclear density.

119

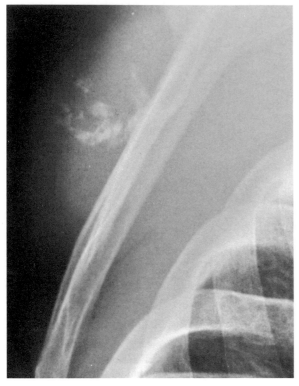

Figure 148
JUXTACORTICAL CHONDROSARCOMA
A 49-year-old woman had noticed a slightly tender, enlarging mass over her scapula. The lesion clearly was in continuity with the cortex of the scapula. (Courtesy of Dr. F.B. Askin, Baltimore, MD.) (Figures 148 and 150 are from the same patient.)

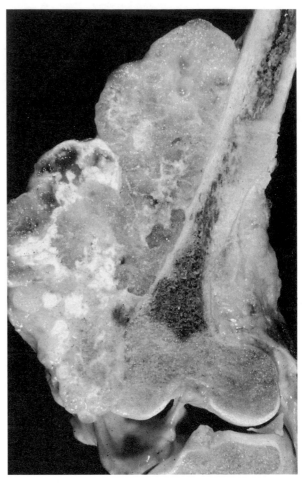

Figure 149
JUXTACORTICAL CHONDROSARCOMA
This large juxtacortical chondrosarcoma involves the distal femur. There is focal extension of this otherwise typical tumor through the thinned cortex of the epiphysis. Microscopically, this was a grade 1 chondrosarcoma. (Courtesy Dr. K.W. Barwick, Jacksonville, FL.)

Sites. The appendicular skeleton, especially the femur is usually involved. Other sites of disease include the humerus, pelvis, and, rarely, the rib or foot. Long bone lesions have a predilection for the metaphysis, with the remainder affecting the diaphysis (139).

Radiographic Appearance. As with periosteal chondroma, the underlying cortex is often sclerotic and shows a saucer-shaped defect which usually has a sharply defined border (138). In some instances, margination is ill defined, with obvious partial cortical destruction (136). A triangular sclerotic spur of cortex is commonly seen at the margin of the tumor. Juxtacortical chondrosarcomas tend to be large tumors. In one series, 6 of 8 were greater than 5 cm in diameter with an average size of 11 cm (138). Bertoni et al. (136), reported tumors ranging from 7 to 17 cm in greatest dimension. There

is a tendency for cartilage-type, "eggshell," or "popcorn" matrix calcifications in juxtacortical chondrosarcomas (fig. 148). This is an uncommon finding in periosteal chondromas.

Gross Findings. The typical juxtacortical chondrosarcoma is a grossly lobulated, gray-white, focally translucent, obviously cartilaginous mass (fig. 149). Areas of calcification are common. The underlying cortex is usually eroded with an irregular sclerotic reaction. Involvement of the medullary cavity is almost invariably absent, but large, otherwise typical lesions may show focal, subcortical extension (fig. 149).

Microscopic Findings. The lobulated appearance seen grossly is confirmed on microscopic examination. The cartilaginous lobules are typically of the well-differentiated, hyaline type (136) and are separated either by thin fibrous bands, or partly or totally encased by metaplastic bone. The stroma may be focally myxoid. By definition, osteoid production by neoplastic cells is lacking (136). Microscopic extension into soft tissue is usually present (138). Applying the grading system used for conventional intramedullary chondrosarcomas, juxtacortical chondrosarcomas are almost always grade 1 or 2 neoplasms (fig. 150) (136,138). Grade 3 tumors are rare, but have been described (136).

Differential Diagnosis. Juxtacortical chondrosarcoma is commonly confused both with a less aggressive lesion, periosteal chondroma, and a more aggressive one, periosteal osteosarcoma. Although juxtacortical chondrosarcoma can usually be distinguished from periosteal chondroma, in some cases the differentiation is admittedly arbitrary. There is an overlap in the radiographic appearances for both lesions, and there is overlap microscopically between cellular chondromas and grade 1 chondrosarcomas. Tumors that are microscopically grade 2 or grade 3 can be designated as chondrosarcoma with confidence, even though these juxtacortical neoplasms rarely metastasize. Mirra (137) noted that juxtacortical chondrosarcomas are usually wider than they are long, a feature that contrasts with periosteal chondromas. A width in excess of 5 cm is highly suggestive of malignancy. Radiographic findings indicating very large size and aggressive growth into the cortex are also helpful for the diagnosis of osteosarcomas.

Periosteal osteosarcoma is a predominately chondroblastic, juxtacortical variant of osteosarcoma that occasionally has a grossly lobular pattern. Some authors have lumped periosteal osteosarcoma and juxtacortical chondrosarcoma together, and their recognition as distinct entities is relatively recent. Unlike the predominantly low-grade cartilage in juxtacortical chondrosarcoma, the chondroid element in periosteal osteosarcoma is usually high grade. By definition, there are areas of osteoid formation by neoplastic cells, although much of the osteoid is immature and may constitute only a minority of the neoplasm. Periosteal osteosarcoma tends to

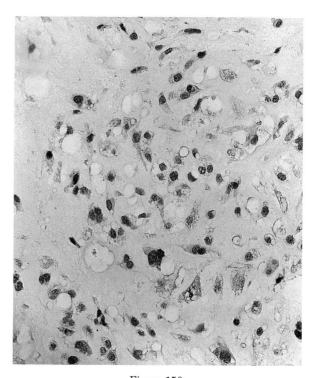

Figure 150
JUXTACORTICAL CHONDROSARCOMA
This juxtacortical chondrosarcoma shows moderate pleomorphism, indicating a grade 2 neoplasm. (Courtesy of Dr. F.B. Askin, Baltimore, MD.)

involve the diaphysis and is characterized by reactive bony trabeculae running perpendicular to the cortex. Juxtacortical chondrosarcoma is a predominantly metaphyseal lesion with reactive bone surrounding cartilaginous lobules in a curved, nonradiating configuration. The diagnosis of grade 3 juxtacortical chondrosarcoma should be approached with caution, especially if the lesion is diaphyseal. Such cases are more likely periosteal osteosarcomas.

Treatment and Prognosis. Two patients with juxtacortical chondrosarcomas treated by local excision had local recurrences and subsequent pulmonary metastases (138). Both were grade 2 neoplasms. Patients treated by resection have a lower rate of recurrence, recurrences are subsequently controlled by resection or amputation. None of the patients reported by Mirra (137) or Bertoni et al. (136) had recurrent or metastatic disease with follow-up periods of 9 and 11 years, respectively.

REFERENCES

Osteochondroma

1. Borges AM, Huvos AG, Smith J. Bursa formation and synovial chondrometaplasia associated with osteochondromas. Am J Clin Pathol 1981;75:648–53.
2. Chrisman OD, Goldenberg RR. Untreated solitary osteochondroma. Report of two cases. J Bone Joint Surg [Am] 1968;50:508–12.
3. Cohen EK, Kressel HY, Frank TS, et al. Hyaline cartilage—origin bone and soft-tissue neoplasms: MR appearance and histologic correlation. Radiology 1988;167:477–81.
4. Dahlin DC, Unni KK. Bone tumors: general aspects and data on 8,542 cases. 4th ed. Springfield, Ill: Charles C. Thomas, 1986:28.
5. D'Ambrosia R, Ferguson AB. The formation of osteochondroma by epiphyseal cartilage transplantation. Clin Orthop 1968;61:103–15.
6. El-Khoury GY, Bassett GS. Symptomatic bursa formation with osteochondromas. AJR Am J Roentgenol 1979;133:895–8.
7. Garrison RC, Unni KK, McLeod RA, Pritchard DJ, Dahlin DC. Chondrosarcoma arising in osteochondroma. Cancer 1982;49:1890–7.
8. Griffiths HJ, Thompson RC Jr, Galloway HR, Everson LI, Suh JS. Bursitis in association with solitary osteochondromas presenting as mass lesions. Skeletal Radiol 1991;20:513–6.
9. Herman TE, McAlister WH, Rosenthal D, Dehner LP. Case report 691. Radiation-induced osteochondromas (RIO) arising from the neural arch and producing compression of the spinal cord. Skeletal Radiol 1991;20:472–6.
10. Libshitz HI, Cohen MA. Radiation-induced osteochondromas. Radiology 1982;142:643–7.
11. Lizama VA, Zerbini MA, Gagliardi RA, Howell L. Popliteal vein thrombosis and popliteal artery pseudoaneurysm complicating osteochondroma of the femur. AJR Am J Roentgenol 1987;148:783–4.
12. Milgram JW. The origins of osteochondromas and enchondromas. Clin Orthop 1983;174:264–84.
13. Paling MR. The "disappearing" osteochondroma. Skeletal Radiol 1983;10:40–2.
14. Perez CA, Vietti T, Ackerman LV, Eagleton MD, Powers WE. Tumors of the sympathetic nervous system in children. An appraisal of treatment and results. Radiology 1967;88:750–60.
15. Unger EC, Gilula LA, Kyriakos M. Case report 430: Ischemic necrosis of osteochondroma of tibia. Skeletal Radiol 1987;16:416–21.

Osteochondromatosis

16. Garrison RC, Unni KK, McLeod RA, Pritchard DJ, Dahlin DC. Chondrosarcoma arising in osteochondroma. Cancer 1982;49:1890–7.
17. Jaffe HL. Tumors and tumorous conditions of the bones and joints. Philadelphia: Lea & Febiger, 1958:150–62.
18. Johnston CE II, Sklar F. Multiple hereditary exostoses with spinal cord compression. Orthopedics 1988;11:1213–6.
19. Masada K, Tsuyuguchi Y, Kawai H, Kawabata H, Noguchi K, Ono K. Operations for forearm deformity caused by multiple osteochondromas. J Bone Joint Surg [Br] 1989;71:24–9.
20. Matsuno T, Ichioka Y, Yagi T, Ishii S. Spindle-cell sarcoma in patients who have osteochondromatosis. A report of two cases. J Bone Joint Surg [Am] 1988;70:137–41.
21. Peterson HA. Multiple hereditary osteochondromata. Clin Orthop 1989;239:222–30.
22. Shapiro F, Simon S, Glimcher MJ. Hereditary multiple exostoses. Anthropometric, roentgenographic, and clinical aspects. J Bone Joint Surg [Am] 1979;61:815–24.
23. Voutsinas S, Wynne-Davies R. The infrequency of malignant disease in diaphyseal aclasis and neurofibromatosis. J Med Genet 1983;20:345–9.

Periosteal Chondroma

24. Bauer TW, Dorfman HD, Latham JT Jr. Periosteal chondroma. A clinicopathologic study of 23 cases. Am J Surg Pathol 1982;6:631–7.
25. Boriani S, Bacchini P, Bertoni F, Campanacci M. Periosteal chondroma. A review of twenty cases. J Bone Joint Surg [Am] 1983;65:205–12.
26. Chacha PB, Tan KK. Periosteal myxoma of the femur. A case report. J Bone Joint Surg [Am] 1972;54:1091–4.
27. de Santos LA, Spjut HJ. Periosteal chondroma: a radiographic spectrum. Skeletal Radiol 1981;6:15–20.
28. Nojima T, Unni KK, McLeod RA, Pritchard DJ. Periosteal chondroma and periosteal chondrosarcoma. Am J Surg Pathol 1985;9:666–77.

Enchondroma

29. Crim JR, Mirra JM. Enchondroma protuberans. Report of a case and its distinction from chondrosarcoma and osteochondroma adjacent to an enchondroma. Skeletal Radiol 1990;19:431–4.
30. Culver JE Jr, Sweet DE, McCue FC. Chondrosarcoma of the hand arising from a preexistent benign solitary enchondroma. Case report and pathological description. Clin Orthop 1975;113:128–31.
31. Dahlin DC, Salvador AH. Chondrosarcomas of bone of the hands and feet—a study of 30 cases. Cancer 1974;34:755–60.
32. Kuur E, Hansen SL, Lindequist S. Treatment of solitary enchondromas in fingers. J Hand Surg [Br] 1989;14:109–12.

33. Mirra JM, Gold R, Downs J, Eckardt JJ. A new histologic approach to the differentiation of enchondroma and chondrosarcoma of the bones. A clinicopathologic analysis of 51 cases. Clin Orthop 1985;201:214–37.
34. Noble J, Lamb DW. Enchondromata of bones of the hand. A review of 40 cases. Hand 1974;6:275–84.
35. Sanerkin NG, Woods CG. Fibrosarcomata and malignant fibrous histiocytomata arising in relation to enchondromata. J Bone Joint Surg [Br] 1979;61:366–72.
36. Smith GD, Chalmers J, McQueen MM. Osteosarcoma arising in relation to an enchondroma. A report of three cases. J Bone Joint Surg [Br] 1986;68:315–9.
37. Takigawa K. Chondroma of the bones of the hand. A review of 110 cases. J Bone Joint Surg [Am] 1971;53: 1591–600.
38. Wu KK, Frost HM, Guise EE. A chondrosarcoma of the hand arising from an asymptomatic benign solitary enchondroma of 40 years' duration. J Hand Surg [Am] 1983;8:317–9.

Enchondromatosis (Ollier Disease)

39. Cannon SR, Sweetnam DR. Multiple chondrosarcomas in dyschondroplasia (Ollier's disease). Cancer 1985; 55:836–40.
40. Goodman SB, Bell RS, Fornasier VL, De Demeter D, Bateman JE. Ollier's disease with multiple sarcomatous transformations. Hum Pathol 1984;15:91–3.
41. Liu J, Hudkins PG, Swee RG, Unni KK. Bone sarcomas associated with Ollier's disease. Cancer 1987;59:1376–85.
42. Mitchell ML, Ackerman LV. Case report 405: Ollier disease (enchondromatosis). Skeletal Radiol 1987;16:61–6.

Maffucci Syndrome

43. Lewis RJ, Ketcham AS. Maffucci's syndrome: functional and neoplastic significance. J Bone Joint Surg [Am] 1973;55:1465–79.
44. Sun TC, Swee RG, Shives TC, Unni KK. Chondrosarcoma in Maffucci's syndrome. J Bone Joint Surg [Am] 1985;67:1214–9.

Chondroblastoma

45. Bertoni F, Unni KK, Beabout JW, Harner SG, Dahlin DC. Chondroblastoma of the skull and facial bones. Am J Clin Pathol 1987;88:1–9.
46. Bloem JL, Mulder JD. Chondroblastoma: a clinical and radiological study of 104 cases. Skeletal Radiol 1985; 14:1–9.
47. Dahlin DC, Ivins JC. Benign chondroblastoma. A study of 125 cases. Cancer 1972;30:401–13.
48. _____, Unni KK. Bone tumors: general aspects and data on 8,542 cases. 4th ed. Springfield, Ill: Charles C. Thomas, 1986:52–67.
49. Fanning CV, Sneige NS, Carrasco CH, Ayala AG, Murray JA, Raymond AK. Fine needle aspiration of chondroblastoma of bone. Cancer 1990;65:1847–63.
50. Huvos AG, Marcove RC. Chondroblastoma of bone. A critical review. Clin Orthop 1973;95:300–12.
51. Kahn LB, Wood FM, Ackerman LV. Malignant chondroblastoma. Report of two cases and review of the literature. Arch Pathol 1969;88:371–6.
52. Karabela-Bouropoulou V, Markaki S, Prevedorou D, Vidali N. A combined immunohistochemical and histochemical approach on the differential diagnosis of giant cell epiphyseal neoplasms. Pathol Res Pract 1989;184:184–7.
53. Kurt AM, Unni KK, Sim FH, McLeod RA. Chondroblastoma of bone. Hum Pathol 1989;20:965–76.
54. Kyriakos M, Land VJ, Penning HL, Parker SG. Metastatic chondroblastoma. Report of a fatal case with a review of the literature on atypical, aggressive, and malignant chondroblastoma. Cancer 1985;55:1770–89.
55. Monda L, Wick MR. S-100 protein immunostaining in the differential diagnosis of chondroblastoma. Hum Pathol 1985;16:287–93.
56. Reyes CV, Kathuria S. Recurrent and aggressive chondroblastoma of the pelvis with late malignant neoplastic changes. Am J Surg Pathol 1979;3:449–55.
57. Riddell RJ, Louis CJ, Bromberger NA. Pulmonary metastases from chondroblastoma of the tibia. Report of a case. J Bone Joint Surg [Br] 1973;55:848–53.
58. Roberts PF, Taylor JG. Multifocal benign chondroblastomas: report of a case. Hum Pathol 1980;11:296–8.
59. Schajowicz F, Gallardo H. Epiphysial chondroblastoma of bone. A clinico-pathological study of sixty-nine cases. J Bone Joint Surg [Br] 1970;52:205–26.
60. Semmelink HJ, Pruszczynski M, Wiersma-van Tilburg A, Smedts F, Ramaekers FC. Cytokeratin expression in chondroblastomas. Histopathology 1990;16:257–63.
61. Sirsat MV, Doctor VM. Benign chondroblastoma of bone. Report of a case of malignant transformation. J Bone Joint Surg [Br] 1970;52:741–5.
62. Sotelo-Avila C, Sundaram M, Kyriakos M, Graviss ER, Tayob AA. Case report 373: diametaphyseal chondroblastoma of the upper portion of the left femur. Skeletal Radiol 1986;15:387–90.
63. Springfield DS, Capanna R, Gherlinzoni F, Picci P, Campanacci M. Chondroblastoma. A review of seventy cases. J Bone Joint Surg [Am] 1985;67:748–55.
64. Steiner GC. Ultrastructure of benign cartilaginous tumors of intraosseous origin. Hum Pathol 1979;10:71–86.
65. Weiss AP, Dorfman HD. S-100 protein in human cartilage lesions. J Bone Joint Surg [Am] 1986;68:521–6.
66. Wirman JA, Crissman JD, Aron BF. Metastatic chondroblastoma: report of an unusual case treated with radiotherapy. Cancer 1979;44:87–93.

Chondromyxoid Fibroma

67. Andrew T, Kenwright J, Woods C. Periosteal chondromyxoid fibroma of the tibia: a case report. Acta Orthop Scand 1982;53:467–70.
68. Bleiweiss IJ, Klein MJ. Chondromyxoid fibroma: report of six cases with immunohistochemical studies. Mod Pathol 1990;3:664–6.
69. Gherlinzoni F, Rock M, Picci P. Chondromyxoid fibroma. The experience at the Istituto Ortopedico Rizzoli. J Bone Joint Surg [Am] 1983;65:198–204.
70. Kreicbergs A, Lönnquist PA, Willems J. Chondromyxoid fibroma. A review of the literature and a report on our own experience. Acta Pathol Microbiol Immunol Scand [A] 1985;93:189–97.
71. Kyriakos M. Soft tissue implantation of chondromyxoid fibroma. Am J Surg Pathol 1979;3:363–72.
72. Rahimi A, Beabout JW, Ivins JC, Dahlin DC. Chondromyxoid fibroma: a clinicopathologic study of 76 cases. Cancer 1972;30:726–36.
73. Schajowicz F, Gallardo H. Chondromyxoid fibroma (fibromyxoid chondroma) of bone. A clinico-pathological study of thirty-two cases. J Bone Joint Surg [Br] 1971;53:198–216.
74. Sehayik S, Rosman MA. Malignant degeneration of a chondromyxoid fibroma in a child. Can J Surg 1975;18:354–60.
75. Ushigome S, Takakuwa T, Shinagawa T, Kishida H, Yamazaki M. Chondromyxoid fibroma of bone. An electron microscopic observation. Acta Pathol Jpn 1982; 32:113–22.
76. van Horn JR, Lemmens JA. Chondromyxoid fibroma of the foot. A report of a missed diagnosis. Acta Orthop Scand 1986;57:375–7.
77. Zillmer DA, Dorfman HD. Chondromyxoid fibroma of bone: thirty-six cases with clinicopathologic correlation. Hum Pathol 1989;20:952–64.

Chondrosarcoma

78. Alho A, Connor JF, Mankin HJ, Schiller AL, Campbell CJ. Assessment of malignancy of cartilage tumors using flow cytometry. A preliminary report. J Bone Joint Surg [Am] 1983;65:779–85.
79. Barnes R, Catto M. Chondrosarcoma of bone. J Bone Joint Surg [Br] 1966;48:729–64.
80. Campanacci M, Guernelli N, Leonessa C, Boni A. Chondrosarcoma: a study of 133 cases, 80 with long-term follow-up. Ital J Orthop Traumatol 1975;1:387–414.
81. Dahlin DC, Salvador AH. Chondrosarcomas of bones of the hands and feet—a study of 30 cases. Cancer 1974; 34:755–60.
82. _____, Unni KK. Bone tumors: general aspects and data on 8,542 cases. 4th ed. Springfield, Ill: Charles C. Thomas, 1986:228.
83. Demetrick DJ, Kneafsey PD, Hwang WS. Signet-ring chondrosarcoma: a new morphologic entity. Hum Pathol 1991;22:1175–9.
84. Eriksson AI, Schiller A, Mankin HJ. The management of chondrosarcoma of bone. Clin Orthop 1980;153:44–66.
85. Evans HL, Ayala AG, Romsdahl MM. Prognostic factors in chondrosarcoma of bone: a clinicopathologic analysis with emphasis on histologic grading. Cancer 1977;40:818–31.
86. Gitelis S, Bertoni F, Picci P, Campanacci M. Chondrosarcoma of bone. The experience at the Istituto Ortopedico Rizzoli. J Bone Joint Surg [Am] 1981;63:1248–57.
87. Henderson ED, Dahlin DC. Chondrosarcoma of bone—a study of two hundred and eighty-eight cases. J Bone Joint Surg [A] 1963;45:1450–8.
88. Hudson TM, Manaster BJ, Springfield DS, Spanier SS, Enneking WF, Hawkins IF Jr. Radiology of medullary chondrosarcoma: preoperative treatment planning. Skeletal Radiol 1983;10:69–78.
89. Huvos AG, Marcove RC. Chondrosarcoma in the young. A clinicopathologic analysis of 79 patients younger than 21 years of age. Am J Surg Pathol 1987;11:930–42.
90. Kreicbergs A, Boquist L, Borssén B, Larsson SE. Prognostic factors in chondrosarcoma: a comparative study of cellular DNA content and clinicopathologic features. Cancer 1982;50:577–83.
91. Kristensen IB, Sunde LM, Jensen OM. Chondrosarcoma. Increasing grade of malignancy in local recurrence. Acta Pathol Microbiol Immunol Scand [A] 1986;94:73–7.
92. Mankin HJ, Cantley KP, Lippiello L, Schiller AL, Campbell CJ. The biology of human chondrosarcoma. I. Description of the cases, grading, and biochemical analyses. J Bone Joint Surg [Am] 1980;62:160–76.
93. _____, Cantley KP, Schiller AL, Lippiello L. The biology of human chondrosarcoma. II. Variation in chemical composition among types and subtypes of benign and malignant cartilage tumors. J Bone Joint Surg [Am] 1980;62:176–88.
94. _____, Connor JF, Schiller AL, Perlmutter N, Alho A, McGuire M. Grading of bone tumors by analysis of nuclear DNA content using flow cytometry. J Bone Joint Surg [Am] 1985;67:404–13.
95. Marcove RC, Huvos AG. Cartilaginous tumors of the ribs. Cancer 1971;27:794–801.
96. _____, Miké V, Hutter RV, et al. Chondrosarcoma of the pelvis and upper end of the femur. An analysis of factors influencing survival time in one hundred and thirteen cases. J Bone Joint Surg [Am] 1972;54:561–72.
97. Mirra JM, Gold R, Downs J, Eckardt JJ. A new histologic approach to the differentiation of enchondroma and chondrosarcoma of the bones. A clinicopathologic analysis of 51 cases. Clin Orthop 1985;201:214–37.
98. Pritchard DJ, Lunke RJ, Taylor WF, Dahlin DC, Medley BE. Chondrosarcoma: a clinicopathologic and statistical analysis. Cancer 1980;45:149–57.
99. Rosenthal DI, Schiller AL, Mankin HJ. Chondrosarcoma: correlation of radiological and histological grade. Radiology 1984;150:21–6.
100. Sanerkin NG. The diagnosis and grading of chondrosarcoma of bone: a combined cytologic and histologic approach. Cancer 1980;45:582–94.
101. _____, Gallagher P. A review of the behaviour of chondrosarcoma of bone. J Bone Joint Surg [Br] 1979; 61:395–400.

102. Schiller AL. Diagnosis of borderline cartilage lesions of bone. Semin Diagn Pathol 1985;2:42–62.

103. Young CL, Sim FH, Unni KK, McLeod RA. Chondrosarcoma of bone in children. Cancer 1990;66:1641–8.

Dedifferentiated Chondrosarcoma

104. Abenoza P, Neumann MP, Manivel JC, Wick MR. Dedifferentiated chondrosarcoma: an ultrastructural study of two cases, with immunocytochemical correlations. Ultrastruct Pathol 1986;10:529–38.

105. Bertoni F, Present D, Bacchini P, et al. Dedifferentiated peripheral chondrosarcomas. A report of seven cases. Cancer 1989;63:2054–9.

106. Campanacci M, Boriani S, Giunti A. Hemangioendothelioma of bone: a study of 29 cases. Cancer 1980;46:804–14.

107. Capanna R, Bertoni F, Bettella G, et al. Dedifferentiated chondrosarcoma. J Bone Joint Surg [Am] 1988; 70:60–9.

108. Dahlin DC, Beabout JW. Differentiation of low-grade chondrosarcomas. Cancer 1971;28:461–6.

109. de Lange EE, Pope TL Jr, Fechner RE. Dedifferentiated chondrosarcoma: radiographic features. Radiology 1986;161:489–92.

110. Dervan PA, O'Loughlin J, Hurson BJ. Dedifferentiated chondrosarcoma with muscle and cytokeratin differentiation in the anaplastic component. Histopathology 1988;12:517–26.

111. Frassica FJ, Unni KK, Beabout JW, Sim FH. Dedifferentiated chondrosarcoma. A report of the clinicopathological features and treatment of seventy-eight cases. J Bone Joint Surg [Am] 1986;68:1197–205.

112. Johnson S, Têtu B, Ayala AG, Chawla SP. Chondrosarcoma with additional mesenchymal component (dedifferentiated chondrosarcoma) I. A clinicopathologic study of 26 cases. Cancer 1986;58:278–86.

113. McCarthy EF, Dorfman HD. Chondrosarcoma of bone with dedifferentiation: a study of eighteen cases. Hum Pathol 1982;13:36–40.

114. Mirra JM, Marcove RC. Fibrosarcomatous dedifferentiation of primary and secondary chondrosarcoma. J Bone Joint Surg [Am] 1974;56:285–96.

115. Sanerkin NG, Woods CG. Fibrosarcomata and malignant fibrous histiocytomata arising in relation to enchondromata. J Bone Joint Surg [Br] 1979;61:366–72.

116. Smith GD, Chalmers J, McQueen MM. Osteosarcoma arising in relation to an enchondroma. A report of three cases. J Bone Joint Surg [Br] 1986;68:315–9.

117. Têtu B, Ordóñez NG, Ayala AG, MacKay B. Chondrosarcoma with additional mesenchymal component (dedifferentiated chondrosarcoma). II. An immunohistochemical and electron microscopic study. Cancer 1986;58:287–98.

118. Wick MR, Siegal GP, Mills SE, Thompson RC, Sawhney D, Fechner RE. Dedifferentiated chondrosarcoma of bone. An immunohistochemical and lectin-histochemical study. Virchows Arch [A] 1987;411:23–32.

Clear Cell Chondrosarcoma

119. Angervall L, Kindblom LG. Clear-cell chondrosarcoma. A light- and electron-microscopic and histochemical study of 2 cases. Virchows Arch [A] 1980;389:27–41.

120. Bjornsson J, Unni KK, Dahlin DC, Beabout JW, Sim FH. Clear cell chondrosarcoma of bone. Observations in 47 cases. Am J Surg Pathol 1984;8:223–30.

121. Faraggiana T, Sender B, Glicksman P. Light- and electron-microscopic study of clear cell chondrosarcoma. Am J Clin Pathol 1981;75:117–21.

122. Present D, Bacchini P, Pignatti G, Picci P, Bertoni F, Campanacci M. Clear cell chondrosarcoma of bone. A report of 8 cases. Skeletal Radiol 1991;20:187–91.

123. Taconis WK. Clear cell chondrosarcoma: report of three cases and review of the literature. Diagn Imag Clin Med 1986;55:219–27.

124. Unni KK, Dahlin DC, Beabout JW, Sim FH. Chondrosarcoma. clear-cell variant. A report of sixteen cases. J Bone Joint Surg [Am] 1976;58:676–83.

Mesenchymal Chondrosarcoma

125. Bertoni F, Picci P, Bacchini P, et al. Mesenchymal chondrosarcoma of bone and soft tissues. Cancer 1983; 52:533–41.

126. Harwood AR, Krajbich JI, Fornasier VL. Mesenchymal chondrosarcoma: a report of 17 cases. Clin Orthop 1981;158:144–8.

127. Hutter RV, Foote FW Jr, Francis KC, Sherman RS. Primitive multipotential primary sarcoma of bone. Cancer 1966;19:1–25.

128. Huvos AG, Rosen G, Dabska M, Marcove RC. Mesenchymal chondrosarcoma. A clinicopathologic analysis of 35 patients with emphasis on treatment. Cancer 1983;51:1230–7.

129. Jacobson SA. Polyhistioma: a malignant tumor of bone and extraskeletal tissues. Cancer 1977;40:2116–30.

130. Martinez-Tello FJ, Navas-Palacios JJ. Ultrastructural study of conventional chondrosarcomas and myxoid- and mesenchymal-chondrosarcomas. Virchows Arch [A] 1982;396:197–211.

131. Nakamura Y, Becker LE, Marks A. S-100 protein in tumors of cartilage and bone. An immunohistochemical study. Cancer 1983;52:1820–4.

132. Nakashima Y, Unni KK, Shives TC, Swee RG, Dahlin DC. Mesenchymal chondrosarcoma of bone and soft tissue. A review of 111 cases. Cancer 1986;57:2444–53.

133. Salvador AH, Beabout JW, Dahlin DC. Mesenchymal chondrosarcoma—observation on 30 new cases. Cancer 1971;28:605–15.

134. Steiner GC, Mirra JM, Bullough PG. Mesenchymal chondrosarcoma. A study of the ultrastructure. Cancer 1973;32:926–39.

135. Swanson PE, Lillemoe TJ, Manivel JC, Wick MR. Mesenchymal chondrosarcoma. An immunohistochemical study. Arch Pathol Lab Med 1990;114:943–8.

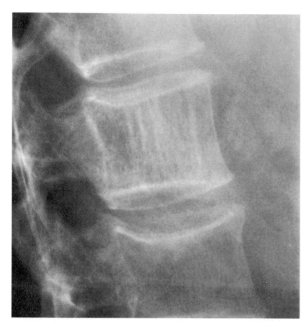

Figure 152
HEMANGIOMA
Typical vertebral hemangioma with prominent vertical trabecular striations results in the "corduroy cloth" pattern. This patient was asymptomatic. (Fig. 1 from Wold LE, Swee RG, Sim FH. Vascular lesions of bone. Pathol Annu 1985;20(Pt 2):101–37.)

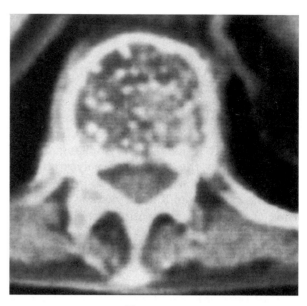

Figure 153
HEMANGIOMA
Computerized tomographic appearance of a vertebral hemangioma exhibiting the diagnostic "polka-dot" appearance due to the remaining trabeculae viewed in cross section. (Fig. 2 from Wold LE, Swee RG, Sim FH. Vascular lesions of bone. Pathol Annu 1985;20(Pt 2):101–37.)

of surgically biopsied or resected bone lesions, the prevalence of these lesions is very high. Nearly 11 percent of vertebral columns contain intraosseous hemangiomas when carefully examined at autopsy (9). Two thirds are solitary lesions and one third are multiple (usually 2 to 5). Clearly, only a small number of intraosseous hemangiomas are symptomatic.

Clinical Features. Intraosseous hemangiomas have been diagnosed in individuals of all ages, but most are found in the fifth decade of life. Females are affected slightly more often than males. Symptomatic lesions are usually painful and may be accompanied by swelling. The calvarial tumors are slowly enlarging, painless masses. Temporal bone hemangiomas may cause facial paralysis by encroaching on the facial nerve (3). The vertebral lesions often present with muscle spasm or neurologic symptoms related to compression fracture or impingement on the nerve roots or spinal cord. Many hemangiomas of the calvarium and spine are incidental findings in radiographs taken for other reasons.

Sacral hemangiomas are sometimes accompanied by multiple congenital abnormalities (6).

Sites. The calvarium is the most common site for surgically treated hemangiomas. Nearly half of the intraosseous hemangiomas reported by the Mayo Clinic involved the calvarium, 25 percent were in the vertebrae (most often the thoracic vertebrae), and 14 percent involved the gnathic bones (10). The ribs, femur, humerus, and pelvis follow in frequency. The small bones of hands and feet are rarely involved (4). Rare intracortical (8) and subperiosteal hemangiomas have been described (13).

Radiographic Appearance. Hemangiomas of the vertebrae characteristically are lytic medullary lesions with intervening thickened vertical striations, which are often referred to as the "corduroy cloth" pattern (fig. 152). On CT scan the striations are seen in cross section, resulting in a polka-dot pattern (fig. 153). The tumor primarily involves the vertebral body, but it may extend into the laminae, pedicles, and transverse or spinous processes. Rarely, there is extension into the intervertebral disc. Arteriography usually shows a highly vascular soft tissue

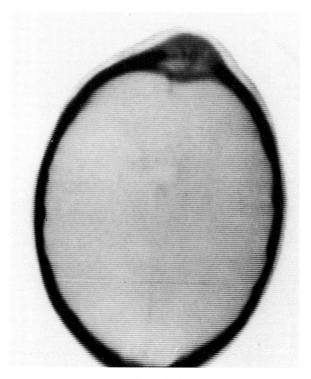

Figure 154
HEMANGIOMA
Computed tomography of skull discloses intralesional new bone formation and bulging of both the inner and outer tables. Because of the cosmetic deformity, the area was excised. (Figures 154 and 155 are from the same patient.)

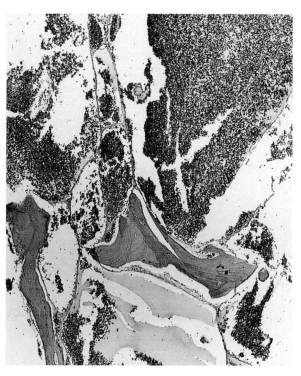

Figure 155
HEMANGIOMA
The more vascular areas of the lesion seen in figure 154 show a cavernous hemangioma with irregularly shaped, large thin-walled vessels.

component, which is invariably present if contiguous vertebrae are involved.

The lesions in the calvarium arise in the diploë and may be lytic or have a "sunburst" appearance with the reactive bone radiating from the center of the hemangioma. The outer table bulges outward, and the inner table, to a lesser degree, may bulge inward (fig. 154) (7).

Periosteal reactions to hemangiomas of the long bones can also have a sunburst pattern, or there may be irregular bone deposition, resulting in a reticulated appearance. Alternately, long bone hemangiomas may be purely lytic and devoid of reactive bone.

A group of subperiosteal hemangiomas has been reported in which there is slight cortical erosion radiographically (13). Intracortical hemangiomas are rare and may be mistaken for osteoid osteomas (8).

Gross Findings. Intact vertebral hemangiomas seen at autopsy are ill-defined, soft, purple or red masses with markedly thickened, vertically arranged bands of bone. The entire lesion usually measures 1 cm or less in size. Resected specimens from the calvarium that have a sunburst radiographic appearance are densely sclerotic, and the radiating spicules of reactive bone are often grossly discernible.

Microscopic Findings. Most intraosseous hemangiomas are of cavernous type, with conglomerates of thin-walled vessels that are often filled with erythrocytes (fig. 155). Mixed capillary and cavernous lesions are second in frequency, and a minority consist only of small capillaries. Occasionally, they are composed of larger, thick-walled arteries or veins and resemble arteriovenous malformations of the soft tissues (11).

The vascular channels of intraosseous hemangioma replace the normal marrow elements. The endothelial cells are small and normal in appearance. Mitotic figures are rarely seen and, when present, have a normal configuration.

Differential Diagnosis. Intraosseous hemangiomas are microscopically indistinguishable from skeletal angiomatosis, and the differentiation is based on the much more extensive nature of the latter. The flattened, normal-appearing endothelial cells of hemangioma are easily distinguished from the larger, more prominent cells of epithelioid hemangioendothelioma and angiosarcoma.

Treatment and Prognosis. Some intraosseous hemangiomas progress slowly over time, and others seem to stabilize. The calvarial hemangiomas lend themselves to surgical excision, but the vertebral lesions are formidable problems from a surgical standpoint. Patients with symptomatic vertebral hemangiomas are perhaps best treated with radiation (5), after which about 80 percent will have complete relief of symptoms. The radiographic appearance of the lesion, however, usually does not change (12).

SKELETAL ANGIOMATOSIS

Definition. A multifocal or diffuse intraosseous proliferation of hemangiomatous, lymphangiomatous, or mixed vascular channels that are lined by normal-appearing endothelial cells. Skeletal angiomatosis is often accompanied by extraosseous vascular malformations.

General Features. This is an uncommon condition with fewer than 100 reported cases. Typically, the term skeletal angiomatosis is applied to widely multifocal or diffuse intraosseous disease, rather than to several discrete intraosseous lesions, each with the features of a solitary hemangioma. Karlin and Brower (15) suggested that multiple hemangiomas be distinguished from angiomatosis because of the better prognosis in the former. Patients with skeletal angiomatosis may be broadly divided into two groups: those with and those without accompanying extraosseous disease.

Clinical Findings. Skeletal angiomatosis, particularly when confined to bone, can be asymptomatic and discovered incidentally on radiographs taken for other reasons. Alternately, patients may present with bone pain, with or without a fracture. Many patients are seen for problems related to associated nonosseous vascular lesions, such as hemorrhagic or chylous effusions, soft tissue hemangiomas, or secondary

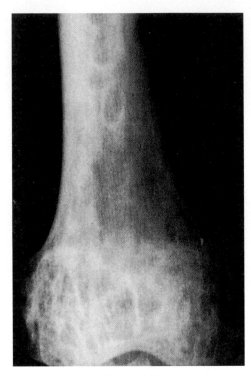

Figure 156
SKELETAL ANGIOMATOSIS
The lower end of the femur has numerous cyst-like lucencies traversed by dense bony trabeculae. A chest radiograph demonstrated similar lesions in the upper end of both humeri. There were no symptoms related to the skeletal lesions. The patient subsequently died and one femur was removed at autopsy. (Fig. 363 (left) from Fascicle 5, 2nd Series.) (Figures 156 and 157 are from the same patient.)

thrombocytopenia. There appears to be a slight male predominance, especially in patients without extraosseous involvement (14). Most patients are diagnosed in the first two decades of life, but a few are over 45 years of age.

Sites. The skull, vertebrae, long bones, ribs, and pelvic bones are most frequently involved. Small bones of the hands and feet are affected less frequently, and the gnathic bones are almost never involved.

Radiographic Appearance. Skeletal angiomatosis produces oval or round lytic defects that sometimes have a slightly sclerotic rim (fig. 156). There may be expansion of the affected bone, but a periosteal reaction is not seen. An involved bone may have multiple, separate lesions or it may be diffusely abnormal. Some lesions stimulate reactive bone formation, resulting in coarse intralesional trabeculations. However, the sunburst pattern of reactive bone seen in hemangiomas is not present in skeletal angiomatosis.

Gross Findings. The marrow cavity is replaced by irregular, dark red or tan cystic areas surrounded by sclerotic bone (fig. 157) (14).

Microscopic Findings. Skeletal angiomatosis is microscopically identical to localized intraosseous hemangioma. There is typically a combination of capillary and cavernous vascular spaces lined with flattened, normal-appearing endothelium. Some vascular lumina are devoid of red blood cells and may be lymphatic channels. The intervening medullary bone may have reactive-appearing, widely broadened trabeculae. The cortex, in contrast, is often thinned with dilated vessels in the haversian spaces.

Differential Diagnosis. The radiographic differential diagnosis includes other multifocal, usually malignant, processes such as metastatic carcinoma or multiple myeloma. Microscopically, the differential diagnosis includes solitary hemangioma and massive osteolysis. The diagnosis is based on the clinical findings because all three lesions are microscopically interchangeable.

Treatment and Prognosis. Skeletal angiomatosis does not seem to undergo malignant transformation. Patients who have only osseous involvement do well, requiring therapy only in the event of fracture. A variety of radiographic alterations in patients followed for many years may be seen. Some lesions remain unchanged, others slowly progress, and still others undergo sclerosis and regression (16). It is unclear whether radiation therapy hastens regression, although it is often employed for individual angiomas that appear at high risk for pathologic fracture. If skeletal angiomatosis is associated with extraosseous lesions, the prognosis is poor, especially for patients with recurrent effusions.

MASSIVE OSTEOLYSIS

Definition. Resorption of most or all of a bone associated with a proliferation of vascular channels. Other terms for this lesion include *phantom bone disease*, *vanishing* or *disappearing bone disease*, and *Gorham disease*.

General Features. Massive osteolysis is thought by some to be related to skeletal angiomatosis because both lesions may be histolog-

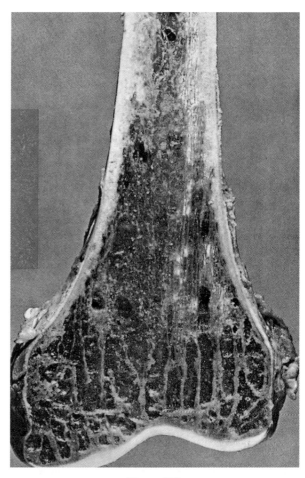

Figure 157
SKELETAL
ANGIOMATOSIS
A sagittal section through the lower end of the femur demonstrates angiomatous areas separated by broad, irregularly arranged trabeculae. Some cystic spaces are also evident. Microscopically, the lesion was a hemangioma. (Fig. 364 from Fascicle 5, 2nd Series.)

ically identical. However, the far greater destructiveness of massive osteolysis and its tendency to involve only a single bone, or at most, a few contiguous bones, are important clinical points of differentiation. The pathogenesis of massive osteolysis is unknown, although some cases seem associated with prior trauma to the affected bone. Fewer than 150 cases have been reported.

Clinical Features. There does not appear to be a sexual predilection. Most cases are diagnosed in children or young adults before 35 years of age, with patients ranging in age from 14 to 59 years. Pain, with or without pathologic fracture, is the presenting symptom.

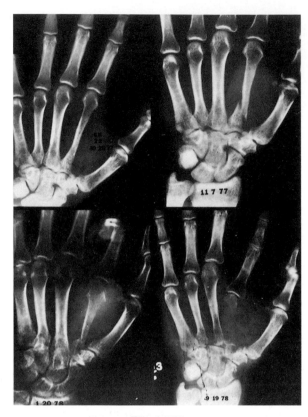

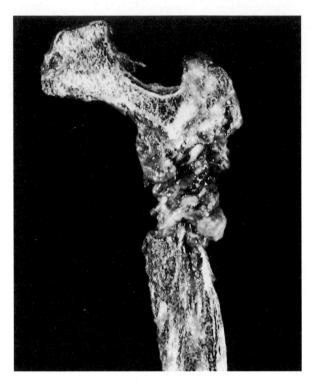

Figure 158
MASSIVE OSTEOLYSIS
Massive osteolysis involves a metacarpal bone. There is progressive rarefaction that began with narrowing or tapering of the bone in October 1977. This was followed by a fracture and subsequent dissolution of the bone by September 1978. (Fig. 8 from Wold LE, Swee RG, Sim FH. Vascular lesions of bone. Pathol Annu 1985;20(Pt 2):101–37.)

Figure 159
MASSIVE OSTEOLYSIS
This 28-year-old woman underwent resection of her proximal femur with total hip arthroplasty for disappearing bone disease. The proximal femur is markedly distorted as a result of this process. (Fig. 9 from Wold LE, Swee RG, Sim FH. Vascular lesions of bone. Pathol Annu 1985;20(Pt 2):101–37.)

Sites. Involvement of almost every bone has been reported. In descending order, there is a predilection for the mandible, ribs, femur, scapula, humerus, and sternum.

Radiographic Appearance. The earliest change is a lucent area in the medullary portion of the bone, or concentric destruction of the cortex, giving rise to a "sucked candy" appearance. Eventually, the entire medullary cavity and then the cortex is destroyed (fig. 158). About 75 percent of cases involve at least one contiguous bone (19).

Gross and Microscopic Findings. Grossly, the affected bone has, at most, a paper-thin cortex enclosing soft red or brown tissue (20). The bone may be totally destroyed and replaced, along with adjacent soft tissues, by an ill-defined, vascular mass (fig. 159) (21). Microscopi-

cally, there is a vascular proliferation with anastomosing thin-walled vessels between the remaining bony trabeculae. As mentioned above, the appearance may be histologically identical to solitary hemangioma or angiomatosis. Despite the rapid loss of bone, osteoclastic activity is usually not conspicuous, although occasionally it is prominent (fig. 160) (18). In some cases, there is no recognizable microscopic abnormality.

Differential Diagnosis. Individuals with Paget disease involving a long bone who develop a pathologic fracture and require immobilization may experience a marked acceleration in the lytic phase of their disease. The intense osteolysis and rarefaction of the underlying bone may somewhat mimic massive osteolysis, and, microscopically, the highly vascular appearance of Paget disease may add to the confusion. Paget disease typically affects much older individuals, however, and the underlying lesion should be present on

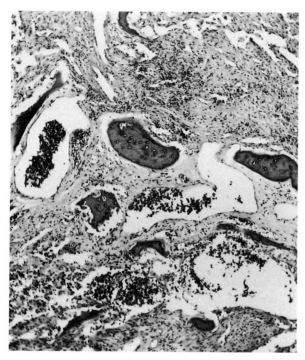

Figure 160
MASSIVE OSTEOLYSIS
This 9-year-old female had a lesion in the proximal femur which showed hypervascular bone indistinguishable from hemangioma. Complete dissolution of the proximal femur ensued over the next 5 1/2 years. (Fig. 10 from Wold LE, Swee RG, Sim FH. Vascular lesions of bone. Pathol Annu 1985;20(Pt 2):101-37.)

the initial radiographs. Furthermore, the irregular, mosaic pattern of osteoid seen in Paget disease is not a feature of massive osteolysis.

Treatment and Prognosis. Embolization, complete resection, bone grafting, and reconstruction with prosthetic devices have been tried with variable results. Radiation therapy has had some apparent benefit (22), although this is difficult to evaluate since some cases spontaneously arrest without any treatment. Regrowth of the bone is rare (17). Death has resulted from respiratory failure due to rib involvement (19).

EPITHELIOID (HISTIOCYTOID) HEMANGIOENDOTHELIOMA

Definition. A borderline or low-grade malignant neoplasm composed of endothelial cells with conspicuous cytoplasm, which impart an epithelioid or histiocytoid appearance. The tumors exhibit different degrees of vasoformative activity, ranging from vacuolization of single cells to well-formed vascular channels.

General Features. Rosai et al. (30) originally described a microscopically distinctive group of vascular tumors from various anatomic sites under the designation of histiocytoid hemangioma. This term was chosen because of the plump, eosinophilic to amphophilic cytoplasm of the neoplastic endothelial cells. Two lesions in that study were of osseous origin. Weiss and Enzinger (33) subsequently used the term epithelioid hemangioendothelioma for a group of soft tissue tumors that included, but was not limited to, vascular neoplasms with the appearance of histiocytoid hemangioma. Six of their 31 cases metastasized, a rate considerably lower than that of typical angiosarcomas.

Thus far, only two reported skeletal epithelioid hemangioendotheliomas have metastasized. Indeed, these "metastases" might be interpreted as separate primary tumors, especially since another patient with multiple cutaneous epithelioid hemangioendotheliomas, as well as a microscopically identical osseous lesion at the time of presentation, had no further evidence of disease spread 5 years later (28). We encountered a similar case of an epithelioid hemangioendothelioma of the humerus and discontinuous, microscopically identical lesions developing in the overlying skin and soft tissues. Patients with skeletal tumors may thus have cutaneous involvement without evidence of progressive disease. This is important to remember, in view of one patient reported by Tsuneyoshi et al. (32) with an osseous epithelioid hemangioendothelioma who developed an abdominal wall "metastasis" 1 year later. The authors view this as a metastasis, but this may be a separate cutaneous primary. One reported patient with visceral "metastases" (multiple pulmonary lesions) is still alive 20 years after diagnosis of an osseous lesion and 18 years after detection of the pulmonary "metastases." Again, the possibility of multiple primary tumors deserves consideration. Epithelioid hemangioendothelioma is well known to primarily involve the lung, often as multiple lesions, where it is often referred to by the older term of *intravascular bronchoalveolar cell tumor* (IVBAT).

Most reports of skeletal angiosarcoma were written before the introduction of the term epithelioid hemangioendothelioma. The published

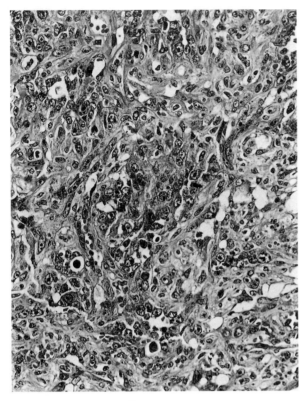

Figure 166
ANGIOSARCOMA
This grade 3 angiosarcoma has only a few discernible vascular channels lined by neoplastic cells. Most of tumor consists of round or ovoid cells with no discernible lumens.

outlook for skeletal angiosarcoma is poor. In one report, 10 of 12 patients died of pulmonary or skeletal metastases, usually within 1 year of diagnosis (36). One patient in that series with pulmonary metastases was alive at 5 years. In another series 20 of 25 died of their tumor (40).

HEMANGIOPERICYTOMA

Definition. A potentially to overtly malignant, vascular neoplasm consisting primarily of pericyte-like spindle cells with associated prominent vascular channels.

General and Clinical Features. Tang and colleagues (43) described four cases of skeletal hemangiopericytoma in 1988 and reviewed 41 previously published examples. These tumors occur in patients between 12 and 90 years of age, although most are between the ages of 30 and 60 years. There is no sexual predominance. Symp-

toms consist primarily of pain or swelling (or both) that ranges in duration from 1 month to more than 1 year. Skeletal hemangiopericytoma is one of the osseous and soft tissue neoplasms that may be associated with hypophosphatemic osteomalacia (42,44).

Sites. The pelvis is the most common location for skeletal hemangiopericytoma, followed by the femur, vertebrae, and mandible. Involvement of the clavicle, humerus, scapula, and fibula has also been reported.

Radiographic Appearance. There is a broad spectrum of radiographic appearances which, in part, reflects the histologic grade. These are predominantly lytic lesions that occasionally have a trabecular, honeycomb, or reticulated appearance similar to that seen in skeletal hemangiomas. The margin varies from sharp and sclerotic to ill defined. The presence of a sharp, sclerotic rim reflects slow growth and is seen in microscopically better differentiated tumors. Conversely, hemangiopericytomas with ill-defined margins tend to be poorly differentiated.

Gross Findings. The gross features of the lesion are nondescript. Curetted or resected tissue is generally solid, firm, and gray or tan.

Microscopic Findings. The microscopic appearance of skeletal hemangiopericytoma is virtually identical to that of its far more common soft tissue counterpart. Microscopic patterns depend on the ratio of thin-walled capillary or sinusoidal vessels and the pericyte-like round, oval, or spindle cells. The more vascular lesions may have irregular, branching vessels, creating a "deer antler" appearance. Other lesions are more cellular with inconspicuous, small capillaries. In such cases, the cells may be arranged in ill-defined bundles or in sheets. Small areas of storiform arrangement are common. The neoplastic cells can be uniform and mildly atypical or display great degrees of nuclear pleomorphism. The mitotic count roughly parallels the degree of nuclear abnormality.

Microscopic Grading. Because of the variation indicated above, hemangiopericytoma lends itself to grading. Grade 1 tumors are hypocellular lesions with oval, uniform nuclei set far apart. Nucleoli are not conspicuous and mitotic figures are absent or fewer than 1 per 10 high-power fields. The deer antler vascular pattern is especially prominent in this grade. Grade

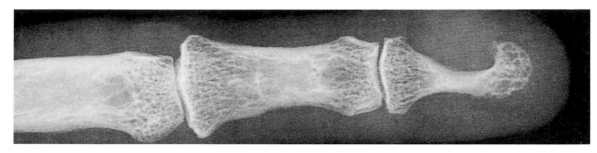

Figure 167
GLOMUS TUMOR
Radiograph of a soft tissue glomus tumor of the distal phalanx discloses smooth deformity of the bone with an intact cortex. (Fig. 425 from Fascicle 5, 2nd Series.) (Figures 167 and 169 are from the same patient.)

2 tumors have greater cellularity, and the cells have larger nuclei. Mitotic figures range from 1 to 5 per 10 high-power fields. Grade 3 tumors are highly cellular lesions with a less conspicuous vascular component. The cells have marked nuclear abnormalities and considerable pleomorphism. Six or more mitotic figures are seen per 10 high-power fields, and may include atypical forms. These most pleomorphic foci have a nondiagnostic, spindle cell appearance and require more typical, lower grade areas to permit diagnosis. Necrosis is seen in both grade 2 and grade 3 lesions (43).

Differential Diagnosis. As in soft tissue, the diagnosis of hemangiopericytoma should be approached with caution, and is essentially one of exclusion. Lesions reported as hemangiopericytomas of the skull more likely represent meningeal hemangiopericytomas secondarily invading bone. Furthermore, meningeal hemangiopericytomas may produce distant osseous metastases, often several years after treatment of the primary tumor (41). The deer antler vascular pattern of hemangiopericytoma can be seen in a wide variety of neoplasms including synovial sarcoma, mesenchymal chondrosarcoma, malignant fibrous histiocytoma, and small cell osteosarcoma (44).

Treatment and Prognosis. Surgical ablation is the usual form of therapy. The role of chemotherapy or radiation is uncertain at this time. All grades are subject to metastases, although metastases are less common in the grade 1 tumors, and may not occur until almost two decades after the initial therapy (44). About half of grade 2 cases develop metastases, as do at least two thirds of patients with grade 3 hemangiopericytomas. The

follow-up in many instances is short. Accordingly, these metastatic rates represent minimal figures, as metastases have appeared as long as 26 years after initial diagnosis (43).

GLOMUS TUMOR

Definition. A benign, often highly vascular tumor composed of small, uniform, specialized smooth muscle cells resembling the smooth muscle component of a vascular glomus body.

Clinical Features. Although cutaneous and soft tissue glomus tumors are relatively common, fewer than 100 such lesions either primarily or secondarily involving bone have been reported. Patients range from 16 to 70 years of age, but most are between 20 and 40 years old. Females are more commonly affected. Glomus tumors involving bone present with extreme pain.

Sites. The tumors almost always occur in the distal phalanx. Rarely, however, other bones such as the ulna or coccyx may be affected (47,48). The latter site is of interest because of the normal presence of a well-formed glomus body in this location (45,47).

Radiographic Appearance. Skeletal involvement by glomus tumors can take three forms, which are best distinguished radiographically. First, there may be a deformity of the bone by an overlying soft tissue glomus tumor that compresses the cortex but does not invade it (fig. 167). Second, glomus tumors, especially those arising in the terminal phalanges, can erode the cortex and thereby become intraosseous by direct extension. This results in a well-demarcated, eccentric defect extending through the cortex, into the medullary bone. Third, glomus

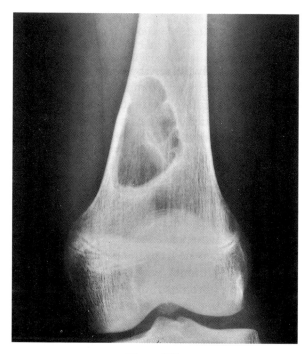

Figure 170
NONOSSIFYING FIBROMA
A 14-year-old boy had an incidentally found nonossifying fibroma when a radiograph was taken following trauma to his knee. The lesion is lytic, irregular in outline, and has a sclerotic rim. Because of the size, the surgeon elected to curette the lesion and pack it with bone chips. (Figures 170 and 171 are from the same patient.)

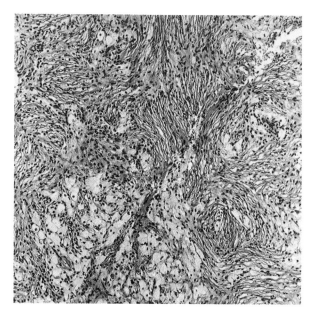

Figure 171
NONOSSIFYING FIBROMA
The fibrous tissue has a storiform pattern, and there are aggregates of foam cells.

remodeling takes place and the remnants of the nonossifying fibroma cease to be visible (11).

Gross Findings. The tissue submitted is almost always in the form of curettings and has varying shades of gray or yellow, depending on the relative proportions of fibrous tissue and foamy histiocytes. The occasional nonossifying fibroma that is an incidental finding in an amputation specimen is sharply rimmed by reactive bone (9).

Microscopic Findings. Fibrous tissue is present in irregular configurations, although there is often a storiform arrangement (fig. 171). Foamy histiocytes, hemosiderin-laden histiocytes, and multinucleated giant cells are present in varying proportions. Reactive new bone may be conspicuous, especially if there has been fracture. Even in the absence of fracture new bone formation may be present if the lesion is spontaneously resolving.

Differential Diagnosis. The distinction between metaphyseal fibrous defects or nonossifying fibromas and benign fibrous histiocytomas, based on clinical and radiographic grounds, is discussed in the section dealing with benign fibrous histiocytoma. The microscopic appearance of this group of lesions is nonspecific and can be encountered as a component of a variety of benign and malignant proliferations. The importance of radiographic correlation cannot be overemphasized.

Desmoplastic fibroma enters into the differential diagnosis if the nonossifying fibroma has a prominent fibrous component to the near exclusion of other cell types. The dense collagenization of desmoplastic fibroma, however, is only focally present or is absent in nonossifying fibroma. Reactive bone in nonossifying fibroma may lead to confusion with fibrous dysplasia, however, the prominent trabecular osteoblastic rimming of the reactive bone is uncommon in fibrous dysplasia, and the latter lesion rarely has a storiform pattern in its fibrous component. The presence of multinucleated giant cells in a cellular background may lead to consideration of giant cell tumor. However, nonossifying fibroma lacks the diffuse giant cell pattern and characteristic mononuclear cell background of that tumor. More importantly, there are critical clinical and radiographic distinctions. Giant cell tumor is a lesion almost exclusively of skeletally mature bone that involves the epiphysis.

Treatment and Prognosis. Resection or curettage with bone graft is curative for nonossifying fibromas requiring treatment. Some lesions have disappeared after an associated fracture that was treated only by immobilization (5). As a general rule, lesions that occupy more than half the diameter of the bone are considered to be at high risk for fracture and may be treated before fracture occurs.

We agree with Kyriakos and Murphy (6) that the association of metaphyseal fibrous defect or nonossifying fibroma with malignant tumors is probably coincidental. One report of a metaphyseal fibrous defect undergoing malignant transformation is not convincing for a preexistent benign lesion (2).

FIBROUS DYSPLASIA

Definition. A benign, monostotic or polyostotic proliferation of fibrous tissue and bone. The osseous component is irregularly distributed and consists predominately of woven bone with inconspicuous osteoblastic rimming. Cartilage is present in about 10 percent of cases.

General Features. Fibrous dysplasia is one of the more common benign proliferations of bone. Although it produces tumorous masses, not all authors agree that the process is truly neoplastic. Hamartomatous proliferation and a localized failure of bone to mature from the woven to the lamellar form are other theories that may account for fibrous dysplasia. Most cases involve a single bone, but about 20 percent of patients have polyostotic involvement, often with extraosseous abnormalities.

Clinical Features. *Monostotic.* Monostotic fibrous dysplasia has been diagnosed in every decade of life from infants to the elderly. However, about 75 percent of patients are diagnosed before 30 years of age, usually between 5 and 20 years of age. Males and females are affected equally. Symptomatology varies with the location of the disease. Involvement of the long bones may present with pain following fracture. Gnathic lesions often result in an obvious deformity but are otherwise asymptomatic. Rib lesions are frequently asymptomatic, incidental findings. Untreated lesions may enlarge or remain stable in their radiographic appearance. Henry (17) stated that most monostotic fibrous dysplasias cease to be active

after puberty, although a few cases first present later in life, and some lesions are reactivated with pregnancy. Patients with fibrous dysplasia having a conspicuous cartilaginous component may have rapid enlargement of the bone during adolescence, and the term *fibrocartilaginous dysplasia* has been applied to these lesions (13).

Polyostotic. Patients with polyostotic fibrous dysplasia often have macular pigmented skin lesions, precocious puberty, and, rarely, multiple fibromyxomatous soft tissue tumors (Albright disease). The multiple skin lesions are often unilateral. Polyostotic disease is usually symptomatic before 10 years of age, due to abnormalities of skeletal development manifested by limp, pain, or fracture. Recurrent fractures may lead to deformities in the lower extremities.

Sites. About one third of monostotic fibrous dysplasias involve the craniofacial bones, another third the femur or tibia, and about 20 percent occur in the ribs (16,17). In patients with polyostotic disease, the femur, tibia, and pelvis are involved in 75 to 90 percent of cases. Small bones of the feet also may be involved, as well as the ribs and skull (16).

Radiographic Appearance. Fibrous dysplasia produces widely variable radiographic images. The radiographic abnormality may be more lucent or more dense than the surrounding normal bone. The latter appearance indicates large amounts of heavily calcified intralesional osteoid or, less commonly, cartilage. Often, there is a "ground glass" appearance with a density similar to that of the surrounding cancellous bone, but lacking a trabecular structure. The affected bone may be greatly expanded, especially when the rib is involved (fig. 172). Fibrous dysplasia may be sharply defined with a sclerotic rim, or lack perilesional sclerosis and fade into the adjacent normal bone. The latter pattern is especially common in craniofacial lesions (fig. 173). Erosion through the cortex may occur, and, if a fracture is present, there is often a prominent periosteal reaction.

Gross Findings. Grossly, fibrous dysplasia is firm, fibrous, white or red tissue with a variably gritty consistency, depending on the amount of mineralized bone (fig. 174). Secondary cyst formation is common, and these are filled with amber or bloody fluid (fig. 175). Cartilage nodules, if present, appear as sharply circumscribed, translucent gray and can measure up to 3 cm.

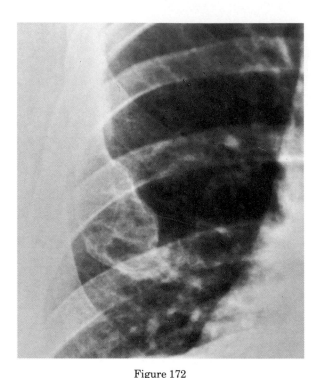

Figure 172
FIBROUS DYSPLASIA
This expanded rib was an incidental finding on the chest radiograph of a 57-year-old man.

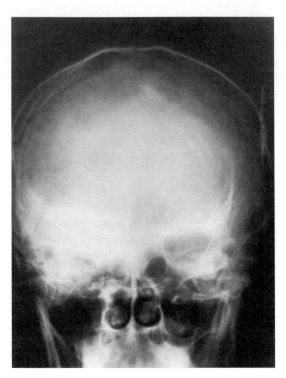

Figure 173
FIBROUS DYSPLASIA
Typical appearance of fibrous dysplasia involving frontal and ethmoid bones. The junction between the lesion and adjacent bone is indistinct, especially along the medial portion. (Fig. 5 from Fechner RE. Problematic lesions of the craniofacial bones. Am J Surg Pathol 1989;13(Suppl 1):17–30.)

Microscopic Findings. Fibrous dysplasia prototypically appears as irregularly shaped trabeculae of woven bone in a background of moderately cellular fibrous tissue. The bony trabeculae assume a variety of shapes, including spheres, "C" shapes, circles, or branching structures (figs. 176, 177). The osteoid is often referred to as metaplastic because it contains interspersed osteoblasts and appears to emerge from the surrounding fibrous background. Even the better formed trabeculae have osteoblasts uniformly distributed within the osteoid. Osteoblasts uniformly aligned along the edges of bony trabeculae (so-called osteoblastic rimming), a characteristic feature of reactive bone, are only occasionally seen and are not conspicuous. The osteoid in fibrous dysplasia is initially woven, that is, it consists of more irregularly distributed collagen, rather than the laminated collagen fibrils of lamellar bone. However, it is usually easy to find foci of lamellar bone formation, including reversal lines, as well as foci of peripheral rimming by osteoblasts. Whether such areas are intrinsic to fibrous dysplasia or represent sec-

ondary reactive changes is often unclear. Calcification is common, and may affect the smallest deposits of osteoid, as well as the more mature-appearing trabeculae (fig. 177). Often, the calcification in an individual bony trabecula is more prominent centrally, leaving unmineralized osteoid at the periphery (fig. 178).

The fibro-osseous tissue infiltrates between trabeculae of normal bone at the periphery of the lesion. This leads to a mixture of reactive bone with prominent osteoblastic rimming and typical fibrous dysplasia near the margin. Such foci should not detract from the diagnosis of fibrous dysplasia.

The fibrous stroma exhibits striking variation in its microscopic appearance. It can be highly cellular with little collagen, sparsely cellular with abundant collagen, or myxomatous. Collagen fibers sometimes connect the osteoid and fibrous tissue at right angles. Multinucleated giant cells, presumably functioning as osteoclasts, are present

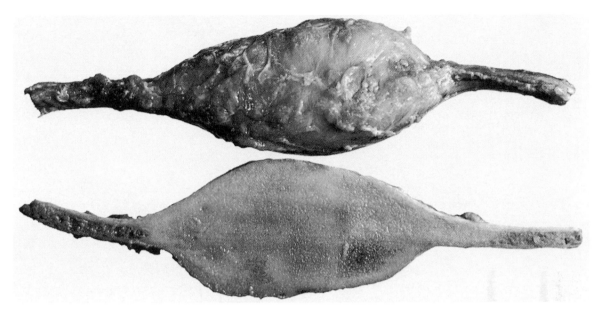

Figure 174
FIBROUS DYSPLASIA
Gross appearance of an expanded rib from a 53-year-old woman with fibrous dysplasia. The cortex is destroyed but the periosteum is intact. The lesion merges into the adjacent normal bone. This was an asymptomatic tumor found on a routine radiograph of the chest. (Fig. 294 from Fascicle 5, 2nd Series.)

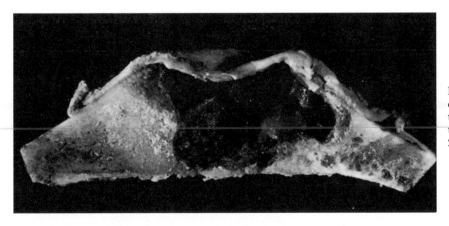

Figure 175
FIBROUS DYSPLASIA
A cross section of an expanded lesion of the calvarium illustrates cystic change. The cyst was partially filled with old blood. The patient was a 17-year-old girl. (Fig. 299 from Fascicle 5, 2nd Series.)

focally along the surface of trabeculae. The fibroblasts usually have plump, ovoid nuclei, but elongated, narrow nuclei are also seen. Multinucleated giant cells are frequently present, albeit in small numbers. Occasionally, they form aggregates in a pattern reminiscent of so-called giant cell reparative granuloma. Nodules of cartilage may be in continuity with the typical fibro-osseous component (fig. 179) and undergo enchondral ossification at their periphery.

The histologic pattern does not appear to change even when the same lesions are sampled over a period of years (16). There are no consistent differences between lesions found in children or adults.

Differential Diagnosis. The differential diagnosis includes osteofibrous dysplasia, well-differentiated intraosseous osteosarcoma, and desmoplastic fibroma. Perhaps the lesion most often confused with fibrous dysplasia is osteofibrous dysplasia. The latter entity almost exclusively involves the tibia and fibula, however, and has clinical and radiographic features that are quite different from those of fibrous dysplasia.

149

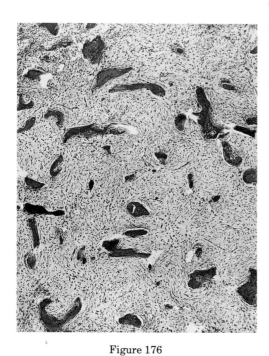

Figure 176
FIBROUS DYSPLASIA
Irregularly shaped trabeculae of bone lie in a moderately cellular, haphazard, fibrous stroma.

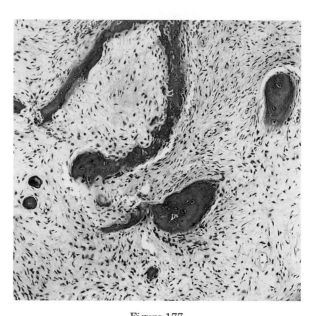

Figure 177
FIBROUS DYSPLASIA
Trabeculae of varying configurations, including small spherical forms, lie in a loosely fibrous stroma.

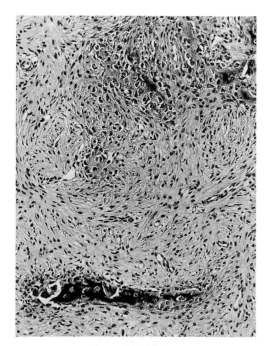

Figure 178
FIBROUS DYSPLASIA
Metaplastic osteoid and bone formation with central calcification is seen at the top. A better developed trabecula with heavy calcification and a thin rim of uncalcified osteoid is present in the lower field.

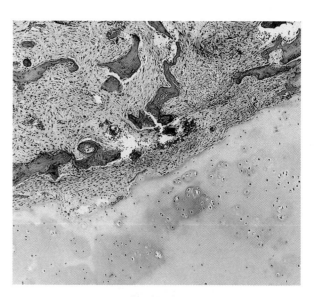

Figure 179
FIBROUS DYSPLASIA
Broad island of cartilage adjacent to typical trabeculae and fibrous background of fibrous dysplasia.

Microscopically, osteofibrous dysplasia displays a much greater tendency for osteoblastic rimming along the bony trabeculae.

Well-differentiated osteosarcoma has short, irregular trabeculae similar to those of fibrous dysplasia. Nonetheless, the fibrous component of well-differentiated osteosarcoma has larger nuclei, and, although the cells are fairly uniform, the enlarged nuclei with their chromatin clumping are more atypical than the smaller fibroblasts of fibrous dysplasia. Radiographic findings may be of equal or greater value in making the distinction between fibrous dysplasia and osteosarcoma (14).

Desmoplastic fibroma enters into the differential diagnosis because fibrous dysplasia may have broad areas devoid of osteoid formation, and, conversely, the infiltrative margin of desmoplastic fibroma may result in closely apposed fibrous tissue and reactive bony trabeculae. Although fibrous dysplasia may be heavily collagenized in areas, it lacks the extensive, uniformly collagenized appearance typical of desmoplastic fibroma. Bony trabeculae in the peripheral portions of desmoplastic fibroma have conspicuous osteoblastic rimming and lack the "metaplastic" appearance of osteoid in fibrous dysplasia.

Treatment and Prognosis. The management of fibrous dysplasia is complex, depending on the bone(s) involved, symptoms, extent of disease, and age of the patient. Recurrence following curettage or marginal resection is common because the extent of disease is often underestimated at the time of surgery. As previously noted, fibrous dysplasia extends between trabeculae of normal bone at the periphery of the lesion, and such extensions may not be clinically recognized.

Malignant transformation is very rare. Yabut et al. (20) recently reviewed 83 apparent examples. Sixty-nine patients had information regarding radiation. In two thirds of cases (46 of 69) there had been no antecedent radiation therapy; the remaining one third had been irradiated as therapy for their disease. In this review 0.4 percent of patients with fibrous dysplasia developed sarcoma. Taconis (19) arrived at a similar figure (0.5 percent) but noted that this frequency was too high because many cases of monostotic fibrous dysplasia remain undiscovered due to mild or absent symptoms. In addition, some published reports of sarcomas arising in "fibrous dysplasia" represent unrecognized intraosseous well-differentiated osteosarcomas with subsequent "dedifferentiation" to a more easily identified high-grade sarcoma.

Sarcoma can occur from 2 to 30 years after the diagnosis of fibrous dysplasia and can occur in a previously undiagnosed lesion as well (18). Males and females are at equal risk. Of the 72 cases in which the information was available, 41 patients had monostotic disease and 31 had polyostotic disease. The gnathic bones were most commonly involved, followed by the femur, tibia, and pelvis. Osteosarcomas comprised just over half the malignancies, followed by fibrosarcoma and chondrosarcoma. Interestingly, many of the patients with osteosarcoma had a prior history of radiation therapy. Only a small proportion of patients with fibrosarcoma and chondrosarcoma had such histories (15). The age at the time the malignancy was diagnosed ranged from 3 to 61 years with an average of 33 years.

OSTEOFIBROUS DYSPLASIA

Definition. A self-limiting, deformity-producing proliferation of bone and fibrous tissue involving the tibia or fibula of infants and children.

General Features. Osteofibrous dysplasia is a rare, clinicopathologically distinct lesion whose variable nomenclature has led to unnecessary confusion. It differs clinically and microscopically from both ossifying fibroma of the jaws and fibrous dysplasia, despite the fact that such terms as *ossifying fibroma of long bones* (25) and *intracortical fibrous dysplasia* have been applied to these lesions. The greatest experience with osteofibrous dysplasia comes from Campanacci and colleagues (21,22) at the Istituto Rizzoli in Bologna, and their studies included only 35 patients. It is unclear whether this is a benign, self-limited, occasionally regressing neoplasm, or a non-neoplastic anomaly related to bone growth, which seems far more likely, given the invariable lack of progression after skeletal maturation. Malignant transformation has not been reported. There is a well-documented but poorly understood relationship between osteofibrous dysplasia and extragnathic adamantinoma (28).

Clinical Features. Osteofibrous dysplasia is almost invariably diagnosed during the first decade of life, usually in the first 5 years, and occasionally shortly after birth. Resnik et al. (27) identified 79 cases, only 4 of which occurred after the age of 16 years (18 to 22 years). There may be a slight male predilection (22). Osteofibrous dysplasia presents as a painless enlargement of the involved bone that can lead to bowing and, occasionally, pseudoarthrosis or pathologic fracture (26).

Sites. To date, well-documented cases have exclusively involved the tibia and fibula. The great majority affect the tibia with fibular involvement being much less common. The process is almost always confined to one tibia, but occasionally the ipsilateral fibula is also involved. Rarely are both tibias or fibulas involved.

Radiographic Appearance. The radiographic appearance of osteofibrous dysplasia is often diagnostic, or at least highly characteristic. There is an expanded, lucent defect centered in the cortex and involving the diaphyseal portion of the bone (fig. 180) (24). The anterior cortical surface is commonly involved. Even when large, the lesion is separated from the medullary cavity by a rim of reactive bone of variable thickness, along the distorted inner cortical margin. The outer cortical bone may be thin or, occasionally, absent. The reactive changes surrounding the lesion often result in considerable perilesional sclerosis. Osteofibrous dysplasia may consist of a single lucent area, but more often there are multiple, confluent, bubble-like lucencies. Rarely, there may be multifocal or diffuse involvement of the entire tibia (22). Tibial disease almost invariably produces a severe anterior bowing deformity. In patients followed into puberty or adulthood the resultant chronic radiographic changes resemble Paget disease (22).

Gross Findings. The lesional tissue is soft, fibrous, and may be white, yellow, or red. If sufficient osteoid is present, there may be a gritty consistency. In rare, completely resected specimens the overlying, reactive periosteum is intact, even if there has been extension beyond the cortex (fig. 181).

Microscopic Findings. Osteofibrous dysplasia is characterized by bony trabeculae showing prominent osteoblastic rimming and a fibrous background (fig. 182). The fibrous tissue is variably cellular with either delicate collagen fiber deposition or more densely packed bands of collagen. There is a spectrum of appearances, depending on the state of lesional maturation.

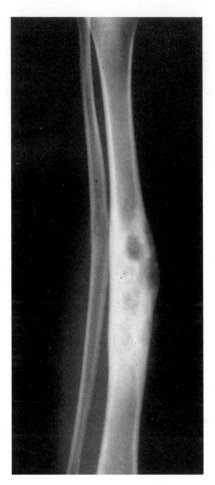

Figure 180
OSTEOFIBROUS DYSPLASIA
A 12-year-old boy had enlargement of the leg in the region of the tibia. The radiograph discloses multiple ill-defined lucencies and bowing deformity. (Figures 180–182 are from the same patient.)

Campanacci and Laus (22) have described a "zonation phenomenon" visible in larger, well-oriented specimens obtained by wedge biopsy. The central portion of the lesion has a predominantly fibroblastic appearance with only occasional, short, thin, immature trabeculae of woven bone. Moving toward the periphery in any direction, there is a progressive widening of trabeculae and conversion to lamellar bone. As the trabeculae become more numerous, they frequently anastomose and ultimately merge with the surrounding reactive cortical bone at the edge of the lesion. Foci of cartilage are rarely seen in the absence of fracture. Plump osteoblasts rimming bony trabeculae are conspicuous

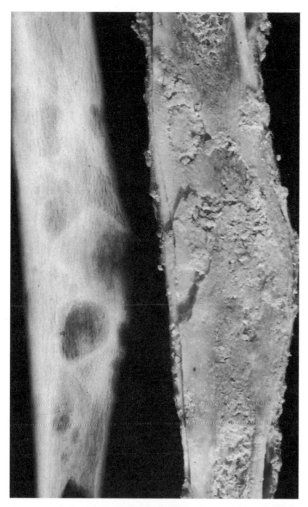

Figure 181
OSTEOFIBROUS DYSPLASIA
A segmental resection shows the cortex to be focally eroded. The lucent areas seen in the specimen radiograph correspond with less mineralized areas rather than representing true cysts.

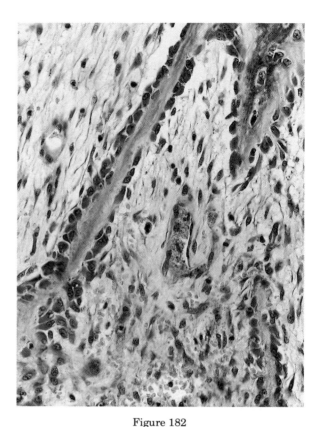

Figure 182
OSTEOFIBROUS DYSPLASIA
Trabeculae are lined by plump osteoblasts. The stroma is loose, moderately cellular fibrous tissue.

in every zone. Osteoclasts are sometimes adjacent to the bone. Focal collections of giant cells may be present in the fibrous stroma, probably in response to microhemorrhages, in a pattern reminiscent of giant cell reparative granuloma. Sweet and colleagues (28) noted that single, cytokeratin-positive cells were present in 93 percent of 30 cases of osteofibrous dysplasia.

Differential Diagnosis. Osteofibrous dysplasia may be confused with fibrous dysplasia or adamantinoma. Fibrous dysplasia tends to occur in older individuals, shows no predilection for the tibia or fibula, and lacks the prominent osteoblastic rimming that surrounds virtually

every trabecula in osteofibrous dysplasia. Radiographically, fibrous dysplasia involves the medullary portion of the bone, whereas osteofibrous dysplasia is an intracortical lesion.

Both osteofibrous dysplasia and adamantinoma show a striking, if not exclusive, predilection for the diaphyseal region of the tibia and fibula. Furthermore, adamantinomas may contain large osteofibrous dysplasia–like areas. In some cases, the epithelial component may be minimal and easily overlooked microscopically. Conversely, as noted above, single cytokeratin-positive cells are very common in osteofibrous dysplasia, and, in the absence of epithelial islands, do not warrant a diagnosis of adamantinoma (28). The low-grade malignancy of adamantinoma, as opposed to the self-limited nature of osteofibrous dysplasia, mandates that this distinction be made. Initial diagnosis of osteofibrous dysplasia in an adolescent should be approached with caution and careful search

153

made for any adamantinoma component. The relationship between adamantinoma and osteofibrous dysplasia is further discussed in the section dealing with adamantinoma.

Treatment and Prognosis. Osteofibrous dysplasia can become stationary or spontaneously regress during childhood, or slowly enlarge to involve most of the tibia. Enlarging lesions do so primarily during the first 10 years of life; progression does not occur after skeletal maturity. Surgical resection is rarely necessary and should be avoided, especially during childhood (22); attempts at surgical treatment prior to 15 years of age nearly always lead to recurrences (21–23). Biopsy is often unnecessary, given the stereotypical clinicoradiographic features. Fractures should be treated by cast immobilization. The bowing deformity may be treated by an osteotomy, and, if the deformity is severe, should be done as soon as feasible (22).

DESMOPLASTIC FIBROMA

Definition. A nonmetastasizing, but often locally aggressive neoplasm composed of nearly normal-appearing fibroblasts and myofibroblasts in an abundantly collagenized stroma.

General Features. Desmoplastic fibroma is the osseous analog of soft tissue aggressive fibromatosis. These are uncommon neoplasms with only about 150 reported cases. They comprised less than 0.1 percent of bone tumors in the Mayo Clinic series (33). As with its soft tissue counterpart, desmoplastic fibroma is capable of exhibiting locally aggressive, infiltrative growth. Because of this, some authors view these lesions as "borderline" rather than purely "benign," even though metastases do not occur. Desmoplastic fibroma is an intramedullary lesion, clearly distinguished from so-called periosteal desmoid, which is a misnomer for the cortical irregularity syndrome (described elsewhere).

Clinical Features. Patients range from 1 to 70 years of age. In one review, 46 percent of cases occurred in the second decade of life, and 78 percent before 40 years of age (37). There is a slight male predominance. Patients present with swelling, sometimes accompanied by pain. About 10 percent have a pathologic fracture. A history of symptoms for 2 or 3 years is common. Desmoplastic fibromas are rarely associated with underlying fibrous dysplasia or Paget disease of bone (32,38).

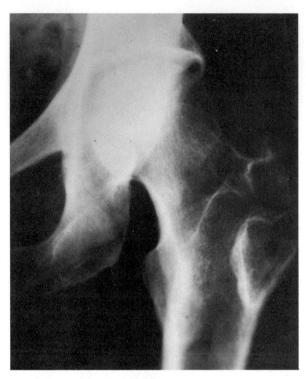

Figure 183
DESMOPLASTIC FIBROMA
A lesion with sclerotic margins is present in the greater trochanter. This 54-year-old woman had mild discomfort in the hip. (Fig. 18-6 from Fechner RE, Spjut HJ, Haggitt RC. Diseases of bones and joints. Based on the proceedings of the 51st Annual Anatomic Pathology Slide Seminar of the American Society of Clinical Pathologists. American Society of Clinical Pathologists Press. Chicago, 1985:93.)

Sites. The mandible is the most common site of disease, followed by the metaphysis of the femur, tibia, or humerus (31). Long bone involvement of the diaphysis and epiphysis is rare, but has been described. The pelvis is another common site of disease, and, less frequently, there may be involvement of the ribs, vertebrae, or small bones of the feet.

Radiographic Appearance. The tumors are lytic, range from 4 to 20 cm in size, and expand the bone, often circumferentially. There typically is a "soap bubble" appearance with irregular trabeculations traversing the lytic areas (29). Periosteal reaction is lacking. The margin is usually sharp (fig. 183), but may be permeative in a few lesions, and the cortex is often destroyed (fig. 184) (33). Computerized tomography may show a much greater soft tissue component than is appreciated on plain radiographs (39).

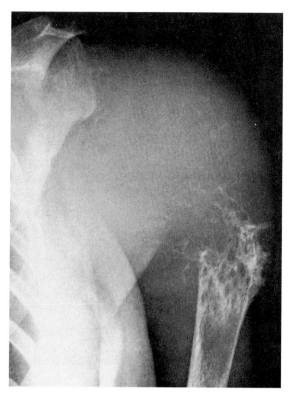

Figure 184
DESMOPLASTIC FIBROMA
This 33-year-old woman had intermittent pain in the region of the right deltoid muscle for 9 years. The proximal portion of the humerus has been destroyed and there is an irregular, sclerotic reaction in the remaining bone. (Fig. 288 from Fascicle 5, 2nd Series.) (Figures 184–186 are from the same patient.)

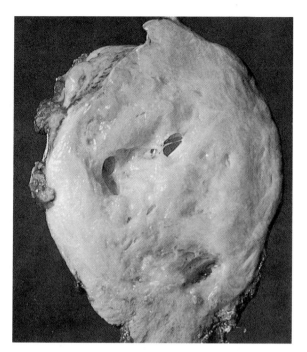

Figure 185
DESMOPLASTIC FIBROMA
The resected tumor forms a well-circumscribed fibrous mass with a few, small cystic areas. (Fig. 289 from Fascicle 5, 2nd Series.)

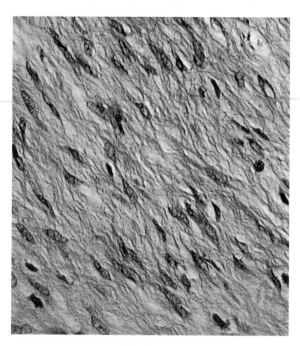

Figure 186
DESMOPLASTIC FIBROMA
Densely collagenized tissue has fibroblasts with uniform nuclei without abnormalities. (Fig. 290 from Fascicle 5, 2nd Series.)

Gross Findings. Desmoplastic fibroma of bone is grossly identical to desmoid tumor of soft tissue. It is firm, gray, and may have a whorled appearance. Occasionally, small cysts are present (fig. 185).

Microscopic Findings. The microscopic appearance is dominated by small spindle cells shown ultrastructurally to have features of fibroblasts, myofibroblasts, and primitive mesenchymal cells (34). The proliferating spindle cells are separated by abundant collagen fibers (fig. 186). The latter may be straight or wavy, loosely or densely distributed, and form delicate strands or extremely broad fibrous bands. Entrapped remnants of bone are often present, some showing evidence of osteoclastic resorption, and others lacking osteoclasts and completely surrounded by the proliferating fibrous tumor. Foci of lymphocytes and mast cells have been described in some cases (30). Desmoplastic fibroma may extend into the soft tissues with infiltration of the adjacent muscle in a fashion microscopically identical to that seen in aggressive fibromatosis of the soft tissues.

By light microscopy, the nuclei of the neoplastic spindle cells vary from somewhat plump and ovoid to elongated, thin, and uniformly hyperchromatic. Nucleoli are absent. Mitotic figures are rare and usually absent. More than an occasional division figure should suggest that the tumor is a well-differentiated fibrosarcoma. The cells of desmoplastic fibroma are arranged in parallel or haphazard arrays and rarely assume a herring-bone or storiform pattern. Although the lesions are generally sparsely cellular, there is variation, even within a single case, from paucicellular to moderately cellular foci in which the cells are separated by minimal collagen. The nuclei tend to be slightly larger in the more cellular areas (36).

Differential Diagnosis. The main consideration in the differential diagnosis is low-grade fibrosarcoma, a tumor that can have considerable collagen production and minimal nuclear atypia. Nonetheless, the cells of low-grade fibrosarcoma have more than an occasional enlarged nucleus with irregular chromatin clumping, the nucleus often possesses a nucleolus, and at least a few mitotic figures are readily identified.

Although it is easy to draw a verbal distinction between desmoplastic fibroma and well-differentiated fibrosarcoma, microscopic images from the two lesions clearly overlap. Furthermore, a well-differentiated fibrosarcoma may appear benign radiographically, with a sharply circumscribed or even sclerotic margin. The classification of a few low-grade fibrous lesions will be arbitrary.

Soft tissue aggressive fibromatosis arising periosteally and secondarily involving the bone is rare. These lesions are radiographically distinct from intramedullary desmoplastic fibroma. Most so-called periosteal desmoids are examples of the cortical irregularity syndrome.

Fibrous dysplasia enters into the differential diagnosis of desmoplastic fibroma, especially in view of the occasionally reported coexistence of the two lesions. Since desmoplastic fibroma has an infiltrative growth, entrapped trabeculae of bone, surrounded by neoplasm, may be seen at the periphery of the lesion. However, the predominately woven bone and more irregularly shaped trabeculae seen in fibrous dysplasia are

missing. Distinction of desmoplastic fibroma from well-differentiated osteosarcoma is briefly discussed under the latter entity.

Treatment and Prognosis. In a review of the literature, Gebhardt et al. (30) found that 26 patients treated with curettage (with or without bone graft) had a recurrence rate of 42 percent. Recurrences were seen in four of their own six patients treated in a similar intralesional manner; there was no recurrence in the two patients treated with marginal excision. Similar results were reported by Bertoni et al. (29). Recurrent tumors have been satisfactorily treated with wide resection. Rabhan and Rosai (36) noted an apparent correlation between the degree of cellularity of the tumor and the likelihood of recurrence. The role of radiation in cases that would otherwise require amputation is not clear, and chemotherapy has not as yet been shown to have a role (35). No desmoplastic fibroma has been reported to metastasize.

EXTRAGNATHIC FIBROMYXOMA

Definition. A benign intraosseous tumor composed of fibrous tissue with a variable myxoid stroma. Lesions with abundant myxoid tissue have been designated as myxomas.

General Features. Fibromyxoma or myxoma of bone is an accepted entity in the jaw. Extragnathic lesions are much less common, and their existence is controversial. Approximately 30 cases have been reported (40–42).

Clinical Features. Extragnathic fibromyxoma occurs over a broad age range, affecting patients from 2 to 74 years of age. Most are between 10 and 20 years or older than 50 years. There is no sexual predilection. Pain is the usual complaint.

Sites. There is a predilection for the metaphysis of long bones. Lesions in the distal or proximal part of the femur comprise about one third of cases, followed by involvement of the proximal or distal tibia, pelvic bones, and other long tubular bones.

Radiographic Appearance. The tumor can be a well-marginated, lytic medullary defect or an expansile, bubbly lesion with cortical destruction and soft tissue extension (41,42). Surrounding reactive bone is typically absent (41).

Gross Findings. The excised tissue is usually gray or white, and varies from fibrous to gelatinous, slimy, or mucoid in consistency. Cystic areas may be noted in completely resected specimens.

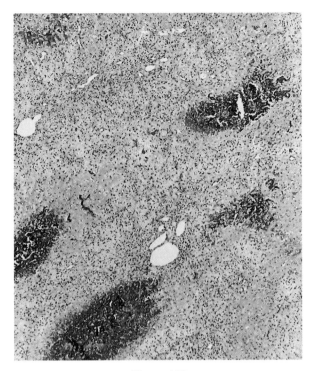

Figure 187
FIBROMYXOMA
Loose myxoid areas alternate with more fibrotic regions. Foci of dystrophic calcification are interspersed. (Courtesy of Dr. M.J. Klein, New York, NY.)

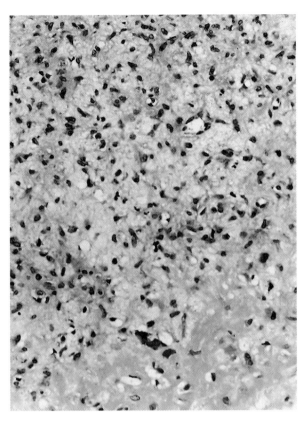

Figure 188
FIBROMYXOMA
Uniform, stellate and spindle shaped cells comprise the characteristic stroma of fibromyxoma. Dense fibrous tissue is also present at the lower right. (Courtesy of Dr. M.J. Klein, New York, NY.)

Microscopic Findings. As its name implies, fibromyxoma is a fibrous and myxoid neoplasm with both elements present to variable degrees (fig. 187). The proliferating stromal cells may be spindle shaped or stellate (fig. 188). Areas of chondroid, osteoid, densely mineralized bone, or dystrophic calcification are often interspersed. The stromal cells associated with such foci do not differ from those in other fibromyxoid areas. In the more myxoid areas, the stroma may be sparsely cellular. The cell nuclei throughout the lesion are uniform and small, without evidence of pleomorphism or mitotic figures (42). Lobulation is not present microscopically, and there is no surrounding fibrous capsule (42). Secondary aneurysmal bone cyst formation may be present (41).

Differential Diagnosis. Predominantly myxoid forms of fibromyxoma may be confused with an intraosseous ganglion, chondromyxoid fibroma, or chondrosarcoma. Unlike fibromyxoma, an intraosseous ganglion is a purely cystic myxoid lesion, lined by a fibrous capsule. The older literature contains several reports of "fibromyxomas" that are probably chondromyxoid fibromas. The lobular pattern of chondromyxoid fibroma with peripheral condensation of stromal cells and well-formed fibrous septa is missing in true fibromyxoma. Chondromyxoid fibroma tends to occur in the second decade of life, whereas fibromyxoma has a much broader age distribution (41), and is distinguished from fibromyxoma on the basis of its atypical stromal cells in the myxoid areas and its more prominent chondroid matrix.

Treatment and Prognosis. Fibromyxoma may recur after curettage, but subsequent curettage is curative. Extension into the adjacent soft tissues may require en bloc excision.

157

FIBROSARCOMA

Definition. A malignant spindle cell neoplasm that exclusively exhibits fibroblastic differentiation, without the production of osseous or chondroid matrix by the neoplastic cells.

General Features. The skeletal distribution is identical to that of osteosarcoma, prompting some authors to consider fibrosarcoma as an osteosarcoma that fails to produce matrix. Indeed, the survival rate of patients with these two tumors in the prechemotherapy era was very similar. However, the age distribution of fibrosarcoma forms an approximately bell-shaped curve in contrast to osteosarcoma with its sharp peak in the second decade. There also appears to be a greater propensity for fibrosarcoma to metastasize to extrapulmonary sites, as compared with osteosarcoma (52).

There is debate as to whether extramedullary fibrosarcoma involving the periosteum should be viewed as an osseous lesion. Some authors prefer to classify such tumors as periosteal (osseous) fibrosarcomas, whereas others view these as soft tissue tumors that abut the bone. Regardless of how one views these extramedullary tumors, it is clear that they differ, prognostically, from intramedullary fibrosarcoma. Huvos and Higinbotham (51) showed that patients with periosteal tumors had a 52 percent 5-year survival, as compared with 27 percent for intramedullary fibrosarcoma. This is comparable to the survival rate of patients with soft tissue fibrosarcoma (53). Taconis and Mulder (54) correlated the radiographic findings with prognosis and found that lesions with the epicenter of the tumor in the periphery of the bone near the cortex had a better prognosis than tumors with the epicenter in the medullary portion of the bone. This raises the possibility that juxtacortical lesions may be soft tissue tumors with secondary osseous involvement. Whichever is the case, and, indeed, both types of tumor may involve the cortical surface, it is important to keep the intramedullary and superficial groups separate because of this prognostic difference. The following discussion deals only with intramedullary fibrosarcoma.

Clinical Features. Fibrosarcoma affects males and females equally. Patients range from 3 months of age to 90 years (43). One case of congenital fibrosarcoma has been reported (46).

The tumor is rare in the first decade of life, however, and then it has a fairly uniform distribution from the second through the seventh decade.

Symptoms typically consist of pain and swelling. About half of the patients give a history of less than 6 months' duration, but some have been symptomatic for more than 3 years (45).

About 25 percent of osseous fibrosarcomas arise secondarily in a preexisting condition such as giant cell tumor, Paget disease, enchondroma, osteochondroma, chronic osteomyelitis, fibrous dysplasia, or a bone infarct (45). The underlying lesion may have been detected and treated many years earlier. For example, one patient developed a fibrosarcoma at the site of a giant cell tumor treated 25 years earlier by surgery alone (49). Many secondary fibrosarcomas may also be viewed as postradiation sarcomas. In fact, the most common scenario for secondary fibrosarcoma is a preexistent giant cell tumor treated with radiation therapy.

Sites. About 50 percent of intramedullary fibrosarcomas occur in the femur, tibia, or humerus, with predilection for the distal femur and proximal tibia. An additional 10 percent occur in the pelvis. Any bone may be affected, although fibrosarcoma involving the bones of the hands and feet is extremely rare (45). Less than 1 percent of fibrosarcomas are multicentric (45,48), but well-documented examples have been reported (50).

Radiographic Appearance. The lytic, destructive appearance of fibrosarcoma is nonspecific (55). The cortex of the metaphysis is almost always eroded, and there is frequently soft tissue extension. Rarely, the tumor extends down to the articular cartilage (fig. 189). The medullary portion of the bone has a permeative growth pattern in most instances. A few tumors have a less destructive appearance with a geographic pattern of lysis and, occasionally, even a thin sclerotic rim (54).

Gross Findings. The gross appearance of the tumor tends to correlate with the microscopic degree of differentiation. Well-differentiated fibrosarcomas with a large quantity of collagen are firm, white lesions, often with well-defined margins (fig. 190). Conversely, high-grade tumors are often gray, yellow, or brown, depending on the amount of necrosis. They typically have indistinct, infiltrative margins, and may contain myxoid areas.

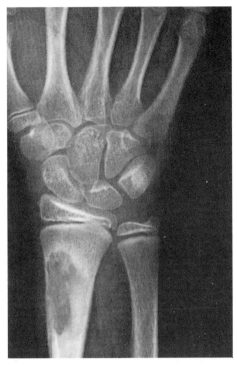

Figure 189
FIBROSARCOMA
A destructive, but relatively well-demarcated lesion is seen in the radius of a 10-year-old girl. (Fig. 306 from Fascicle 5, 2nd Series.) (Figures 189 and 190 are from the same patient.)

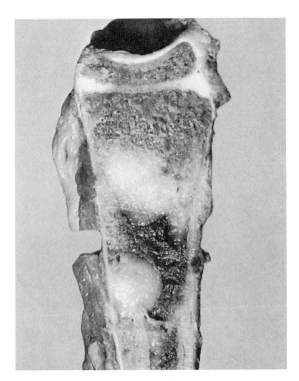

Figure 190
FIBROSARCOMA
A well-circumscribed tumor is replacing marrow space and destroying cortex in this sagittal section of the radius. The hemorrhagic area between tumor nodules represents the site of previous curettage. (Fig. 307 from Fascicle 5, 2nd Series.)

Microscopic Findings. The microscopic spectrum is broad, ranging from heavily collagenized tumors with uniform cells that are difficult to differentiate from desmoplastic fibroma (fig. 191) to bizarre, spindle cells with negligible collagen production. The consistent feature is the arrangement of spindle cells in interlacing fascicles that have a herring-bone pattern, at least focally (fig. 192). A storiform arrangement of fibroblasts can also occur.

By dividing fibrosarcoma into grades, the microscopic variation can be better appreciated. In one review, grade 1 lesions made up approximately 5 percent of fibrosarcomas, grade 2 lesions accounted for 65 percent of cases, and 30 percent were grade 3 (45). Grade 1 tumors have little nuclear pleomorphism. The cells are the size of normal fibroblasts, and there is abundant collagen (fig. 191). Bertoni et al. (44) found between 1 and 4 mitotic figures per 10 high-power fields in the grade 1 tumors. Grade 2 tumors have larger cells with mild nuclear pleomorphism, numerous

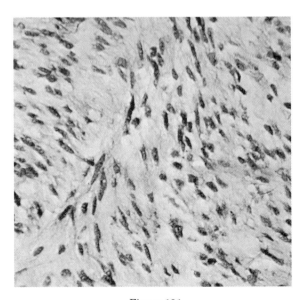

Figure 191
FIBROSARCOMA
This well-differentiated fibrosarcoma is moderately cellular and has only a few mildly atypical nuclei. (Fig. 305 from Fascicle 5, 2nd Series.)

159

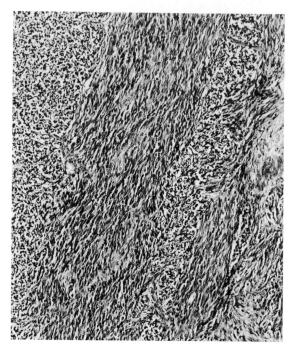

Figure 192
FIBROSARCOMA

This grade 2 fibrosarcoma is highly cellular with the typical herring-bone arrangement of tumor cells. Although the cellularity in this case is identical to that of grade 3 lesions, the degree of nuclear pleomorphism is not as great as in figure 193.

mitotic figures, and less collagen (fig. 192). Nonetheless, collagen can be abundant, and there may be extensive areas of hypocellular collagen. Grade 3 fibrosarcomas have an even greater degree of nuclear pleomorphism, with an increased mitotic rate and many atypical forms (fig. 193). The cells have hyperchromatic nuclei and prominent nucleoli. Areas of hemorrhagic necrosis may be present. Collagen is uniformly sparse, and myxoid areas may be seen. When the latter component predominates, the term *myxoid fibrosarcoma* has been used (48).

Differential Diagnosis. The distinction between well-differentiated fibrosarcoma and desmoplastic fibroma is covered under the latter entity. Osteosarcoma, malignant fibrous histiocytoma, dedifferentiated chondrosarcoma, and metastatic carcinoma may contain microscopic areas morphologically indistinguishable from fibrosarcoma. The absence of osteoid production by neoplastic cells eliminates osteosarcoma from the differential diagnosis, and the absence of a low-grade cartilaginous component eliminates dedifferentiated chondrosarcoma. Malignant fibrous histiocytoma has at least some cells with a more epithelioid, "histiocyte"-like appearance.

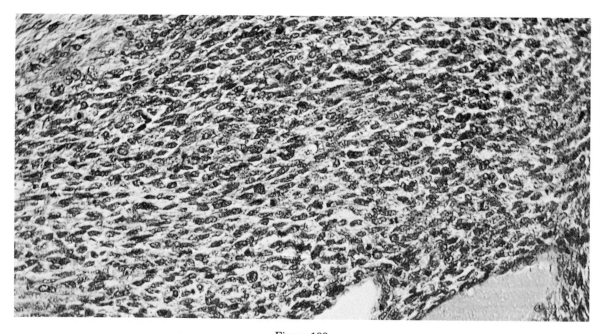

Figure 193
FIBROSARCOMA
This grade 3 fibrosarcoma has markedly atypical nuclei. (Fig. 316 from Fascicle 5, 2nd Series.)

Although some fibrosarcomas contain multinucleated giant cells, these have the appearance of osteoclasts rather than neoplastic giant cells. The fascicular, herring-bone pattern that predominates in fibrosarcoma is only focally present in some malignant fibrous histiocytomas.

Metastatic spindle cell neoplasms often can be differentiated utilizing immunohistochemical methods. Antibodies directed against S-100 protein, and the monoclonal antibody HMB-45, stain spindle cell malignant melanomas. Spindle cell carcinomas, typically of renal origin, usually but not invariably stain for epithelial membrane antigen and cytokeratin.

Treatment and Prognosis. Before chemotherapy, approximately 75 percent of patients died of disease (47). The role of radiation therapy and chemotherapy in the treatment of this tumor is in a state of evolution, and their value remains to be better determined.

Prognosis and histologic grade are strongly correlated for intraosseous fibrosarcoma. Eighty-three percent of patients with grade 1 lesions were 10-year survivors (44). In contrast, only 34 percent of patients with high-grade lesions survived. There is an appreciable local recurrence rate for all fibrosarcomas, especially the high-grade lesions. Recurrence is seen not only in patients who have undergone limb salvage procedures, but also in individuals treated initially with amputation (44).

Frassica et al. (48) found that the proportion of myxomatous change correlated with prognosis. Patients with small myxoid foci had a survival rate of 45 percent, whereas none of the patients in which the myxomatous area predominated survived beyond 21 months. There were only three patients in this category, however, and the overall histologic grade seems to correlate with the quantity of myxoid change, so this may not be an independent variable.

BENIGN FIBROUS HISTIOCYTOMA

Definition. A tumor of fibroblasts and mono- or multinucleated cells that resemble histiocytes. Lipid-filled cells may be conspicuous and occasionally are the major component. The term *xanthoma* or *fibroxanthoma* is often given to the latter lesions (57), which we consider to be within the broad category of benign fibrous histiocytoma.

General Features. From a purely histologic standpoint, benign fibrous histiocytoma has the same appearance as nonossifying fibroma (metaphyseal fibrous defect, fibrous cortical defect). Most pathologists do not consider nonossifying fibromas or metaphyseal fibrous defects as neoplastic, because they are self-limited processes in virtually every instance.

Benign fibrous histiocytoma differs from nonossifying fibroma on clinical and radiographic grounds, rather than histologic findings. Benign fibrous histiocytoma is painful, even in the absence of fracture, whereas nonossifying fibroma is painless unless fractured. The distribution of involved bones differs. Many benign fibrous histiocytomas involve the ribs or ilium, bones that are never involved by nonossifying fibroma. If a long bone is involved, benign fibrous histiocytoma is frequently centered in the diaphysis. When it has a metaphyseal center, extension into the epiphysis is common. Lesions centered in the epiphysis are also seen. Unlike nonossifying fibroma, benign fibrous histiocytoma has a tendency to recur and occasionally behave in an aggressive fashion (59,60).

Clinical Features. Patients range from 5 to 75 years of age (61,63). Magliato and Nastasi (63) documented a lesion in the ilium of a 5-year-old child that grew over 3 1/2 years and was accompanied by pain. Although it was diagnosed microscopically as a nonossifying fibroma, it had the clinical features of benign fibrous histiocytoma. These lesions also originate in adults (58), with males and females equally affected. Patients complain of pain of a few weeks' to 2 years' duration. A few lesions have presented with pathologic fractures (62).

Sites. The wing of the ilium is the most common site of involvement followed by the femur (Table 8). The xanthomas reported by Bertoni et al. (57) included three lesions in the skull, a site not reported by other authors for benign fibrous histiocytoma. In common with more typical benign fibrous histiocytomas, however, the ilium is the most common site for xanthoma.

Radiographic Appearance. Benign fibrous histiocytomas are lytic and usually have sharply defined margins. A sclerotic rim may be present and trabeculation is sometimes seen (59). Rarely, there is an ill-defined margin with destruction of the cortex and invasion into adjacent soft tissues (65).

Table 8

DISTRIBUTION OF 70 BENIGN FIBROUS HISTIOCYTOMAS AND XANTHOMAS REPORTED IN THE LITERATURE

Ilium	17
Femur	12
Vertebra	7
Tibia	7
Rib	6
Hand/Foot	3
Fibula	3
Skull	3
Humerus	3
Mandible	2
Other (one each):	
Sacrum, radius, patella, ulna, scapula, clavicle, ischium	

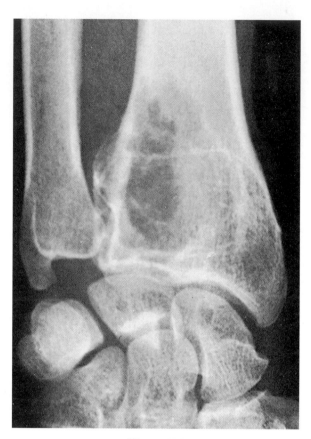

Figure 194
BENIGN FIBROUS HISTIOCYTOMA
This well-demarcated, lytic lesion of the radius is from a 48-year-old man who complained of discomfort. The epiphyseal portion of the bone is involved, as well as the metaphysis. (Fig. 504 from Fascicle 5(Suppl), 2nd Series.) (Figures 194–196 are from the same patient.)

In long bones, the metaphysis, epiphysis, or diaphysis may be involved. Metaphyseal involvement may be in continuity with the epiphysis (fig. 194), or have a conspicuous epiphyseal component (67).

Gross Findings. The gross appearance depends on the amount of lipid, fibrous tissue, and hemorrhage. The tissue may be yellow, gray, white or red, soft or firm. A cystic component has been described at the time of surgery (59).

Microscopic Findings. There are variable proportions of fibrous tissue, multinucleated giant cells, and foam cells (fig. 195). The fibrous tissue often has a storiform pattern. Occasionally, the foam cells are numerous (fig. 196). With rare exceptions, there is no cytologic atypia (see below). Cholesterol clefts and hemosiderin deposits may be evident. Occasional mitotic figures are seen, but there are no atypical forms. Reactive new bone formation may be present, but it is not an intrinsic part of the lesion.

A few benign fibrous histiocytomas have had cells with cytologically abnormal nuclei. Some of these have been treated aggressively (66) without further evidence of disease. Others have not recurred after minimal therapy (56). These lesions are best considered as atypical benign fibrous histiocytomas, rather than extremely well-differentiated malignant fibrous histiocytomas.

Differential Diagnosis. The mixture of histiocytic cells and fibrous tissue is not specific for benign fibrous histiocytoma. Many other lesions contain an identical fibrohistiocytic component that is presumably reactive. This component is seen in broad areas of benign lesions such as giant cell tumor, giant cell reparative granuloma, and eosinophilic granuloma, as well as in malignant neoplasms such as osteosarcoma or malignant fibrous histiocytoma. In effect, the diagnosis of benign fibrous histiocytoma is one of exclusion. In one study, three of five epiphyseal lesions originally diagnosed as benign fibrous histiocytoma were reclassified as giant cell tumors when small foci of typical giant cell tumor were found on review (64).

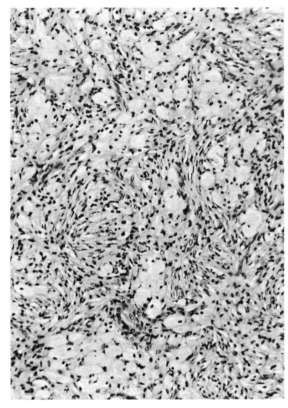

Figure 195
BENIGN FIBROUS HISTIOCYTOMA
Fibrous tissue with focal storiform pattern is interspersed with foam cells. (Fig. 502 from Fascicle 5(Suppl), 2nd Series.)

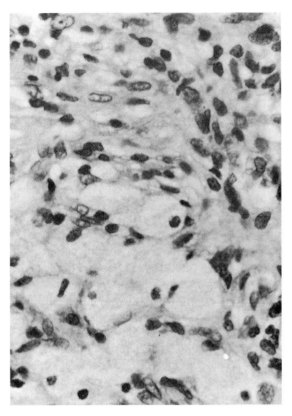

Figure 196
BENIGN FIBROUS HISTIOCYTOMA
Nuclei of the fibrous tissue and foam cells are bland, although there is variation in size. (Fig. 503 from Fascicle 5(Suppl), 2nd Series.)

Treatment and Prognosis. Most benign fibrous histiocytomas have initially been treated with curettage. Three of eight patients reported by Clarke et al. (59) developed recurrences. One had multiple recurrences with soft tissue extension, eventuating in amputation. Most histologic features, including mitotic rate, do not appear to correlate with recurrence. However, none of the 21 cases reported as xanthomas by Bertoni et al. (57) recurred, in contrast to the common recurrence of benign fibrous histiocytoma with fewer xanthoma cells.

One of 10 patients with benign fibrous histiocytoma reported by Dahlin and Unni (60) developed pulmonary metastases 2 years after a local recurrence in the distal femur that required amputation. Histologic findings are not described in detail for this case.

MALIGNANT FIBROUS HISTIOCYTOMA

Definition. A sarcoma of fibroblasts, myofibroblasts, and cells resembling histiocytes under light microscopy. Distinction from osteosarcoma is based on the absence of osteoid production. The microscopic pattern is nonspecific and the diagnosis requires exclusion of other diagnostic features, including preexisting low-grade neoplasms that may have "dedifferentiated."

General Features. The term malignant fibrous histiocytoma was introduced in the 1960s for soft tissue tumors. In 1972 skeletal malignant fibrous histiocytoma was described (73), followed shortly by detailed pathologic studies (80,82). Several subsequent studies retrospectively identified osseous lesions originally classified as osteosarcomas or pleomorphic fibrosarcomas. Dahlin and associates (71) reported 35 cases of

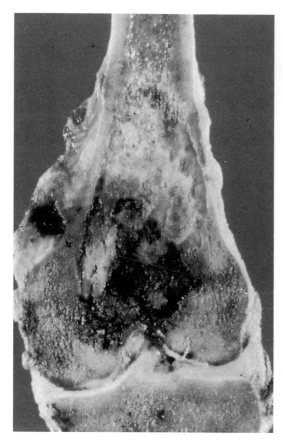

Figure 199
MALIGNANT FIBROUS HISTIOCYTOMA
This resection specimen shows a grossly variegated malignant fibrous histiocytoma in the distal femur. There is cortical erosion on the left with soft tissue extension. (Fig. 3B from Frierson HF Jr, Fechner RE, Stallings RG, Wang GJ. Malignant fibrous histiocytoma in bone infarct. Association with sickle cell trait and alcohol abuse. Cancer 1987;59:496–500.)

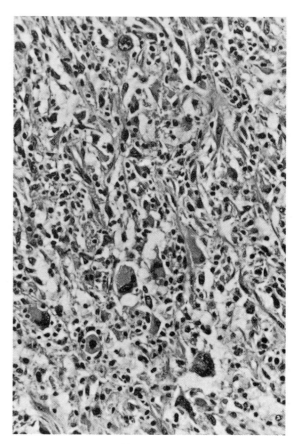

Figure 200
MALIGNANT FIBROUS HISTIOCYTOMA
The haphazard mixture of malignant fibroblasts and histiocytes is typical of malignant fibrous histiocytoma. A prominent lymphocytic component is scattered throughout the tumor. (Fig. 490 from Fascicle 5(Suppl), 2nd Series.)

spindle cells in a pattern identical to that of myxoid malignant fibrous histiocytoma of soft tissues.

The histiocytic cells of malignant fibrous histiocytoma are mono- or multinucleated. The nuclei in the multinucleated cells are usually randomly distributed, but occasionally they resemble Touton or Langhans giant cells. Nuclei range from bland to bizarre. They may be vesicular, lobulated, convoluted, or grooved. One or more prominent nucleoli are the rule. Dense, eosinophilic nucleoli often have clearing of the perinucleolar chromatin and resemble Reed-Sternberg cells. The cytoplasm is usually finely granular or powdery, but may be vacuolated or foamy. The nuclei of the foamy cells, whether mononuclear or multinuclear, tend to be small, bland, and uniform. These may be true,

reactive histiocytes. The mitotic rate varies greatly, but counts of 25 mitotic figures per 50 high-power fields are common. Abnormal configurations are frequent and are most often found in histiocytic cells.

Some malignant fibrous histiocytomas have a conspicuous, branching vascular component that resembles the staghorn blood vessels found in hemangiopericytomas (fig. 204). Inflammation is often prominent, with lymphocytes as the predominant cells. Neutrophils are frequent in areas of necrosis, and may be common in intact tumor. Plasma cells and eosinophils vary from scarce to focally conspicuous (82). Non-neoplastic fragments of bone surrounded by tumor may either retain their nuclei or be necrotic. If the necrotic bone is accompanied by dystrophic calcium deposits in the marrow, it may be the remnant of a bone infarct.

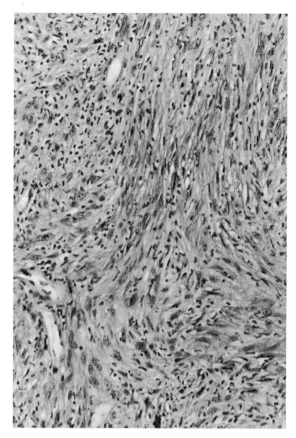

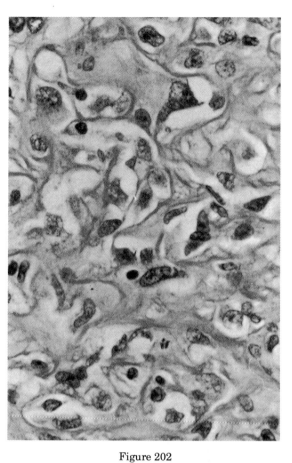

Figure 201
MALIGNANT FIBROUS HISTIOCYTOMA

Fibroblasts dominate this image. Fascicles of fibroblasts intersect in the center of the field to form a storiform pattern. This appearance may be very focal in malignant fibrous histiocytoma and, conversely, can be commonly encountered in other spindle cell neoplasms. (Fig. 491 from Fascicle 5 (Suppl), 2nd Series.)

Figure 202
MALIGNANT FIBROUS HISTIOCYTOMA

Irregular deposits of noncalcified collagen surround neoplastic cells. These foci closely resemble osteosarcoma. (Fig. 492 from Fascicle 5(Suppl), 2nd Series.)

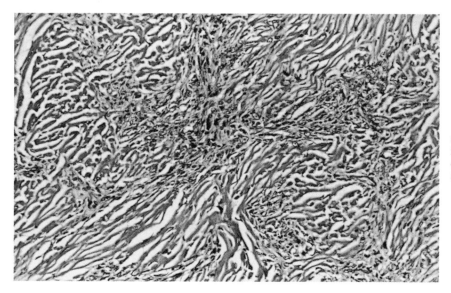

Figure 203
MALIGNANT FIBROUS
HISTIOCYTOMA

This broad area of collagen deposition is sparsely cellular. The storiform arrangement of the collagen is discernible. (Fig. 493 from Fascicle 5(Suppl), 2nd Series.)

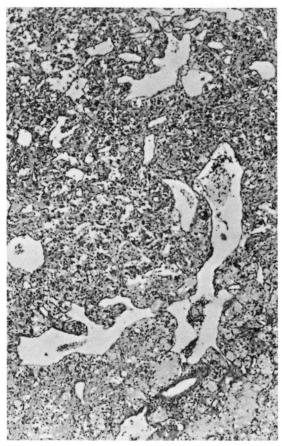

Figure 204
MALIGNANT FIBROUS HISTIOCYTOMA
This markedly vascular tumor contains "staghorn" vascular spaces identical to those seen in hemangiopericytoma. The intervening tumor cells, however, are fibroblasts and histiocytes rather than pericytes. (Fig. 496 from Fascicle 5(Suppl), 2nd Series.)

The broad spectrum of atypia and mitotic activity in malignant fibrous histiocytoma suggests the possibility of microscopically grading these tumors. Detailed criteria for grading do not exist, however, and the value of grading remains to be clearly defined. Moreover, a single lesion can vary cytologically from bland and sparsely cellular to extraordinarily bizarre and pleomorphic (75). Thus, the grade of a small biopsy is likely to be nonrepresentative.

Differential Diagnosis. The differential diagnosis includes fibrosarcoma and osteosarcoma, categories that were the former diagnostic repositories for these tumors. Fibrosarcoma is distinguished by a predominant fascicular (herringbone) pattern of rather monomorphic spindle cells with minimal evidence of storiform configurations. Distinguishing osteosarcoma may be more nebulous. Osteosarcomas with abundant, heavily mineralized osteoid may also have broad areas identical to malignant fibrous histiocytoma. When a tumor has an almost exclusively malignant fibrous histiocytoma–like appearance and only a few areas of unequivocal osteoid formation, it is, perhaps, arbitrary whether one considers it as a malignant fibrous histiocytoma or an osteosarcoma. We believe that a few isolated high-power fields of nonmineralized osteoid need not detract from the diagnosis of malignant fibrous histiocytoma.

Metastatic spindle cell carcinoma must also be considered in the differential diagnosis. This distinction is discussed in the section on metastases to bone. It is worth mentioning here, however, that cytokeratin has been found in some malignant fibrous histiocytomas (85).

Treatment and Prognosis. The survival of patients treated by surgery alone is about 18 percent, the same as for osteosarcoma (76). Adjuvant chemotherapy may be of benefit after adequate surgical resection (68). Some patients treated with multiple drugs before resection had no viable-appearing tumor in the resected specimen (80).

It has been suggested that patients with low-grade malignant fibrous histiocytomas have a better prognosis (69,77). However, not all long-term survivors had low-grade tumors, and Dahlin et al. (71) found no correlation between tumor grade and prognosis. The presence or absence of an osteoid-like matrix does not correlate with survival either (79). The survival rates for tumors arising in preexisting osseous abnormalities are significantly poorer than those for malignant fibrous histiocytomas arising in normal bone (69,77). Neither the age of the patient nor the bone of origin appears related to prognosis.

REFERENCES

Metaphyseal Fibrous Defect and Nonossifying Fibroma

1. Arata MA, Peterson HA, Dahlin DC. Pathological fractures through non-ossifying fibromas. Review of the Mayo Clinic experience. J Bone Joint Surg [Am] 1981;63:980–8.

2. Bhagwandeen SB. Malignant transformation of a non-osteogenic fibroma of bone. J Pathol Bacteriol 1966; 92:562–4.

3. Caffey J. On fibrous defects in cortical walls of growing tubular bones: their radiologic appearance, structure, prevalence, natural course and diagnostic significance. Adv Pediatr 1955;7:13–51.

4. Campanacci M, Laus M, Boriani S. Multiple non-ossifying fibromata with extraskeletal anomalies: a new syndrome? J Bone Joint Surg [Br] 1983;65:627–32.

5. Drennan DB, Maylahn DJ, Fahey JJ. Fractures through large non-ossifying fibromas. Clin Orthop 1974;103:82–8.

6. Kyriakos M, Murphy WA. Concurrence of metaphyseal fibrous defect and osteosarcoma. Report of a case and review of the literature. Skeletal Radiol 1981;6:179–86.

7. Mirra JM, Gold RH, Rand F. Disseminated nonossifying fibromas in association with café-au-lait spots (Jaffe-Campanacci syndrome). Clin Orthop 1982;168:192–205.

8. Moser RP Jr, Sweet DE, Haseman DB, Madewell JE. Multiple skeletal fibroxanthomas: radiologic-pathologic correlation of 72 cases. Skeletal Radiol 1987;16:353–9.

9. Mubarak S, Saltzstein SL, Daniel DM. Non-ossifying fibroma. Report of an intact lesion. Am J Clin Pathol 1974;61:697–701.

10. Ritschl P, Hajek PC, Pechmann U. Fibrous metaphyseal defects. Magnetic resonance imaging appearances. Skeletal Radiol 1989;18:253–9.

11. _____, Karnel F, Hajek P. Fibrous metaphyseal defects—determination of their origin and natural history using a radiomorphological study. Skeletal Radiol 1988;17:8–15.

12. Young JW, Levine AM, Dorfman HD. Case report 293. Diagnosis: nonossifying fibroma (NOF) of the upper tibial diametaphysis, with considerable increase in size over a three-year period. Skeletal Radiol 1984;12:294–7.

Fibrous Dysplasia

13. Drolshagen LF, Reynolds WA, Marcus NW. Fibrocartilaginous dysplasia of bone. Radiology 1985;156:32.

14. Fechner RE. Problematic lesions of the craniofacial bones. Am J Surg Pathol 1989;13(Suppl 1):17–30.

15. Halawa M, Aziz AA. Chondrosarcoma in fibrous dysplasia of the pelvis. A case report and review of the literature. J Bone Joint Surg [Br] 1984;66:760–4.

16. Harris WH, Dudley HR Jr, Barry RJ. The natural history of fibrous dysplasia. J Bone Joint Surg [Am] 1962;44:207–33.

17. Henry A. Monostotic fibrous dysplasia. J Bone Joint Surg [Br] 1969;51:300–6.

18. Huvos AG, Higinbotham NL, Miller TR. Bone sarcomas arising in fibrous dysplasia. J Bone Joint Surg [Am] 1972;54:1047–56.

19. Taconis WK. Osteosarcoma in fibrous dysplasia. Skeletal Radiol 1988;17:163–70.

20. Yabut SM Jr, Kenan S, Sissons HA, Lewis MM. Malignant transformation of fibrous dysplasia. A case report and review of the literature. Clin Orthop 1988;228:281–9.

Osteofibrous Dysplasia

21. Campanacci M. Osteofibrous dysplasia of long bones: a new clinical entity. Ital J Orthop Traumatol 1976;2:221–37.

22. _____, Laus M. Osteofibrous dysplasia of the tibia and fibula. J Bone Joint Surg [Am] 1981;63:367–75.

23. Campbell CJ, Hawk T. A variant of fibrous dysplasia (osteofibrous dysplasia). J Bone Joint Surg [Am] 1982;64:231–6.

24. Castellote A, García-Peña P, Lucaya J, Lorenzo J. Osteofibrous dysplasia. A report of two cases. Skeletal Radiol 1988;17:483–6.

25. Kempson RL. Ossifying fibroma of the long bones. A light and electron microscopic study. Arch Pathol 1966; 82:218–33.

26. Nakashima Y, Yamamuro T, Fujiwara Y, Kotoura Y, Mori E, Hamashima Y. Osteofibrous dysplasia (ossifying fibroma of long bones). A study of 12 cases. Cancer 1983;52:909–14.

27. Resnik CS, Young JW, Levine AM, Aisner SC. Case report 604. Osteofibrous dysplasia (ossifying fibroma) of tibia. Skeletal Radiol 1990;19:217–9.

28. Sweet DE, Vinh TN, Devaney K. Cortical osteofibrous dysplasia of long bone and its relationship to adamantinoma. A clinicopathologic study of 30 cases. Am J Surg Pathol 1992;16:282–90.

Desmoplastic Fibroma

29. Bertoni F, Calderoni P, Bacchini P, Campanacci M. Desmoplastic fibroma of bone. A report of six cases. J Bone Joint Surg [Br] 1984;66:265–8.

30. Gebhardt MC, Campbell CJ, Schiller Al, Mankin HJ. Desmoplastic fibroma of bone. A report of eight cases and review of the literature. J Bone Joint Surg [Am] 1985;67:732–47.

31. Graudal N. Desmoplastic fibroma of bone. Case report and literature review. Acta Orthop Scand 1984;55:215–9.

32. Hillmann JS, Mesgarzadeh M, Tang CK, Bonakdarpour A, Reyes TG. Case report 481. Benign intraosseous fibroma (desmoplastic fibroma) associated with Paget disease of the iliac bone. Skeletal Radiol 1988;17:356–9.

33. Inwards CY, Unni KK, Beabout JW, Sim FH. Desmoplastic fibroma of bone. Cancer 1991;68:1978–83.

34. Lagacè R, Delage C, Bouchard HL, Seemayer TA. Desmoplastic fibroma of bone. An ultrastructural study. Am J Surg Pathol 1979;3:423–30.

35. Marks KE, Bauer TW. Fibrous tumors of bone. Orthop Clin North Am 1989;20:377–93.

36. Rabhan WN, Rosai J. Desmoplastic fibroma. Report of ten cases and review of the literature. J Bone Joint Surg [Am] 1968;50:487–502.

37. Sugiura I. Desmoplastic fibroma. Case report and review of the literature. J Bone Joint Surg [Am] 1976;58:126–30.

38. West R, Huvos AG, Lane JM. Desmoplastic fibroma of bone arising in fibrous dysplasia. Am J Clin Pathol 1983;79:630–3.

39. Young JW, Aisner SC, Levine AM, Resnik CS, Dorfman HD. Computed tomography of desmoid tumors of bone: desmoplastic fibroma. Skeletal Radiol 1988;17:333–7.

Extragnathic Fibromyxoma

40. Abdelwahab IF, Hermann G, Klein MJ, Kenan S, Lewis MM. Fibromyxoma of bone. Skeletal Radiol 1991; 20:95–8.

41. Marcove RC, Lindeque BG, Huvos AG. Fibromyxoma of the bone. Surg Gynecol Obstet 1989;169:115–8.

42. McClure DK, Dahlin DC. Myxoma of bone. Report of three cases. Mayo Clinic Proc 1977;52:249–53.

Fibrosarcoma

43. Bernadò L, Admella C, Lucaya J, Sanchez de Toledo J, Bosch J. Infantile fibrosarcoma of femur. Pediatr Pathol 1987;7:201–7.

44. Bertoni F, Capanna R, Calderoni P, Patrizia B, Campannaci M. Primary central (medullary) fibrosarcoma of bone. Semin Diagn Pathol 1984;1:185–98.

45. Campanacci M, Olmi R. Fibrosarcoma of bone. A study of 114 cases. Ital J Orthop Traumatol 1977;3:199–206.

46. Dahlin DC. Case report 189. Infantile fibrosarcoma (congenital fibrosarcoma-like fibromatosis). Skeletal Radiol 1982;8:77–8.

47. Eyre-Brook AL, Price CH. Fibrosarcoma of bone. Review of fifty consecutive cases from the British Bone Tumour Registry. J Bone Joint Surg [Br] 1969;51:20–37.

48. Frassica FJ, Sim FH, Wold LE. Case report 462. Grade 2 myxoid fibrosarcoma of femur. Skeletal Radiol 1988;17:77–80.

49. Gitelis S, Wang JW, Quast M, Schajowicz F, Templeton A. Recurrence of a giant-cell tumor with malignant transformation to a fibrosarcoma twenty-five years after primary treatment. A case report. J Bone Joint Surg [Am] 1989;71:757–61.

50. Hernandez FJ, Fernandez BB. Multiple diffuse fibrosarcoma of bone. Cancer 1976;37:939–45.

51. Huvos AG, Higinbotham NL. Primary fibrosarcoma of bone. A clinicopathologic study of 130 patients. Cancer 1975;35:837–47.

52. Jeffree GM, Price CH. Metastatic spread of fibrosarcoma of bone: a report on forty-nine cases, and a comparison with osteosarcoma. J Bone Joint Surg [Br] 1976;58:418–25.

53. Pritchard DJ, Soule EH, Taylor WF, Ivins JC. Fibrosarcoma—a clinicopathologic and statistical study of 199 tumors of the soft tissues of the extremities and trunk. Cancer 1974;33:888–97.

54. Taconis WK, Mulder JD. Fibrosarcoma and malignant fibrous histiocytoma of long bones: radiographic features and grading. Skeletal Radiol 1984;11:237–45.

55. _____, van Rijssel TG. Fibrosarcoma of long bones: A study of the significance of areas of malignant fibrous histiocytoma. J Bone Joint Surg [Br] 1985; 67:111–6.

Benign Fibrous Histiocytoma

56. Bertoni F, Calderoni P, Bacchini P, et al. Benign fibrous histiocytoma of bone. J Bone Joint Surg [Am] 1986; 68:1225–30.

57. _____, Unni KK, McLeod RA, Sim FH. Xanthoma of bone. Am J Clin Pathol 1988;90:377–84.

58. Clark TD, Stelling CB, Fechner RE. Case report 328. Benign fibrous histiocytoma of the left 8th rib. Skeletal Radiol 1985;14:149–51.

59. Clarke BE, Xipell JM, Thomas DP. Benign fibrous histiocytoma of bone. Am J Surg Pathol 1985;9:806–15.

60. Dahlin DC, Unni KK. Bone tumors: general aspects and data on 8,542 cases. 4th ed. Springfield, Ill: Charles C. Thomas, 1986:141–8.

61. Destouet JM, Kyriakos M, Gilula LA. Fibrous histiocytoma (fibroxanthoma) of a cervical vertebra. A report with a review of the literature. Skeletal Radiol 1980;5:241–6.

62. Hermann G, Steiner GC, Sherry HH. Case report 465. Benign fibrous histiocytoma (BFH). Skeletal Radiol 1988;17:195–8.

63. Magliato HJ, Nastasi A. Non-osteogenic fibroma occurring in the ilium. Report of a case. J Bone Joint Surg [Am] 1967;49:384–6.

64. Matsuno T. Benign fibrous histiocytoma involving the ends of long bone. Skeletal Radiol 1990;19:561–6.

65. Roessner A, Immenkamp M, Weidner A, Hobik HP, Grundmann E. Benign fibrous histiocytoma of bone. Light- and electron-microscopic observations. J Cancer Res Clin Oncol 1981;101:191–202.

66. Saito R, Caines MJ. Atypical fibrous histiocytoma of the humerus: a light and electron microscopic study. Am J Clin Pathol 1977;68:409–15.

67. Spjut HJ, Fechner RE, Ackerman LV. Tumors of bone and cartilage (Suppl). Atlas of Tumor Pathology, 2nd Series, Fascicle 5. Washington, D.C.: Armed Forces Institute of Pathology, 1981, 16–23.

Malignant Fibrous Histiocytoma

68. Bacci G, Springfield D, Capanna R, Picci P, Bertoni F, Campanacci M. Adjuvant chemotherapy for malignant fibrous histiocytoma in the femur and tibia. J Bone Joint Surg [Am] 1985;67:620–5.

69. Capanna R, Bertoni F, Bacchini P, Bacci G, Guerra A, Campanacci M. Malignant fibrous histiocytoma of bone. The experience at the Rizzoli Institute: report of 90 cases. Cancer 1984;54:177–87.

70. Chen KT. Multiple fibroxanthosarcoma of bone. Cancer 1978;42:770–3.

71. Dahlin DC, Unni KK, Matsuno T. Malignant (fibrous) histiocytoma of bone—fact or fancy? Cancer 1977; 39:1508–16.

72. den Heeten GJ, Koops HS, Kamps WA, Oosterhuis JW, Sleijfer DT, Oldhoff J. Treatment of malignant fibrous histiocytoma of bone: a plea for primary chemotherapy. Cancer 1985;56:37–40.

73. Feldman F, Norman D. Intra- and extraosseous malignant histiocytoma (malignant fibrous xanthoma). Radiology 1972;104:497–508.

74. Finci R, Günhan Ö, Uçmakli E, Sarlak Ö. Multiple and familial malignant fibrous histiocytoma of bone. A report two cases. J Bone Joint Surg [Am] 1990;72:295–8.

75. Frierson HF Jr, Fechner RE, Stallings RG, Wang GJ. Malignant fibrous histiocytoma in bone infarct. Association with sickle cell trait and alcohol abuse. Cancer 1987;59:496–500.

76. Ghandur-Mnaymneh L, Zych G, Mnaymneh W. Primary malignant fibrous histiocytoma of bone: report of six cases with ultrastructural study and analysis of the literature. Cancer 1982;49:698–707.

77. Huvos AG, Heilweil M, Bretsky SS. The pathology of malignant fibrous histiocytoma of bone. A study of 130 patients. Am J Surg Pathol 1985;9:853–71.

78. Martorell M, Calabuig C, Peydro-Olaya A, Llombart-Bosch A, Terrier-Lacombe MJ, Contesso G. Fibroblast and myofibroblast participation in malignant fibrous histiocytoma (MFH) of bone. Ultrastructural study of eight cases with immunohistochemical support. Pathol Res Pract 1989;184:582–90.

79. McCarthy EF, Matsuno T, Dorfman HD. Malignant fibrous histiocytoma of bone: a study of 35 cases. Hum Pathol 1979;10:57–70.

80. Mirra JM, Bullough PG, Marcove RC, Jacobs B, Huvos AG. Malignant fibrous histiocytoma and osteosarcoma in association with bone infarcts: report of four cases, two in caisson workers. J Bone Joint Surg [Am] 1974;56:932–40.

81. Roessner A, Vassallo J, Vollmer E, Zwadlo G, Sorg C, Grundmann E. Biological characterization of human bone tumors. X. The proliferation behaviour of macrophages is compared to fibroblastic cells in malignant fibrous histiocytoma and giant cell tumor of bone. J Cancer Res Clin Oncol 1987;113:559–62.

82. Spanier SS. Malignant fibrous histiocytoma of bone. Orthop Clin North Am 1977;8:947–61.

83. , Enneking WF, Enriquez P. Primary malignant fibrous histiocytoma of bone. Cancer 1975; 36:2084–98.

84. Troop JK, Mallory TH, Fisher DA, Vaughn BK. Malignant fibrous histiocytoma after total hip arthroplasty. A case report. Clin Orthop 1990;253:297–300.

85. Weiss SW, Bratthauer GL, Morris PA. Postirradiation malignant fibrous histiocytoma expressing cytokeratin. Implications for the immunodiagnosis of sarcomas. Am J Surg Pathol 1988;12:554–8.

86. Wigger HJ, Mitsudo SM. Fibrous histiocytoma simulating congenital fibromatosis: a light-, electron microscopic and tissue culture study. Virchows Arch [A] 1976;370:255–66.

✧✧✧

GIANT CELL LESIONS

GIANT CELL TUMOR

Definition. A benign but often locally aggressive neoplasm characterized by large numbers of uniformly distributed, osteoclast-like giant cells and a more diagnostically pertinent background population of plump, epithelioid to spindle mononuclear cells.

General Features. Giant cell tumor accounts for about 5 percent of biopsied primary bone tumors and about 20 percent of benign bone tumors (9), making it the sixth most common primary osseous neoplasm. Because many bone tumors contain a prominent giant cell component, the diagnosis of giant cell tumor requires careful clinicoradiologic correlation and microscopic evaluation of the mononuclear component to exclude other diagnostic elements. Giant cell tumors rarely give rise to pulmonary metastases, and those that occur are usually clinically indolent. Proliferations with large numbers of giant cells developing as a complication of preexisting Paget disease of bone (17,19,41) are interpreted by most authors as true giant cell tumors, although some consider these to be giant cell reparative granulomas. Giant cell tumors may undergo sarcomatous transformation, either spontaneously or in response to radiation therapy. The term malignant giant cell tumor has been inconsistently used and should probably be abandoned in favor of more descriptive terminology.

Several studies have documented intranuclear virus-like inclusions in giant cell tumors with and without associated Paget disease (1,30,40,45). Abelanet et al. (1) noted that 21 of 43 giant cell tumors of bone had intranuclear paramyxovirus-like inclusions in the tumor giant cells, but not in the mononuclear stromal cells. In contrast, 50 other bone lesions with prominent giant cells and osteoclasts from 20 samples of normal bone lacked viral inclusions. In other studies, the virus-like inclusions have been less frequent and more difficult to find: in one study they were noted in 2 of 13 giant cell tumors (40). Their significance is not known.

Flow cytometry studies of 60 giant cell tumors showed that 70 percent were diploid, 27 percent were aneuploid, and 3 percent were tetraploid

(39). Although there was a slightly higher relapse rate in the aneuploid group, the authors believed that this was primarily related to the mode of therapy, rather than ploidy status. It was concluded that DNA analysis had limited value in predicting the biologic behavior of giant cell tumor.

Cytogenetic analysis by Bridge et al. (6) of 20 giant cell tumors showed random chromosomal abnormalities in 14 and clonal abnormalities in 6. Chromosomal abnormalities were detected in all but 1 of the 10 tumors that were locally aggressive, recurrent, or metastatic; 3 of 4 nonaggressive tumors lacked chromosomal abnormalities. These findings prompted the authors to suggest that chromosomal analysis might be of value in predicting the behavior of giant cell tumor. In another study, a locally aggressive giant cell tumor (stage 2) was noted to have cells with a consistent t(12;19)(q13;q13) translocation (31).

The differentiation exhibited by the mononuclear and multinuclear cells of giant cell tumor has been the subject of multiple ultrastructural, histochemical, and immunohistochemical studies. Several studies have supported monocytic (histiocytic) differentiation for the mononuclear cells of giant cell tumor (5,7,24,34,47), and some of these have suggested similar differentiation for the multinucleated component (5,24,34,47). The latter observation supports the concept that the multinucleated cells of giant cell tumor form by fusion of the mononuclear component. Histiocytes and osteoclasts have also been shown to share immunohistochemical features. Other studies, however, have suggested that the mononuclear cells are derived from nonhematopoietic stromal cells that differ from the osteoclast-like giant cell component (2,14).

Clinical Features. Giant cell tumor almost always affects the mature skeleton with closed epiphyseal plates. Approximately 10 to 15 percent of patients are younger than 20 years of age, but almost all are skeletally mature. Less than 2 percent occur adjacent to open epiphyses (32). The diagnosis of giant cell tumor in a skeletally immature patient is, thus, highly suspect. The peak incidence is in the third decade of life with a gradual decrease into late adulthood. Occurrence

Giant cell reparative granuloma has been described as a secondary lesion in a patient with polyostotic fibrous dysplasia (51). It has also been suggested that many of the giant cell proliferations that develop in preexisting Paget disease are giant cell reparative granulomas, rather than true giant cell tumors (65). This remains controversial, although it is recognized that giant cell lesions in Paget disease appear to be less aggressive than de novo giant cell tumors.

Sites. Most giant cell reparative granulomas of the hands and feet involve the phalanges, metatarsals, and metacarpals. Occurrence in the wrist and tarsal bones is less common. The phalanges are most commonly involved in the hand lesions whereas in the foot the metatarsals are most commonly involved (62). Multiple lesions have rarely been reported (49). Giant cell reparative granuloma of the long bones is quite rare (51,64) and may be associated with a preexistent lesion (51). In these locations, more likely diagnoses such as giant cell tumor or aneurysmal bone cyst should be excluded.

Radiographic Appearance. Typically, there is a radiolucent, fusiform expansion centered in the diaphysis or metaphysis, although often the small tubular bones of the hands and feet are entirely involved. The majority of cases show evidence of fine to coarse trabeculation. The cortex is thin but characteristically intact (fig. 215). Extension into the surrounding soft tissues is distinctly uncommon. As with giant cell tumor, there is no sclerosis of the surrounding bone. The ends of the lesion are typically well demarcated and a permeative growth pattern is not present. The epiphysis was spared in all but one of the cases reported by Lorenzo and Dorfman (58). Periosteal reaction has been generally absent (54,62), but was described in almost 25 percent of patients in one study (67).

Gross Findings. Curetted tissue samples from giant cell reparative granulomas typically appear as nondescript, pink-tan to grey-brown, friable material. Cystic components may be noted at the time of surgery (58).

Microscopic Findings. There is a prominent, fibroblastic stroma containing giant cells, often centered around zones of stromal hemorrhage (fig. 216). In some areas, the giant cells may be more diffusely distributed, but focal aggregates are usually present (fig. 217). Most of

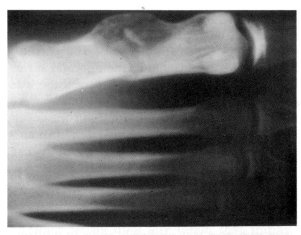

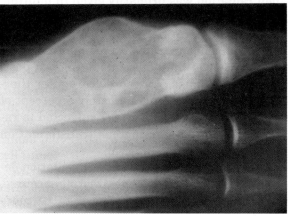

Figure 215
GIANT CELL REPARATIVE GRANULOMA
Enlarging expansile destructive lesion in the metatarsal of a 17-year-old boy. The interval between the initial (top) and subsequent (bottom) radiographs is 1 month.

the giant cells are smaller and contain fewer nuclei than those of giant cell tumor. Some contain phagocytized blood cells and hemosiderin. Giant cells are often seen in vascular spaces (fig. 216). The stromal fibroblasts vary in appearance from spindled to ovoid and form both hypercellular zones and zones of prominent collagenization with few cells. Stromal mitotic figures may be frequent but are usually fewer in number than in giant cell tumor. The giant cells never contain mitotic figures. Trabeculae of reactive osteoid and bone are a common feature of giant cell reparative granuloma, being present in at least 75 percent of cases. The bony trabeculae can be lined by osteoblasts, or lack osteoblastic rimming and resemble "metaplastic" bone (58). Cartilaginous foci are not seen in the absence of

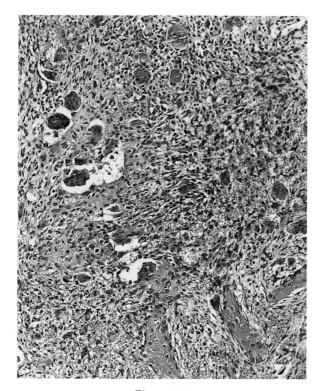

Figure 216
GIANT CELL REPARATIVE GRANULOMA
The background is fibrous stroma with scattered giant cells, some of which lie within small vascular spaces. Reactive bone is present at the lower right.

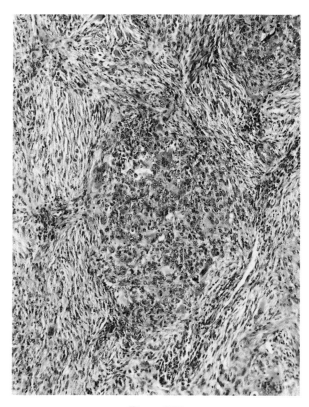

Figure 217
GIANT CELL REPARATIVE GRANULOMA
Occasionally the giant cells are present in well-defined, granuloma-like aggregates.

fracture. Foci of secondary aneurysmal bone cyst are seen both in initial lesions and recurrences (54,58). Lymphocytes and plasma cells are commonly present in the stroma.

Ultrastructurally, the stromal cells of giant cell reparative granuloma have features of fibroblasts (58). Immunohistochemical studies of giant cell reparative granuloma of the jaws have shown positivity of both mononuclear stromal cells and giant cells for alpha-1-antitrypsin and alpha-1-antichymotrypsin, suggesting histiocytic (macrophagic) differentiation (63). The giant cell component also expresses the additional macrophage marker, lysozyme (muramidase) (63).

Differential Diagnosis. *"Brown Tumor" of Hyperparathyroidism.* Giant cell reparative granuloma, regardless of its location, is histologically indistinguishable from the so-called "brown tumor" of hyperparathyroidism (58). Because of this, all patients with suspected giant cell reparative granuloma should have serum calcium,

phosphate, and alkaline phosphatase levels determined to exclude the possibility of hyperparathyroidism. Since there have been rare reports of "normocalcemic" hyperparathyroidism, serum parathyroid hormone levels should be determined when calcium levels are at the upper limits of normal.

Giant Cell Tumor. It is important to separate giant cell reparative granuloma from giant cell tumor, because the latter exhibits more locally aggressive behavior, occasionally produces "benign metastases" to the lung, and may undergo sarcomatous transformation. Distinguishing features are discussed in the section on giant cell tumors (p. 179).

Aneurysmal Bone Cyst. "Solid areas" in aneurysmal bone cyst may be microscopically indistinguishable from giant cell reparative granuloma (67). Furthermore, giant cell reparative granuloma may have a secondary aneurysmal bone cyst component. It seems likely that these are closely related reactive lesions. By convention, at least in the bones of the hands and feet, the presence of foci of giant cell reparative granuloma precludes a primary diagnosis of aneurysmal bone cyst (54).

Nonossifying Fibroma. Mirra (60) found giant cell reparative granuloma of the jaws to be indistinguishable, at least microscopically, from nonossifying fibroma, and he recommends that the jaw lesions be relabeled as nonossifying fibromas. This does not address the nomenclature of their counterparts involving the hands and feet, however. Giant cell reparative granulomas of the hands and feet also may contain microscopic fields with prominent foam cells indistinguishable from nonossifying fibroma. However, their predominantly fibrous stroma and granuloma-like aggregates of giant cells are not typical features of nonossifying fibroma. Moreover, the latter tumors are quite rare in the hands and feet and have a distinctive radiographic appearance with often marked perilesional sclerosis.

Treatment and Prognosis. Curettage, with or without bone grafting, is currently considered adequate therapy. Occasional lesions may be large enough to almost completely destroy a short tubular bone and, in such cases, resection or digital amputation may be necessary. The recurrence rate for curetted giant cell reparative granulomas of the hands and feet is variable. Prior to the paper by Lorenzo and Dorfman (58), there were no recurrences in the 13 reported cases. These authors, however, reported that 4 of 8 patients developed one or more recurrences. In subsequent studies totaling 37 cases, 16 patients developed recurrences (49,54,59,61,67). The mean time from initial treatment to recurrence was 15 months, with a range of from 3 months to 4 years. All recurrences were initially treated with curettage, with or without bone grafting (62). Curettage is considered appropriate therapy for recurrent lesions, most of which will be cured by this second procedure. Giant cell reparative granulomas have not been documented to produce "benign metastases" or undergo sarcomatous transformation, as has been described with giant cell tumor.

REFERENCES

Giant Cell Tumor

1. Abelanet R, Daudet-Monsac M, Laoussadi S, Forest M, Vacher-Lavenu MC. Frequency and diagnostic value of virus-like filamentous intranuclear inclusions in giant cell tumor of bone, not associated with Paget's disease. A study of 43 cases. Virchows Arch [A] 1986;410:65–8.
2. Aqel NM, Pringle JA, Horton MA. Cellular heterogeneity in giant cell tumor of bone (osteoclastoma): an immunohistochemical study of 16 cases. Histopathology 1988;13:675–85.
3. Bertoni F, Present D, Enneking WF. Giant cell tumor of bone with pulmonary metastases. J Bone Joint Surg [Am] 1985;67:890–900.
4. _____, Present D, Sudanese A, Baldini N, Bacchini P, Campanacci M. Giant-cell tumor of bone with pulmonary metastases. Six case reports and a review of the literature. Clin Orthop 1988;237:275–85.
5. Brecher ME, Franklin WA, Simon MA. Immunohistochemical study of mononuclear phagocyte antigens in giant cell tumor of bone. Am J Pathol 1986;125:252–7.
6. Bridge JA, Neff JR, Bhatia PS, Sanger WG, Murphey MD. Cytogenetic findings and biologic behavior of giant cell tumors of bone. Cancer 1990;65:2697–703.
7. Brooks JP, Pascal RR. Malignant giant cell tumor of bone: ultrastructural and immunohistologic evidence of histiocytic origin. Hum Pathol 1984;15:1098–100.
8. Dahlin DC, Cupps RE, Johnson EW Jr. Giant cell tumor: a study of 195 cases. Cancer 1970;25:1061–70.
9. _____, Unni KK. Bone tumors: general aspects and data on 8,542 cases. 4th ed. Springfield, Ill: Charles C. Thomas, 1986:119–40.
10. Dyke SC. Metastasis of the "benign" giant-cell tumor of bone (osteoclastoma). J Pathol Bacteriol 1931;34:259–63.
11. Enneking WF. Musculoskeletal tumor surgery. New York: Churchill Livingstone, 1983:87–8.
12. Glass TA, Mills SE, Fechner RE, Dyer R, Martin W III, Armstrong P. Giant-cell reparative granuloma of the hands and feet. Radiology 1983;149:65–8.
13. Goldenberg RR, Campbell CJ, Bonfiglio M. Giant-cell tumor of bone. An analysis of two hundred and eighteen cases. J Bone Joint Surg [Am] 1970;52:619–64.
14. Goldring SR, Roelke MS, Petrison KK, Bhan AK. Human giant cell tumors of bone. Identification and characterization of cell types. J Clin Invest 1987;79:483–91.
15. Harwood AR, Fornasier VL, Rider WD. Supervoltage irradiation in the management of giant cell tumor of bone. Radiology 1977;125:223–6.
16. Herendeen RE. Results in the röentgen-ray therapy of giant-cell tumors of bone. Ann Surg 1931;93:398–411.
17. Hutter RV, Foote FW Jr, Frazell EL, Francis KC. Giant cell tumors complicating Paget's disease of bone. Cancer 1963;16:1044–56.
18. Huvos AG. "Benign" metastasis in giant cell tumor of bone [Letter]. Hum Pathol 1981;12:1151.

19. Jacobs TP, Michelsen J, Polay JS, D'Adamo AC, Canfield RE. Giant cell tumor in Paget's disease of bone. Familial and geographic clustering. Cancer 1979; 44:742–7.

20. Jaffe HL, Lichtenstein L, Portis RB. Giant cell tumor of bone. Its pathologic appearance, grading, supposed variants, and treatment. Arch Pathol 1940;30:993–1031.

21. Joly MA, Vázquez JJ, Martinez A, Guillen FJ. Blood-borne spread of a benign giant cell tumor from the radius to the soft tissue of the hand. Cancer 1984;54:2564–7.

22. Katz E, Nyska M, Okon E, Zajicek G, Robin G. Growth rate analysis of lung metastases from histologically benign giant cell tumor of bone. Cancer 1987;59:1831–6.

23. Ladanyi M, Traganos F, Huvos AG. Benign metastasizing giant cell tumors of bone. A DNA flow cytometric study. Cancer 1989;64:1521–6.

24. Ling L, Klein MJ, Sissons HA, Steiner GC. Lysozyme and alpha 1-antitrypsin in giant-cell tumor of bone and in other lesions that contain giant cells. Arch Pathol Lab Med 1986;110:713–8.

25. Maloney WJ, Vaughan LM, Jones HH, Ross J, Nagel DA. Benign metastasizing giant-cell tumor of bone. Report of three cases and review of the literature. Clin Orthop 1989;243:208–15.

26. Marcove RC, Lyden JP, Huvos AG, Bullough PG. Giant-cell tumors treated by cryosurgery. A report of 25 cases. J Bone Joint Surg [Am] 1973;55:1633–44.

27. _____, Weis LD, Vaghaiwalla MR, Pearson R, Huvos AG. Cryosurgery in the treatment of giant cell tumors of bone. A report of 52 consecutive cases. Cancer 1978;41:957–69.

28. Matsuno T. Benign fibrous histiocytoma involving the ends of long bone. Skeletal Radiol 1990;19:561–6.

29. Meis JM, Dorfman HD, Nathanson SD, Haggar AM, Wu KK. Primary malignant giant cell tumor of bone: "dedifferentiated" giant cell tumor. Mod Pathol 1989; 2:541–6.

30. Mirra JM, Bauer FC, Grant TT. Giant cell tumor with viral-like intranuclear inclusions associated with Paget's disease. Clin Orthop 1981;158:243–51.

31. Noguera R, Llombart-Bosch A, Lopez-Gines C, Carda C, Fernandez C. Giant cell tumor of bone, stage II, displaying translocation t(12;19)(q13;q13). Virchows Arch [A] 1989;415:377–82.

32. Picci P, Manfrini M, Zucchi V, et al. Giant-cell tumor of bone in skeletally immature patients. J Bone Joint Surg [Am] 1983;65:486–90.

33. Present D, Bertoni F, Hudson T, Enneking WF. The correlation between the radiologic staging studies and histopathologic findings in aggressive stage 3 giant cell tumor of bone. Cancer 1986;57:237–44.

34. Regezi JA, Zarbo RJ, Lloyd RV. Muramidase, alpha-1 antitrypsin, alpha-1 antichymotrypsin, and S-100 protein immunoreactivity in giant cell lesions. Cancer 1987;59:64–8.

35. Rock MG, Pritchard DJ, Unni KK. Metastases from histologically benign giant-cell tumor of bone. J Bone Joint Surg [Am] 1984;66:269–74.

36. _____, Sim FH, Unni KK, et al. Secondary malignant giant-cell tumor of bone. Clinicopathological assessment of nineteen patients. J Bone Joint Surg [Am] 1986;68:1073–9.

37. Rosai J. Carcinoma of pancreas simulating giant cell tumor of bone. Electron-microscopic evidence of its acinar cell origin. Cancer 1968;22:333–44.

38. Sanerkin NG. Malignancy, aggressiveness, and recurrence in giant cell tumor of bone. Cancer 1980;46:1641–9.

39. Sara AS, Ayala AG, El-Naggar A, Ro JY, Raymond AK, Murray JA. Giant cell tumor of bone. A clinicopathologic and DNA flow cytometric analysis. Cancer 1990; 66:2186–90.

40. Schajowicz F, Ubios AM, Araujo ES, Cabrini RL. Virus-like intranuclear inclusions in giant cell tumor of bone. Clin Orthop 1985;201:247–50.

41. Scully RE, Mark EJ, McNeely BU, eds. Case records of the Massachusetts General Hospital. Case 1-1986. N Engl J Med 1986;314:105–13.

42. Seider MJ, Rich TA, Ayala AG, Murray JA. Giant cell tumor of bone. Treatment with radiation therapy. Radiology 1986;161:537–40.

43. Sim FH, Dahlin DC, Beabout JW. Multicentric giant-cell tumor of bone. J Bone Joint Surg [Am] 1977; 59:1052–60.

44. Sladden RA. Intravascular osteoclasts. J Bone Joint Surg [Br] 1957;39:346–57.

45. Welsh RA, Meyer AT. Nuclear fragmentations and associated fibrils in giant cell tumor of bone. Lab Invest 1970;22:63–72.

46. Wold LE, Swee RG. Giant cell tumor of the small bones of the hands and feet. Semin Diagn Pathol 1984;1:173–84.

47. Yoshida H, Akeho M, Yumoto T. Giant cell tumor of bone. Enzyme histochemical, biochemical, and tissue culture studies. Virchows Arch [A] 1982;395:319–30.

Giant Cell Reparative Granuloma

48. Ackerman LV, Spjut HJ. Tumors of bone and cartilage. Atlas of Tumor Pathology, Section II—Fascicle 4. Washington, D.C.: Armed Forces Institute of Pathology, 1962:282,344–5.

49. Caskey PM, Wolf MD, Fechner RE. Multicentric giant cell reparative granuloma of the small bones of the hand. A case report and review of the literature. Clin Orthop 1985;193:199–205.

50. D'Alonzo RT, Pitcock JA, Milford LW. Giant-cell reaction of bone. Report of two cases. J Bone Joint Surg [Am] 1972;54:1267–71.

51. De Smet AA, Travers H, Neff JR. Case report 207. Giant cell reparative granuloma of left femur arising in polyostotic fibrous dysplasia. Skeletal Radiol 1982;8:314–8.

52. Fechner RE, Fitz-Hugh GS, Pope TL Jr. Extraordinary growth of giant cell reparative granuloma during pregnancy. Arch Otolaryngol 1984;110:116–9.

53. Franklin CD, Craig GT, Smith CJ. Quantitative analysis of histologic parameters in giant cell lesions of the jaws and long bones. Histopathology 1979;3:511–22.

54. Glass TA, Mills SE, Fechner RE, Dyer R, Martin W III, Armstrong P. Giant-cell reparative granuloma of the hands and feet. Radiology 1983;149:65–8.

55. Hamner JE III, Ketcham AS. Cherubism: an analysis of treatment. Cancer 1969;23:1133–43.

56. Hirschl S, Katz A. Giant cell reparative granuloma outside the jaw bone. Diagnostic criteria and review of the literature with the first case described in the temporal bone. Hum Pathol 1974;5:171–81.

57. Jaffe HL. Giant-cell reparative granuloma, traumatic bone cyst, and fibrous (fibro-osseous) dysplasia of the jawbones. Oral Surg Oral Med Oral Pathol 1953;6:159–75.

58. Lorenzo JC, Dorfman HD. Giant-cell reparative granuloma of short tubular bones of the hands and feet. Am J Surg Pathol 1980;4:551–63.

59. Merkow RL, Bansal M, Inglis AE. Giant cell reparative granuloma in the hand: report of three cases and review of the literature. J Hand Surg [Am] 1985;10:733–9.

60. Mirra JM. Bone tumors: clinical, radiologic, and pathologic correlations. Philadelphia: Lea & Febiger, 1989: 733–5.

61. Picci P, Baldini N, Sudanese A, Boriani S, Campanacci M. Giant cell reparative granuloma and other giant cell lesions of the bones of the hands and feet. Skeletal Radiol 1986;15:415–21.

62. Ratner V, Dorfman HD. Giant-cell reparative granuloma of the hand and foot bones. Clin Orthop 1990; 260: 251–8.

63. Regezi JA, Zarbo RJ, Lloyd RV. Muramidase, alpha-1 antitrypsin, alpha-1 antichymotrypsin, and S-100 protein immunoreactivity in giant cell lesions. Cancer 1987;59:64–8.

64. Thomas IH, Chow CW, Cole WG. Giant cell reparative granuloma of the humerus. J Pediatr Orthop 1988; 8:596–8.

65. Upchurch KS, Simon LS, Schiller AL, Rosenthal DI, Campion EW, Krane SM. Giant cell reparative granuloma of Paget's disease of bone: a unique clinical entity. Ann Intern Med 1983;98:35–40.

66. Waldron CA, Shafer WG. The central giant cell reparative granuloma of the jaws. An analysis of 38 cases. Am J Clin Pathol 1966;45:437–47.

67. Wold LE, Dobyns JH, Swee RG, Dahlin DC. Giant cell reaction (giant cell reparative granuloma) of the small bones of the hands and feet. Am J Surg Pathol 1986; 10:491–6.

SMALL CELL SARCOMAS

EWING SARCOMA OF BONE

Definition. A primary osseous neoplasm composed of small, round, relatively uniform cells with no microscopic evidence of matrix production.

General Features. The existence of a distinctive group of highly malignant small cell neoplasms of bone was first recognized by Lucke in 1866 (21). It was not until 1921 that James Ewing described his experience with the tumor that he labeled a diffuse endothelioma of bone (9). By 1929, this neoplasm was being referred to as Ewing sarcoma and is now known exclusively by this name. Ewing sarcoma comprises approximately 6 to 10 percent of biopsied primary malignant bone tumors and is the fourth most common primary malignancy of bone, following myeloma, osteosarcoma, and chondrosarcoma.

In the second series Fascicle on bone tumors, published in 1971, Ewing sarcoma was said to apparently arise "...from immature reticulum cells or the primitive mesenchyme of the medullary cavity" (37). Although two decades have elapsed, our understanding of this enigmatic tumor and its relationship to other small cell neoplasms such as the newly described neuroectodermal tumor of bone, has only recently improved on this earlier conjecture. This enhanced understanding is due in large part to the application of immunohistochemical, genetic, and molecular biologic techniques. Ewing sarcoma is now thought to be the least differentiated of a group of small cell neoplasms with varying degrees of neuroectodermal differentiation.

The concept that Ewing sarcoma might have neuroectodermal features is not new. Indeed, Willis (48) steadfastly maintained that Ewing sarcoma was simply metastatic neuroblastoma. Our current knowledge indicates that although Ewing sarcoma may be part of a spectrum of neuroectodermal differentiation, the lesions in this group are distinct from metastatic neuroblastoma.

Cells of Ewing sarcoma grown in culture normally display no evidence of differentiation. However, when these cells are stimulated by the application of differentiation-inducing chemicals such as cyclic adenosine monophosphate (c-AMP) they develop clear-cut neural features (6). These features are manifested by ultrastructural findings of elongated cell processes, cytoplasmic filaments, microtubules, and dense core granules (6). Immunohistochemically, these stimulated cells also express high levels of neuron specific enolase, neurofilament triplet protein, and cholinesterase (6).

Multiple cytogenetic studies of Ewing sarcoma, beginning with the works of Aurias et al. (2) and Turc-Carel et al. (44), have clearly documented a characteristic t(11;22)(q24;q12) chromosomal translocation in the cells of Ewing sarcoma which is present in about 85 percent of cases (30,43). A smaller number of cases manifest a deletion from chromosome 22, del(22)(q12). Identical genetic abnormalities have been found in neuroectodermal tumor of bone, the so-called "small cell tumor of the thoracopulmonary region," also known as the Askin tumor, and small cell osteosarcoma (30).

Patterns of proto-oncogene expression in Ewing sarcoma include c-*myc*, N-*myc*, c-*myb*, and c-*mil*/*raf*-1, which are similar to those seen in peripheral neuroectodermal tumor (23). In contrast, neuroblastoma has a different pattern of proto-oncogene expression, often including high levels of N-*myc* expression, especially in high-stage tumors such as those metastatic to bone (41).

It thus seems likely that Ewing sarcoma represents the most undifferentiated end of a spectrum of neuroectodermal neoplasms that also includes neuroectodermal tumor of bone and peripheral soft tissue lesions such as so-called Askin tumor and peripheral neuroepithelioma (41). This group of lesions seems to be distinct from metastatic neuroblastoma.

Clinical Features. Of all patients with primary malignant bone tumors, those with Ewing sarcoma have the youngest average age (7). Eighty percent occur in the first two decades of life, with a median age of about 13 years (29). Patients over the age of 30 years are uncommon (36). Although Ewing sarcoma has been described in children as young as 18 months, children under 5 years of age with small cell neoplasms of bone should be carefully evaluated to exclude metastatic neuroblastoma. Ewing sarcoma has a definite predilection for males (1.5 to 1) (7) and is uncommon in blacks.

Localized pain and a mass are the most common symptoms. Most patients give a history of pain for several months prior to the presence of swelling. Generalized symptoms include an increased sedimentation rate, fever, anemia with or without leukocytosis, and malaise. Such findings usually indicate disseminated disease. About 10 percent have multiple bone involvement at the time of presentation, which probably represents metastases from a single primary, although multiple primaries cannot be excluded. About 70 percent of patients have disseminated disease, with involvement of additional osseous sites later in their course.

Sites. Any portion of any bone may be affected. There is a predilection for long tubular bones, and the femur is the single most common site. Ewing sarcoma has been said to be typically diaphyseal, but in several large series metaphyseal lesions predominate. Epiphyseal Ewing sarcoma is quite rare. The pelvis and ribs are the most common flat bone sites. Relatively uncommon sites include the hands, toes, upper vertebral column, skull, sternum, and ulna.

Radiographic Appearance. The radiographic features are nonspecific, although often suggestive when considered in conjunction with the clinical features. Typically, there is an obviously malignant, ill-defined, lytic lesion of the medullary cavity with an "onionskin" (fig. 218) or "sunburst" periosteal reaction and an extraosseous component (46). Identical periosteal reactions may be seen in osteosarcoma, traumatic periostitis, and osteomyelitis, although Mirra (25) suggests that the periosteal bone in Ewing sarcoma is often delicate and thinner than the intervening soft tissue, while the reactive bone in these other conditions tends to be thicker with smaller intervening lucent areas. The onionskin periosteal reaction is frequent in tumors involving the diaphysis (37). However, even large expansile neoplasms may lack periosteal reaction altogether (fig. 219). Predominantly sclerotic lesions may be seen occasionally in the metaphyseal region, but are quite rare in diaphyseal Ewing sarcoma.

Ewing sarcoma is often extensive, but pathologic fractures are uncommon (occurring in approximately 5 percent). The entire shaft is often involved, although radiographic changes may suggest a considerably smaller lesion (fig. 220).

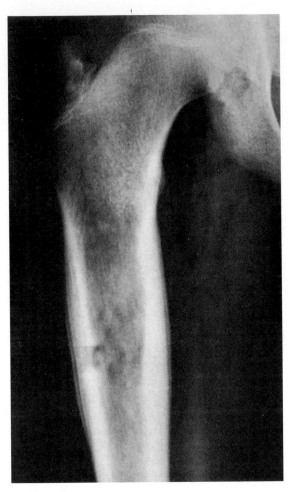

Figure 218
EWING SARCOMA
Radiograph of the upper end of the femur demonstrates the characteristic onionskin periosteal reaction. The medullary cavity shows mottling with mixed lytic and sclerotic areas. The latter indicates reactive bone. (Fig. 233 from Fascicle 5, 2nd Series.)

The soft tissue mass has ill-defined borders and no calcification.

Rarely, Ewing produces a benign-appearing radiograph of an expansile, noninfiltrative lytic lesion that may mimic a bone cyst or eosinophilic granuloma. A few Ewing sarcomas are almost completely periosteal or subperiosteal in location with no involvement of the medullary cavity (4). Such tumors may produce a "saucerization" of the external cortex as is seen in periosteal osteosarcoma (fig. 221).

Gross Findings. The intraosseous component is firm, grey-white, moist and glistening.

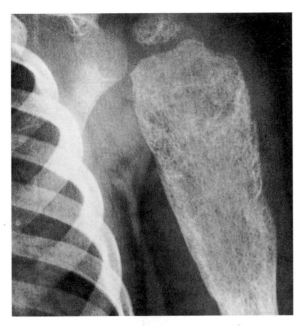

Figure 219
EWING SARCOMA
Radiograph from a 2-year-old boy. There is diffuse loss of the normal contour of bone and destruction of the cortex. At operation, a large hemorrhagic, cystic cavity was encountered. Curettings from the wall revealed Ewing sarcoma. (Fig. 235 from Fascicle 5, 2nd Series.)

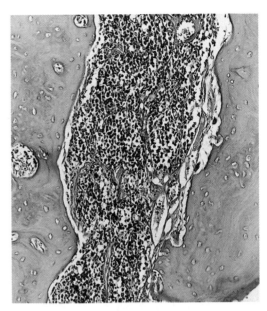

Figure 220
EWING SARCOMA
Tumor extends between normal trabeculae of bone. This section was taken from a radiographically normal-appearing area adjacent to the tumor.

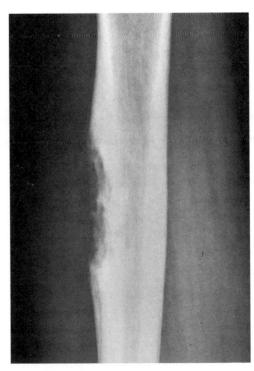

Figure 221
EWING SARCOMA
A 15-year-old boy fractured his distal femur (not shown) playing football. An incidental finding included a subperiosteal defect (saucerization) that proved to be Ewing sarcoma on biopsy.

The almost invariably present extraosseous component may be softer and more friable. Hemorrhagic and cystic degeneration may be present in either location. In amputation specimens, the extraosseous component may be considerably larger than the intraosseous tumor. Diffuse involvement of the medullary cavity is often obvious.

Microscopic Findings. Classic Ewing sarcoma consists of broad sheets and large nests of uniform, small, polygonal cells with scanty pale cytoplasm and indistinct cell borders (figs. 222, 223). The nuclei are round to oval with finely dispersed chromatin (fig. 223), some hyperchromasia, and a variable number of mitotic figures. In areas of necrosis, recognizable neoplasm often forms distinctive perivascular cuffs. About 10 percent of cases contain rosette-like structures that, in reality, represent necrotic cell "drop out" of a central cell mass. Reticulin is typically scant, except around blood vessels (fig. 224).

Schajowicz (35) emphasized the presence of cytoplasmic glycogen as a helpful diagnostic feature for Ewing sarcoma (fig. 225). About 75 percent

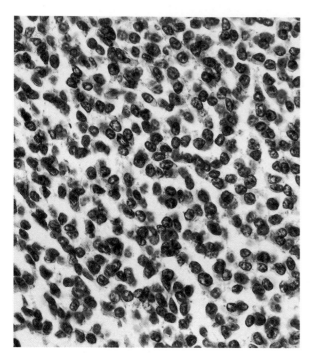

Figure 222
EWING SARCOMA
The typical small cell Ewing sarcoma consists of cells having nuclei that are fairly uniform in size and shape; some are hyperchromatic. The cytoplasm is scanty and indistinct.

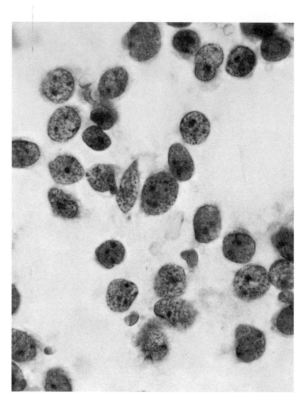

Figure 223
EWING SARCOMA
This touch imprint from a biopsy of Ewing sarcoma demonstrates that the cytoplasm is scanty to practically nonexistent. Nucleoli are small and not readily distinguishable from chromocenters. (Fig. 241 from Fascicle 5, 2nd Series.)

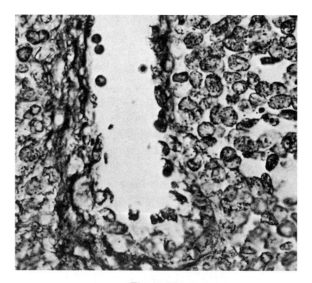

Figure 224
EWING SARCOMA
Wilder reticulin stain shows reticulin in the vessel wall but not around tumor cells. (Fig. 242 from Fascicle 5, 2nd Series.)

of Ewing sarcomas have prominent cytoplasmic glycogen with the PAS technique; about 10 percent are negative. Fixation in 80 percent ethanol, rather than formalin, may allow more consistent staining.

In 1980, Nascimento et al. (27) described 20 cases of Ewing sarcoma composed of larger cells with more marked variation in nuclear size and shape, a clear or vesicular nucleus, and prominent nucleoli (fig. 226). This "large cell variant" can be easily confused, microscopically, with large cell lymphoma, but the glycogen positivity, reticulin pattern, immunohistochemical features, and ultrastructural findings are similar to those of typical Ewing sarcoma. There are no radiographic or clinical features to distinguish this large cell variant from typical Ewing sarcoma, and there is no definite difference in biologic behavior.

Hartman et al. (13) divided Ewing sarcoma into microscopically typical and atypical forms. Histologic features of the typical form include: 1) round cells with varying proportions of large, clear cells and smaller hyperchromatic cells; 2) a filigree pattern; 3) larger tumor cells ("large cell

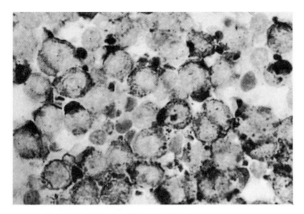

Figure 225
EWING SARCOMA
PAS stain shows diastase-digestible aggregates of glycogen that appear dark gray to black in the photograph. (Fig. 243 from Fascicle 5, 2nd Series.)

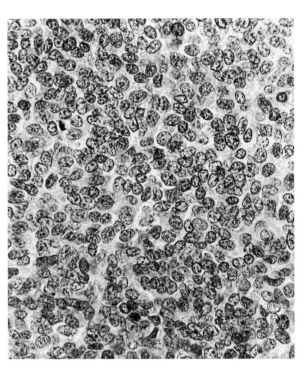

Figure 226
EWING SARCOMA
Large cell variant of Ewing sarcoma has vesicular nuclei and conspicuous nucleoli.

variant"); 4) hemorrhage with vascular lakes or sinuses; 5) geographic necrosis with perivascular sparing; and 6) metaplastic bone or cartilage formation. Tumors are excluded from the typical category if they have: 1) a lack of glycogen, based on negative PAS stains, unless glycogen was confirmed by electron microscopy; 2) intercellular stroma; 3) spindle cell cytology; 4) single cell differentiation (myoblasts, ganglion cells, etc); 5) a lobular architecture with cohesive cells, clear evidence of vascular differentiation, or rosettes.

Atypical tumors resemble Ewing sarcoma, but have any of the following atypical characteristics: 1) lack of glycogen by PAS stain (unless glycogen is seen by electron microscopy); 2) a lobular architecture, increased extracellular matrix, or an alveolar pattern with no evidence of myoblastic differentiation; 3) evidence of neoplastic vascular formation; 4) increased mitoses (more than two per high-power field) and cellular pleomorphism; or 5) some spindle cells, predominantly at the tumor margin, but not a diffuse spindle cell pattern. The prognostic significance of atypical Ewing sarcoma is discussed below.

Telles et al. (40) emphasized that the uniform histologic appearance of classic Ewing sarcoma may be altered by therapy. In their autopsy study of patients treated with radiation and chemotherapy, many tumors had a more pleomorphic appear-

ance than was seen initially. These tumors had large, vesicular nuclei with prominent nuclear folding and more prominent nucleoli. Some resembled the large cell variant of Ewing sarcoma, but others were more bizarre with large cellular forms and multinucleated cells. Despite their marked cytologic transformation, neoplasms that were initially PAS positive, retained PAS positivity in these more pleomorphic cells.

Ultrastructural Features. The cells of Ewing sarcoma seldom exhibit ultrastructural evidence of even abortive differentiation (fig. 227). Nonetheless, this is a valuable technique for the exclusion of light microscopically similar lesions. The most characteristic ultrastructural feature is the presence of varying amounts of particulate glycogen (fig. 227) (22). Many tumors have large cytoplasmic glycogen lakes. Cell organelles are generally sparse and consist of scattered mitochondria, short fragments of rough endoplasmic reticulum, free ribosomes, occasional lipid vacuoles, and poorly developed Golgi complexes. Intermediate filaments

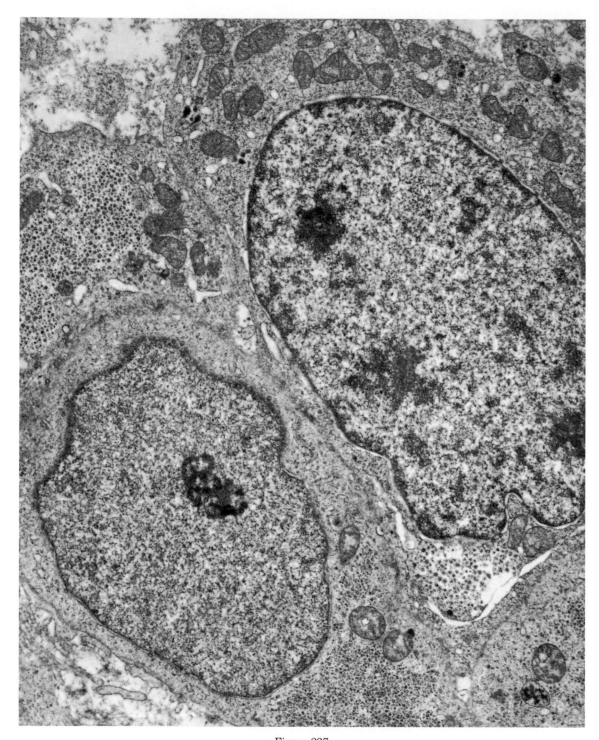

Figure 227
EWING SARCOMA
Electron micrograph of Ewing sarcoma illustrates slight nuclear irregularity, small nucleoli, and few organelles.
Glycogen granules are prominent (X11,900). (Fig. 244 from Fascicle 5, 2nd Series.)

may occasionally be seen, and, rarely, these may be recognized as tonofilaments (11). By definition, cell processes and dense core granules are absent (11). Occasional primitive intercellular junctions are present (28). The nuclei of Ewing sarcoma typically have smooth nuclear contours, abundant finely granular chromatin (euchromatin), and nucleoli with well-developed nucleolonema (28).

Immunohistochemical Features. Ewing sarcoma is, at least currently, noted more for its lack of immunologic staining, than for any characteristic positivity, although this perception is undergoing change. The immunohistochemical profile has been the subject of many studies, and was recently reviewed by Steiner (38). Vimentin expression is present to varying degrees in the majority, if not all, cases (26). Occasional cases may express cytokeratin, usually in a minority of cells (11,26,38). Neurofilaments are not typically present (38). Neuron specific enolase and Leu-7, sensitive but not highly specific markers of neuroectodermal differentiation, are usually absent from typical Ewing sarcoma, at least by the conventional peroxidase-antiperoxidase technique (26,38,41). Their presence in large quantities in a small blue cell tumor should suggest that the lesion is more likely a neuroectodermal tumor (38,41). This approach is by no means universally accepted, however (8,45). Furthermore, with the improved sensitivity of the avidin-biotin complex technique for immunoperoxidase staining, neuron specific enolase, Leu-7, as well as the more neural-specific marker, synaptophysin, are being reported as present in greater numbers of otherwise apparently typical Ewing sarcoma cells (41,42). Additional studies have documented high levels of the neural marker, choline acetyltransferase, in both Ewing sarcoma and neuroectodermal tumor (23). These tumors lack the high levels of adrenergic hormones epinephrine and norepinephrine seen in neuroblastoma (41).

Typical Ewing sarcoma cells are negative for leukocyte common antigen, surface immunoglobulins, lysozyme, alpha-1-antitrypsin, alpha-1-antichymotrypsin, myosin, myoglobin, desmin, and factor VIII–related antigen (38).

Both Ewing sarcoma and neuroectodermal tumor share an overexpression of the pseudoautosomal gene MIC2, located on the short arms of the sex chromosomes, with the resultant production of large amounts of a specific surface glycoprotein, which can be detected by monoclonal antibody HBA-71 (1,18). In a large study of a variety of neoplasms, this antigen was not detected in tumors originating outside of the central nervous system, except for trace staining in a single pancreatic insulinoma (1). Importantly, 12 neuroblastomas lacked staining for this antigen.

Hara et al. (12) reported the development of a monoclonal antibody, 5C11, which is directed against an 81,000 dalton molecular weight cell surface protein in Ewing sarcoma and appears to distinguish the tumor from all other small cell tumors, including neuroectodermal tumor, in preliminary studies. Unfortunately, the antigen reactivity is lost during formalin fixation and paraffin embedding, and frozen sections must be used.

Differential Diagnosis. *Small Cell Osteosarcoma and Mesenchymal Chondrosarcoma.* Distinction of Ewing sarcoma from small cell osteosarcoma and mesenchymal chondrosarcoma is based primarily on the demonstration of the corresponding matrix in close association with and apparently produced by otherwise nondescript small, blue cells. Clinical and radiographic features are often helpful in making this distinction; radiographic evidence of clear-cut matrix production by tumor is not a feature of Ewing sarcoma. Both tumors typically occur in somewhat older patients. To date, immunohistochemical markers have not been of demonstrated value in distinguishing these tumors from Ewing sarcoma.

Lymphoma. The distinction of Ewing sarcoma from intraosseous lymphoma, once a potentially vexing problem, is now straightforward with the advent of sensitive and specific lymphoid markers such as leukocyte common antigen, which may be applied to formalin-fixed, paraffin-embedded tissue. The distinction can often be made or at least strongly suggested by clinical and light microscopic features. Primary intraosseous lymphoma is more often encountered in older patients. Microscopically, there is often a biphasic mixture of small and large lymphocytes with prominent nuclear convolutions and clefts, unlike the smooth nuclear contours of Ewing sarcoma cells.

Metastatic Neuroblastoma. Neuroblastoma may present as an osseous metastasis, often to the skull, from a clinically occult primary site. Patients are typically 5 years of age or younger and have elevated urinary levels of catecholamine metabolites. Light microscopic clues include Homer

Wright rosettes, a fibrillary intercellular background, and tapering cytoplasmic processes, but these microscopic features also may be present, usually to a lesser degree, in neuroectodermal tumor of bone. Immunohistochemically, the cells of neuroblastoma exhibit strong staining for neuron specific enolase, neurofilaments, synaptophysin, vimentin, and with Leu-7. Occasionally, otherwise typical Ewing sarcomas may show neuron specific enolase and Leu-7 staining, but they are typically negative for neurofilaments (38,41) and synaptophysin. Ewing sarcomas have also been reported to express both neurofilaments and synaptophysin (39,42,45), and all of the neural markers listed above may also be expressed by neuroectodermal tumor of bone. Ultrastructurally, neuroblastomas show well-formed, neuritic cell processes containing neurofilaments, neural tubules, and dense core granules, features lacking in Ewing sarcoma (20,41), but seen to varying degrees in neuroectodermal tumor of bone.

Neuroectodermal Tumor of Bone. Given their close association, the validity of distinguishing Ewing sarcoma from neuroectodermal tumor of bone is questioned. For the moment, at least, their distinction seems justified, based on several studies suggesting a higher frequency of metastases at diagnosis, an adverse response to treatment, and a resultant poorer prognosis for tumors with clear-cut neural differentiation as compared to Ewing sarcoma (13,41). Distinguishing features are discussed in the section on neuroectodermal tumor of bone.

Treatment and Prognosis. With the advent of multiagent chemotherapy, new forms of imaging, innovations in radiation therapy, and the development of limb-sparing surgical resections, the treatment of Ewing sarcoma has undergone considerable evolution. Although, in the recent past, radiation therapy was the mainstay of local disease control, surgical resection has re-emerged as an important treatment factor (15). This is due, in part, to the increasing recognition of late recurrences and secondary malignancies following local radiation (31). Currently, surgical resection is recommended wherever feasible, often following preoperative chemotherapy. Lesions of ribs, fibula, and other expendable bones are usually easy to resect. Proximal extremity and, particularly, pelvic lesions are considerably

more difficult. Younger children experience significant decrease in limb growth following radiation-induced closure of an active growth plate. If such asymmetry will result in important functional abnormalities, as in the lower extremity, amputation should be strongly considered.

Prognosis is usually determined by the outcome of metastatic disease, rather than local control of tumor. Prior to the use of chemotherapy, 5-year survival for Ewing sarcoma was in the range of 16 percent, and about one fourth of these patients subsequently died of disease (33). Chemotherapy is significantly altering these figures, and reported 5-year survivals for patients with localized disease at presentation now range from 54 percent to an estimated 74 percent, using surgery and/or radiation plus multidrug chemotherapy (31,32,34). The European Cooperative Trial for the treatment of Ewing sarcoma utilized a four-drug combination chemotherapy prior to local control of disease with either radiation or surgery (16). The overall disease-free survival for 93 patients was 60 percent at 36 months and 55 percent at 69 months.

For patients with metastatic disease at the time of diagnosis, the 5-year survival rate is determined by the nature of the metastases and is currently approximately 30 percent (5). Lanza and colleagues (19) demonstrated that patients undergoing successful resection of metastases confined to the lungs had a significantly improved survival, as compared to those who were not surgically rendered disease free. They also noted that 3 of 19 patients (16 percent) thought to have pulmonary metastases radiographically, in fact had benign disease (organizing pneumonia, hamartoma), emphasizing the importance of microscopic confirmation before initiating additional therapy.

A variety of clinical and pathologic factors have been shown to have prognostic value in Ewing sarcoma. Patients younger than 10 years of age at the time of diagnosis appear to have higher response and survival rates than older patients (5). In patients with localized disease at presentation, the site of tumor is an important prognostic factor. Several studies have demonstrated that patients with pelvic Ewing have a poorer prognosis than those with distal extremity disease (3,17,31). Bacci et al. (3) studied 144 cases for a minimum of 5 years and noted a continuous, disease-free survival for pelvic Ewing sarcoma of only 23 percent, as compared to 46 percent for other tumor sites. Tumor volume has also been shown to predict survival. In one study, patients with lesions having a volume of less than 100 ml had an estimated disease-free, 3-year survival of 80 percent, as compared to 31 percent for those with larger tumors (16). Tumors greater than 8 cm in maximum dimension were shown to have a poorer 3-year disease-free survival than smaller tumors (14). As a corollary to tumor size, gross soft tissue extension has also been associated with a worsened prognosis. In one study of 28 patients, the 5-year survival rate for patients presenting with localized disease was 87 percent for lesions grossly confined to bone and 20 percent for those with extraosseous extension (24).

Other features associated with poorer prognosis for localized Ewing sarcoma include elevated white cell count in the peripheral blood (14) and increased sedimentation rate (47). Serum lactic dehydrogenase (LDH) levels have been variably championed as a prognostic indicator for Ewing sarcoma and as a marker for recurrent disease. Although several studies have refuted this, serum LDH does appear to be a moderately sensitive marker for recurrent Ewing sarcoma, especially multifocal recurrence, where it is 80 percent sensitive (10).

Microscopically, a filigree growth pattern, defined as bicellular strands of tumor separated by stroma, has been associated with a lower survival rate than diffuse or lobular patterns (17). Using the microscopic criteria of Hartman et al. (13), as described above under Microscopic Findings, patients with typical Ewing sarcoma are less likely to have high-stage disease at the time of diagnosis than those with atypical Ewing sarcoma. Lesions with a filigree growth pattern are considered to be within the spectrum of "typical Ewing sarcoma." In one study, the prognosis was increasingly poor with increasing degrees of necrosis (8).

For patients undergoing surgical resection, response to preoperative chemotherapy, assessed microscopically, has been shown to be a powerful prognostic predictor. Patients having less than 10 percent viable tumor had a 79 percent 3-year survival, as compared to a 31 percent 3-year survival for patients with more than 10 percent viable tumor (16).

NEUROECTODERMAL TUMOR OF BONE

Definition. A primary malignancy of bone which closely resembles Ewing sarcoma clinically, radiologically, light microscopically, and at the molecular biologic level. The distinction from Ewing sarcoma is based on the demonstration of clear-cut neuroectodermal differentiation by light microscopic, ultrastructural, or immunohistochemical means.

General Features. Although a primitive, peripheral neuroectodermal tumor of soft tissues has been recognized under a variety of names for many years, neuroectodermal tumor of bone was first distinguished from Ewing sarcoma by Jaffe et al. in 1984 (52). Prior to that time, these tumors had undoubtedly been included with cases of Ewing sarcoma. Jaffe and colleagues stated that: "Any clear evidence of differentiation would be incompatible with a diagnosis of Ewing sarcoma, even though the category of Ewing sarcoma may undergo progressive attrition as newer techniques are applied." Indeed, as immunohistochemical techniques have progressed, an increasing number of otherwise typical "Ewing sarcomas" have shown at least some immunohistochemical evidence of neuroectodermal differentiation. How to classify such relatively common cases is currently unclear.

Although current studies advocate distinguishing these closely related lesions, exact diagnostic criteria for neuroectodermal tumor of bone and what, if any, neuroectodermal features are "allowed" in Ewing sarcoma have not been generally agreed upon.

The frequency of currently detectable neuroectodermal differentiation can be estimated from a study of 11 small cell tumors with cytogenetic changes seen in both Ewing sarcoma and neuroectodermal tumor of bone (55). Five of the 11 cases showed morphologic or immunohistochemical evidence of neural differentiation.

Jürgens et al. (53) suggested that criteria for the diagnosis of neuroectodermal tumor should include immunohistochemical positivity for neuron specific enolase, in conjunction with clear-cut Homer Wright–type rosettes and/or ultrastructural demonstration of dense core granules. Using this approach, neuron specific enolase positivity alone would not be sufficient for exclusion from the category of Ewing sarcoma. Given the often seemingly nonspecific staining encountered with antibodies to neuron specific enolase, we concur with this approach. However, definite positivity for newer, more specific neural antigens such as synaptophysin or neurofilaments is, in the authors' opinion, sufficient to place a light microscopically undifferentiated but otherwise compatible small cell tumor in the neuroectodermal category.

As discussed in the section on Ewing sarcoma, neuroectodermal tumors and Ewing sarcomas share a number of cytogenetic and molecular biologic features, which indicate that the tumors are very closely related. Both tumors have a characteristic t(11;22)(q24;q12) chromosomal translocation. Oncogene studies have documented similar patterns of oncogene expression, including overexpression of the pseudoautosomal gene MIC2. As described below, there are also many clinical similarities. Justification for separating Ewing sarcoma and neuroectodermal tumor of bone is based on the poorer prognosis for the latter neoplasm.

Clinical Features. The clinical features of patients with neuroectodermal tumor of bone are similar in most respects to those of patients with Ewing sarcoma. Median age is approximately 15 years, with patients ranging from less than 1 year to 32 years of age (53,58,60). Most patients are in their first or second decades of life. There is a male predominance of 2–3 to 1. About half present with fever or other systemic symptoms, and about one third have pathologic fractures (60). Unlike Ewing sarcoma, between one half (60) and one fourth (53) of patients with neuroectodermal tumor of bone have clinically detectable metastases at the time of initial diagnosis. Metastases primarily involve bone, lung, and liver, with lymph nodes less commonly involved.

Sites. Many, if not most, so-called "Askin tumors" of the chest wall represent peripheral neuroectodermal tumors with osseous involvement. If these cases are considered primary osseous neoplasms, then neuroectodermal tumor of bone most commonly involves the ribs, sternum, and vertebrae of the chest. Aggregate cases from several series, excluding rib and chest lesions, had the following distribution: fibula, 26 percent; tibia, 19 percent; pelvis, 19 percent; scapula, 10 percent; with femur, metatarsal, humerus, and radius, 6.5 percent each (57,58,60,66). The predilection for the fibula and less common involvement of the femur and humerus is unusual for osseous neoplasia.

Radiographic Appearance. Neuroectodermal tumor of bone, like Ewing sarcoma, produces a highly variable, nondiagnostic radiographic image. Typically, the radiographic appearance is that of an aggressive, poorly demarcated tumor with cortical destruction, periosteal reaction, and soft tissue invasion (60). The lesion may be centered in either the diaphyseal or metaphyseal regions, and there is often epiphyseal extension. Of 13 cases described by Rousselin et al. (60), 8 were central, 4 were eccentric, and 1 was centered in the cortex. None showed saucerization of the outer cortex, but 11 demonstrated obvious cortical destruction, 12 showed periosteal reactions, and 5 formed Codman triangles. Soft tissue involvement was present in all 13 cases.

Gross Findings. Neuroectodermal tumor of bone is grossly indistinguishable from Ewing sarcoma. The tumor is typically soft, fleshy, and hemorrhagic, often with areas of cystic degeneration (66). A soft tissue component is virtually always present. Despite the neuroectodermal features, direct connection to a nerve root is not seen (66).

Microscopic Findings. The microscopic appearance depends, in part, on how the lesion is defined. It is clear that some tumors lacking differentiation on light microscopy and indistinguishable from Ewing sarcoma, may exhibit ultrastructural and immunohistochemical evidence of neuroectodermal differentiation. Typically, such "undifferentiated" areas are composed of small "blue cells" with scant cytoplasm, round to oval nuclei with evenly dispersed chromatin, and one or more distinct nucleoli (66). Glycogen, as demonstrated by PAS stains, may be present in the neoplastic cells, but tends to be less than is typical of Ewing sarcoma (52,66,67).

Most neuroectodermal tumors of bone, as currently described, exhibit at least some light microscopic evidence of differentiation, however. Several studies have reported focal Homer Wright rosettes in all cases (fig. 228) (52,53,58, 62,66), often in association with a fibrillary intercellular background (fig. 229) (58). A lobular growth pattern is also common (52,58), and is best seen with reticulin stains that show reticular

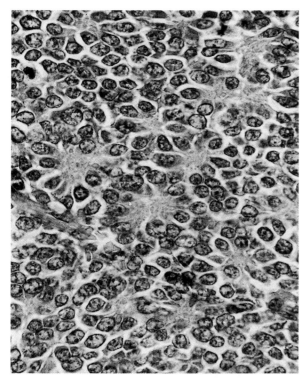

Figure 228
NEUROECTODERMAL TUMOR OF BONE
This osseous neoplasm has well-formed Homer Wright rosettes and larger, more vesicular nuclei than are seen in figure 229.

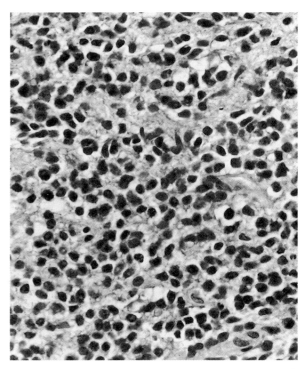

Figure 229
NEUROECTODERMAL TUMOR OF BONE
A 15-year-old with a lytic lesion in the femur has a tumor composed of cells with small, dense nuclei and a fibrillary background.

fibers surrounding large groups of cells in a "basket-like" distribution. There is a tendency for cells at the periphery of lobules to be somewhat larger and exhibit evidence of ganglion cell differentiation (52,66). Ganglion cell differentiation may also be present in metastases.

Ultrastructural Findings. Many areas in neuroectodermal tumor of bone appear undifferentiated, even at the ultrastructural level. Clumps of glycogen may be prominent, as in Ewing sarcoma (54,58,63). Occasional, often poorly formed cell junctions of intermediate type may be present (58,66). Cell processes range from rare and poorly formed to numerous dendrite-like structures with microtubules, neurofilaments, and groups of dense core granules (61). Ultrastructurally, the Homer Wright rosettes, when encountered, consist of a central core of tangled cytoplasmic processes (58). True rosettes were described in one tumor (59). Scattered dense core granules may also be present in the central cyto-

plasm and typically measure 50 to 200 nm in diameter. Llombart-Bosch et al. (58) also described basal lamina surrounding the cells of neuroectodermal tumor of bone with long spacing collagen (Luse bodies) within the interstitium. Neural differentiation was noted in a cultured cell line from a neuroectodermal tumor (51).

Immunohistochemical Findings. Results of immunohistochemical staining have been somewhat variable owing to differences in technique and progressive improvement in available antibodies and methodology. Results also vary depending on whether immunohistochemical findings are used to define neuroectodermal tumors, or the tumors are defined by light microscopic, ultrastructural, or molecular biologic techniques, and then studied for their immunohistochemical profile.

The results of several studies are shown in Table 9 (52,53,58,64,66). All cases studied with antibodies to vimentin have been uniformly positive. Stains for glial fibrillary acidic protein

(GFAP), cytokeratin, desmin, and leukocyte common antigen have been uniformly negative. As discussed in the section on Ewing sarcoma, both the latter tumor and neuroectodermal tumor of bone have been shown by immunohistochemistry to express a specific surface glycoprotein, the product of the pseudoautosomal gene MIC2, which is detected by monoclonal antibody HBA-71 (49).

Differential Diagnosis. The distinction between neuroectodermal tumor of bone and small cell osteosarcoma, mesenchymal chondrosarcoma, and lymphoma is typically straightforward. The distinguishing features described in the chapter on Ewing sarcoma apply equally well to neuroectodermal tumor.

Metastatic Neuroblastoma. Neuroectodermal tumor of bone must be distinguished from metastatic neuroblastoma. The latter tumors tend to occur in children 5 years of age or younger, show a strong tendency to metastasize to the skull, and are associated with high levels of urinary catecholamine metabolites. Urinary catecholamine metabolites are normal or, rarely, mildly elevated, in patients with neuroectodermal tumor of bone. The two tumors show considerable light microscopic, ultrastructural, and immunohistochemical overlap. In general, however, the degree of neural differentiation in metastatic neuroblastoma greatly exceeds that in neuroectodermal tumor of bone. Metastatic neuroblastoma has been shown to have high levels of N-*myc* gene expression and this is not seen in neuroectodermal tumor of bone (50,65).

Ewing Sarcoma. The relationship between Ewing sarcoma and neuroectodermal tumor of bone has been the subject of numerous publications. Although in many instances, Ewing sarcoma and neuroectodermal tumor of bone can be distinguished on immunohistochemical and ultrastructural grounds, in some cases the distinction is arbitrary, and where the "line is drawn" varies from study to study (65,66). This difficulty was clearly noted by Jaffe et al. (52) in their initial description of neuroectodermal tumor of bone and its distinction from Ewing sarcoma. According to these authors: "It remains to be shown that the two tumors are clearly and reproducibly separable; it certainly cannot be done on previously published criteria. Ewing sarcoma may be the most undifferentiated form of the neuroectodermal tumor."

Table 9

IMMUNOHISTOCHEMICAL STUDY RESULTS FOR NEUROECTODERMAL TUMORS*

Marker	No. Studied	No. Positive
Neuron specific enolase	71	61
Leu-7	28	14
Synaptophysin	14	11
Neurofilaments	18	3
Chromogranin	4	3
S-100	18	1

*From data compiled from references 52,53,58,64,66.

Clearly, studies of Ewing sarcoma prior to the recognition of neuroectodermal tumor have included these tumors. In one review of 261 "Ewing sarcoma cases" 54 were shown to have structures suggestive of pseudorosettes (56). Another study noted that 16 of 42 neuroectodermal tumors had been originally diagnosed as Ewing sarcoma (53).

Typical Ewing sarcoma lacks any light microscopic, ultrastructural, and, in most cases, immunohistochemical evidence of differentiation. In contrast, the neuroectodermal tumor of bone may be light microscopically identical to Ewing sarcoma, at least by some definitions, but, ultrastructurally, typically contains at least scattered dense core granules in the perinuclear cytoplasm, often with abortive cell processes (65). Immunohistochemically, it expresses some neuroectodermal differentiation in the form of positive staining for neuron specific enolase, synaptophysin, or Leu-7. As described above, so-called atypical Ewing sarcoma is a provisional diagnosis for a tumor that seems to occupy an intermediate position in this spectrum.

Whether Ewing sarcoma and neuroectodermal tumor of bone will ultimately be "lumped" under a single category remains to be seen. For the present, although treatment regimens are highly similar for both groups, it has been suggested that the lesions be separated, when possible, to allow for better study of their natural history and response to therapy (65).

Treatment and Prognosis. Patients with neuroectodermal tumor of bone are treated similarly to individuals with Ewing sarcoma. Local control of disease is attempted through surgery and/or radiation therapy, with multidrug chemotherapy for control of distant metastases. The role of surgery in local control, a subject of current controversy for Ewing sarcoma, has not been as well defined for neuroectodermal tumor, but local recurrence is also a problem with these neoplasms, suggesting an augmented role for aggressive surgical resections.

Several studies have noted an apparently poorer prognosis for neuroectodermal tumor of bone, as compared to Ewing sarcoma, suggesting that their distinction is clinically warranted, at least at this time. In the study by Llombart-Bosch et al. (58), 6 of 14 patients had metastases at the time of diagnosis, 5 of which were to bone. Median survival was 25 months following radiation and chemotherapy. The only survivor had a metatarsal lesion treated with surgery and chemotherapy. Seven of the 14 patients developed local recurrence, and 9 had distant metastases.

In a series by Rousselin et al. (60) only 1 of 13 patients (7.6 percent) was alive at 5 years, a poorer prognosis than the 30 percent survival for their Ewing sarcoma patients. Metastases were present at the time of diagnosis in 53 percent, as compared to 18 percent of Ewing sarcomas. The incidence of local recurrence was the same for both tumors.

Tsuneyoshi et al. (66) reported four patients with neuroectodermal tumor of bone and seven patients with Ewing sarcoma who had been treated similarly. Three of the four patients with neuroectodermal tumor died within 16 months of initial treatment, whereas four of the seven Ewing sarcoma patients were alive, with long follow-up (17 years) for two of them. The authors concluded: "Long-term survival is more likely for patients with Ewing's sarcoma of bone."

REFERENCES

Ewing Sarcoma of Bone

1. Ambros IM, Ambros PF, Strehl S, Kovar H, Gadner H, Salzer-Kuntschik M. MIC2 is a specific marker for Ewing's sarcoma and peripheral primitive neuroectodermal tumors. Evidence for a common histogenesis of Ewing's sarcoma and peripheral primitive neuroectodermal tumors from MIC2 expression and specific chromosome aberration. Cancer 1991;67:1886–93.
2. Aurias A, Rimbaut C, Buffe D, Dubousset J, Mazabraud A. Chromosomal translocations in Ewing's sarcoma [Letter]. N Engl J Med 1983;309:496–7.
3. Bacci G, Toni A, Avella M, et al. Long-term results in 144 localized Ewing's sarcoma patients treated with combined therapy. Cancer 1989;63:1477–86.
4. Bator SM, Bauer TW, Marks KE, Norris DG. Periosteal Ewing's sarcoma. Cancer 1986;58:1781–4.
5. Cangir A, Vietti TJ, Gehan EA, et al. Ewing's sarcoma metastatic at diagnosis. Results and comparisons of two intergroup Ewing's sarcoma studies. Cancer 1990; 66:887–93.
6. Cavazzana AO, Miser JS, Jefferson J, Triche TJ. Experimental evidence for a neural origin of Ewing's sarcoma of bone. Am J Pathol 1987;127:507–18.
7. Dahlin DC, Unni KK. Bone tumors: general aspects and data on 8,542 cases. 4th ed. Springfield, Ill: Charles C. Thomas, 1986:322–36.
8. Daugaard S, Kamby C, Sunde LM, Myhre-Jensen O, Schiødt T. Ewing's sarcoma. A retrospective study of histological and immunohistochemical factors and their relation to prognosis. Virchows Arch [A] 1989; 414:243–51.
9. Ewing J. Diffuse endothelioma of bone. Proc NY Pathol Soc 1921;21:17–24.
10. Farley FA, Healey JH, Caparros-Sison B, Godbold J, Lane JM, Glasser DB. Lactase dehydrogenase as a tumor marker for recurrent disease in Ewing's sarcoma. Cancer 1987;59:1245–8.
11. Greco MA, Steiner GC, Fazzini E. Ewing's sarcoma with epithelial differentiation: fine structural and immunocytochemical study. Ultrastruct Pathol 1988; 12:317–25.
12. Hara S, Ishii E, Tanaka S, et al. A monoclonal antibody specifically reactive with Ewing's sarcoma. Br J Cancer 1989;60:875–9.
13. Hartman KR, Triche TJ, Kinsella TJ, Miser JS. Prognostic value of histopathology in Ewing's sarcoma. Long-term follow-up of distal extremity primary tumors. Cancer 1991;67:163–71.
14. Hayes FA, Thompson EI, Meyer WH, et al. Therapy for localized Ewing's sarcoma of bone. J Clin Oncol 1989; 7:208–13.
15. Horowitz ME, Neff JR, Kun LE. Ewing's sarcoma. Radiotherapy versus surgery for local control. Pediatr Clin North Am 1991;38:365–80.

16. Jürgens H, Exner U, Gadner H, et al. Multidisciplinary treatment of primary Ewing's sarcoma of bone. A 6-year experience of a European Cooperative Trial. Cancer 1988;61:23–32.

17. Kissane JM, Askin FB, Foulkes M, Stratton LB, Shirley SF. Ewing's sarcoma of bone: clinicopathologic aspects of 303 cases from the Intergroup Ewing's Sarcoma Study. Hum Pathol 1983;14:773–9.

18. Kovar H, Dworzak M, Strehl S, et al. Overexpression of the pseudoautosomal gene MIC2 in Ewing's sarcoma and peripheral primitive neuroectodermal tumor. Oncogene 1990;5:1067–70.

19. Lanza LA, Miser JS, Pass HI, Roth JA. The role of resection in the treatment of pulmonary metastases from Ewing's sarcoma. J Thorac Cardiovasc Surg 1987;94:181–7.

20. Llombart-Bosch A, Blache R, Peydro-Olaya A. Ultrastructural study of 28 cases of Ewing's sarcoma: typical and atypical forms. Cancer 1978;41:1362–73.

21. Lucke A. Beitrage zur geschwulstlehre. Virchows Arch Pathol Anat 1866;35:524–39.

22. Mahoney JP, Alexander RW. Ewing's sarcoma. A light- and electron-microscopic study of 21 cases. Am J Surg Pathol 1978;2:283–98.

23. McKeon C, Thiele CJ, Ross RA, et al. Indistinguishable patterns of protooncogene expression in two distinct but closely related tumors: Ewing's sarcoma and neuroepithelioma. Cancer Res 1988;48:4307–11.

24. Mendenhall CM, Marcus RB Jr, Enneking WF, Springfield DS, Thar TL, Million RR. The prognostic significance of soft tissue extension in Ewing's sarcoma. Cancer 1983;51:913–7.

25. Mirra JM. Bone tumors: clinical, radiologic, and pathologic correlations. Philadelphia: Lea & Febiger, 1989;1087–117.

26. Moll R, Lee I, Gould VE, Berndt R, Roessner A, Franke WW. Immunocytochemical analysis of Ewing's tumors. Patterns of expressions of intermediate filaments and desmosomal proteins indicate cell type heterogeneity and pluripotential differentiation. Am J Pathol 1987;127:288–304.

27. Nascimento AG, Unni KK, Pritchard DJ, Cooper KL, Dahlin DC. A clinicopathologic study of 20 cases of large-cell (atypical) Ewing's sarcoma of bone. Am J Surg Pathol 1980;4:29–36.

28. Navas-Palacios JJ, Aparicio-Duque R, Valdés MD. On the histogenesis of Ewing's sarcoma. An ultrastructural, immunohistochemical, and cytochemical study. Cancer 1984;53:1882–901.

29. Nesbit ME Jr, Gehan EA, Burgert EO Jr, et al. Multimodal therapy for the management of primary, nonmetastatic Ewing's sarcoma of bone. A long-term follow-up of the First Intergroup Study. J Clin Oncol 1990;8:1664–74.

30. Noguera R, Navarro S, Triche TJ. Translocation (11;22) in small cell osteosarcoma. Cancer Genet Cytogenet 1990;45:121–4.

31. O'Connor MI, Pritchard DJ. Ewing's sarcoma. Prognostic factors, disease control, and the reemerging role of surgical treatment. Clin Orthop 1991;262:78–87.

32. Pilepich MV, Vietti TJ, Nesbit ME. Radiotherapy and combination chemotherapy in advanced Ewing's sarcoma—intergroup study. Cancer 1981;47:1930–6.

33. Pritchard DJ, Dahlin DC, Dauphine RT, Taylor WF, Beabout JW. Ewing's sarcoma. A clinicopathological and statistical analysis of patients surviving five years or longer. J Bone Joint Surg [Am] 1975;57:10–6.

34. Rosen G, Caparros B, Mosende C, McCormick B, Huvos AG, Marcove RC. Curability of Ewing's sarcoma and considerations for future therapeutic trials. Cancer 1978;41:888–99.

35. Schajowicz F. Ewing's sarcoma and reticulum-cell sarcoma of bone. With special reference to the histochemical demonstration of glycogen as an aid to the differential diagnosis. J Bone Joint Surg [Am] 1959;41:349–56.

36. Siegel RD, Ryan LM, Antman KH. Adults with Ewing's sarcoma. An analysis of 16 patients at the Dana-Farber Cancer Institute. Am J Clin Oncol 1988;11:614–7.

37. Spjut HJ, Dorfman HD, Fechner RE, Ackerman LV. Tumors of the bone and cartilage. Atlas of Tumor Pathology, 2nd Series, Fascicle 5. Washington, D.C.: Armed Forces Institute of Pathology, 1971, 216–29.

38. Steiner GC. Neuroectodermal tumor versus Ewing's sarcoma—immunohistochemical and electron microscopic observations. Curr Top Pathol 1989;80:1–29.

39. Swanson PE, Wick MR, Hagan KA, Dehner LP. Synaptophysin in small round cell tumors [Abstract]. Am J Clin Pathol 1987;88:523.

40. Telles NC, Rabson AS, Pomeroy TC. Ewing's sarcoma: an autopsy study. Cancer 1978;41:2321–9.

41. Triche T, Cavazzana A. Round cell tumors of bone. In: Unni KK, ed. Bone tumors. New York: Churchill Livingstone, 1988:199–223.

42. Tsuneyoshi M, Yokoyama R, Hashimoto H, Enjoji M. Comparative study of neuroectodermal tumor and Ewing's sarcoma of the bone. Histopathologic, immunohistochemical and ultrastructural features. Acta Pathol Jpn 1989;39:573–81.

43. Turc-Carel C, Aurias A, Mugneret F, et al. Chromosomes in Ewing's sarcoma. I. An evaluation of 85 cases of remarkable consistency of t(11;22)(q24;q12). Cancer Genet Cytogenet 1988;32:229–38.

44. _____, Philip I, Berger MP, Philip T, Lenoir GM. Chromosomal translocations in Ewing's sarcoma [Letter]. N Engl J Med 1983;309:497–8.

45. Ushigome S, Shimoda T, Takaki K, et al. Immunocytochemical and ultrastructural studies of the histogenesis of Ewing's sarcoma and putatively related tumors. Cancer 1989;64:52–62.

46. Vohra VG. Roentgen manifestations in Ewing's sarcoma. A study of 156 cases. Cancer 1967;20:727–33.

47. Wilkins RM, Pritchard DJ, Burgert EO Jr, Unni KK. Ewing's sarcoma of bone. Experience with 140 patients. Cancer 1986;58:2551–5.

48. Willis RA. Metastatic neuroblastoma in bone presenting the Ewing syndrome, with a discussion of "Ewing's sarcoma." Am J Pathol 1940;16:317–32.

Neuroectodermal Tumor of Bone

49. Ambros IM, Ambros PF, Strehl S, Kovar H, Gadner H, Salzer-Kuntschik M. MIC2 is a specific marker for Ewing's sarcoma and peripheral primitive neuroectodermal tumors. Evidence for a common histogenesis of Ewing's sarcoma and peripheral primitive neuroectodermal tumors from MIC2 expression and specific chromosome aberration. Cancer 1991;67:1886–93.

50. Hartman KR, Triche TJ, Kinsella TJ, Miser JS. Prognostic value of histopathology in Ewing's sarcoma. Long-term follow-up of distal extremity primary tumors. Cancer 1991;67:163–71.

51. Isayama T, Iwasaki H, Kikuchi M, Yoh S, Takagishi N. Neuroectodermal tumor of bone. Evidence for neural differentiation in a cultured cell line. Cancer 1990; 65:1771–81.

52. Jaffe R, Santamaria M, Yunis EJ, et al. The neuroectodermal tumor of bone. Am J Surg Pathol 1984;8:885–98.

53. Jürgens H, Bier V, Harms D, et al. Malignant peripheral neuroectodermal tumors. A retrospective analysis of 42 patients. Cancer 1988;61:349–57.

54. Kawaguchi K, Koike M. Neuron-specific enolase and Leu-7 immunoreactive small round-cell neoplasm. The relationship to Ewing's sarcoma in bone and soft tissue. Am J Clin Pathol 1986;86:79–83.

55. Ladanyi M, Heinemann FS, Huvos AG, Rao PH, Chen Q, Jhanwar SC. Neural differentiation in small round cell tumors of bone and soft tissue with the translocation t(1;22)(q24;q12). An immunohistochemical study of 11 cases. Hum Pathol 1990;21:1245–51.

56. Llombart-Bosch A, Contesso G, Henry-Amar M, et al. Histopathological predictive factors in Ewing's sarcoma of bone and clinicopathological correlations. A retrospective study of 261 cases. Virchows Arch [A] 1986;409:627–40.

57. _____, Lacombe MJ, Contesso G, Peydro-Olaya A. Small round blue cell sarcoma of bone mimicking atypical Ewing's sarcoma with neuroectodermal features. An analysis of five cases with immunohistochemical and electron microscopic support. Cancer 1987;60:1570–82.

58. _____, Lacombe MJ, Peydro-Olaya A, Perez-Bacete M, Contesso G. Malignant peripheral neuroectodermal tumours of bone other than Askin's neoplasm: characterization of 14 new cases with immunohistochemistry and electron microscopy. Virchows Arch [A] 1988;412:421–30.

59. Parham DM, Thompson E, Fletcher B, Meyer WH. Metastatic small cell tumor of bone with "true" rosettes and glial fibrillary acidic protein positivity. Am J Clin Pathol 1991;95:166–71.

60. Rousselin B, Vanel D, Terrier-Lacombe MJ, Istria BJ, Spielman M, Masselot J. Clinical and radiologic analysis of 13 cases of primary neuroectodermal tumors of bone. Skeletal Radiol 1989;18:115–20.

61. Schmidt D, Mackay B, Ayala AG. Ewing's sarcoma with neuroblastoma-like features. Ultrastruct Pathol 1982; 3:143–51.

62. Steiner GC. Neuroectodermal tumor versus Ewing's sarcoma—immunohistochemical and electron microscopic observations. Curr Top Pathol 1989;80:1–29.

63. _____, Graham S, Lewis MM. Malignant round cell tumor of bone with neural differentiation (neuroectodermal tumor). Ultrastruct Pathol 1988;12:505–12.

64. Swanson PE, Wick MR, Hagan KA, Dehner LP. Synaptophysin in small round cell tumors [Abstract]. Am J Clin Pathol 1987;88:523.

65. Triche T, Cavazzana A. Round cell tumors of bone. In: Unni KK, ed. Bone tumors. New York: Churchill Livingstone, 1988:199–223.

66. Tsuneyoshi M, Yokoyama R, Hashimoto H, Enjoji M. Comparative study of neuroectodermal tumor and Ewing's sarcoma of the bone. Histopathologic, immunohistochemical and ultrastructural features. Acta Pathol Jpn 1989;39:573–81.

67. Ushigome S, Shimoda T, Takaki K, et al. Immunocytochemical and ultrastructural studies of the histogenesis of Ewing's sarcoma and putatively related tumors. Cancer 1989;64:52–62.

◇◇◇

MISCELLANEOUS MESENCHYMAL LESIONS

INTRAOSSEOUS LIPOMA

Definition. A benign tumor of mature adipocytes arising in the medullary canal.

General and Clinical Features. This is a rare tumor of medullary bone with approximately 100 to 150 reported cases. A few parosteal lipomas have also been described but are not included in this section. Patients with intraosseous lipomas have ranged from 5 to 85 years of age (4). The tumor is rare in the first decade of life and has a fairly even age distribution by decade after that. There is a slight male predominance. Approximately 70 percent of patients complain of minor, aching pain, ranging in duration from a few days to as long as 16 years (1). About 20 percent have swelling, with or without pain, and the remainder have lesions found incidentally on radiograph.

Sites. Most intraosseous lipomas occur in the long bones, with a propensity for the proximal femur, fibula, and tibia. Ribs, calvarium, gnathic bones, and sacrum are other frequent sites. Skeletal lipomas are rarely multiple (5).

Radiographic Appearance. Radiographically, these are lytic, benign-appearing lesions with sharply demarcated borders, often surrounded by a zone of sclerosis, reflecting their slow growth (5). Lipomas involving small diameter bones such as the fibula and rib are often expansile (fig. 230) (3). Goldman et al. (2) noted that lipomas often are ovoid with a wedge shape at the end of the diaphyseal component. There may be round or ovoid opacities in the central portions of the lesion, reflecting areas of necrosis and dystrophic calcification (fig. 231). Rarely, there may be extension through the cortex.

Gross Findings. There is a discrete, lobulated lesion consisting of yellow, grossly normal-appearing fat. Areas of dystrophic calcification, usually located centrally, may be grossly visible. Extensive fat necrosis may result in secondary cyst formation (5).

Microscopic Findings. Most of the lesion is mature adipose tissue. Trabeculae of bone are almost always widely scattered within the fat. Dystrophic calcium may be found in areas of fat

necrosis (fig. 232), and dense aggregates of dystrophic calcification can have a Liesegang ring–like configuration. In some instances, the majority of the tumor is necrotic, with or without calcification. The calcified areas may contain trabeculae of necrotic bone, presumably representing the trabeculae that were widely scattered in the original lipoma.

Treatment and Prognosis. Curettage, usually accompanied by bone grafting, is curative and recurrences have not been reported (3). However, two skeletal lipomas were followed by the development of malignant fibrous histiocytoma at the site of the original lesions (6). This appears

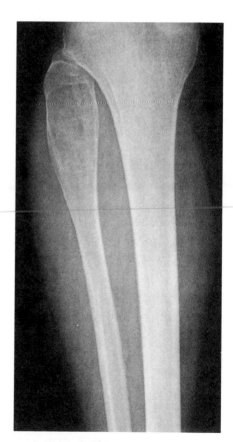

Figure 230
INTRAOSSEOUS LIPOMA
A 57-year-old woman had cramp-like pain for 4 to 5 months. This radiograph reveals an expanding radiolucent lesion of the fibula. (Fig. 2 from Smith WE, Fienberg R. Intraosseous lipoma of bone. Cancer 1957;10:1151–2.)

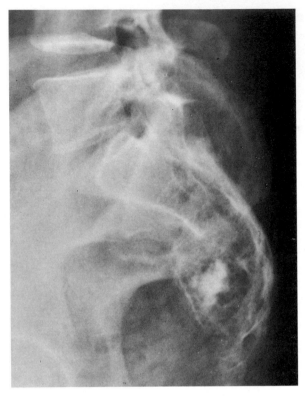

Figure 231
INTRAOSSEOUS LIPOMA
A 52-year-old woman fell on her coccyx and experienced severe pain. This radiograph was taken immediately after the fall and shows no abnormality in the coccyx. However, the sacrum is markedly expanded and has irregular deposits of calcium. Because the radiograph was interpreted as a cartilaginous neoplasm, the sacrum was resected. (Figures 231 and 232 are from the same patient.)

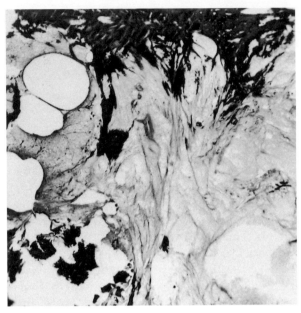

Figure 232
INTRAOSSEOUS LIPOMA
Numerous sections disclose broad areas of dystrophic calcification and fibrosis. A few necrotic adipocytes are discernable.

analogous to the phenomenon of "dedifferentiation" described in soft tissue lipomas, as well as other osseous lesions.

LIPOSARCOMA OF BONE

Definition. A rare sarcoma of bone composed of malignant mesenchymal cells exhibiting lipogenesis, without evidence of other forms of differentiation.

General and Clinical Features. Addison and Payne (7) described a primary intramedullary liposarcoma in 1982, accepting only six examples as unequivocal from previous literature. Patients range from 15 to 53 years of age with most being 25 to 45 years old. Pain is the usual presenting complaint.

Sites. Intraosseous liposarcomas have involved primarily the long bones, including the humerus, femur, and tibia.

Radiographic Appearance. The radiographic findings are nonspecific but indicative of malignancy. There is typically a large, lytic defect with destructive growth and ill-defined margins (fig. 233).

Gross and Microscopic Findings. Tumors may be yellow, gray, or white, and firm or gelatinous. Microscopically, most liposarcomas have been of the high-grade, pleomorphic type (fig. 234) (8,9,11). These tumors often have signet ring cells with a large, single globule of lipid filling the cytoplasm. One myxoid liposarcoma has been described (10).

Differential Diagnosis. The differential diagnosis includes malignant fibrous histiocytoma, malignant mesenchymoma, and metastases. Liposarcoma may contain "dedifferentiated" areas that microscopically resemble malignant fibrous histiocytoma. However, the latter tumors lack the conspicuous lipid-filled cells seen, at least focally, in liposarcomas. Malignant mesenchymoma is excluded because, by definition, it contains more than one form of sarcoma. It seems likely that

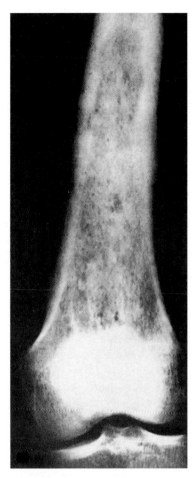

Figure 233
LIPOSARCOMA
The distal femur of a 28-year-old woman shows irregular, lytic destruction of the medullary and cortical bone. There is no soft tissue component. (Fig. 216A from Fascicle 5, 2nd Series.) (Figures 233 and 234 are from the same patient.)

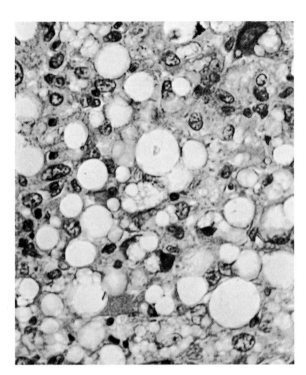

Figure 234
LIPOSARCOMA
This pleomorphic liposarcoma has neoplastic cells with varying degrees of lipogenic differentiation. Signet ring cells are evident. (Fig. 217 from Fascicle 5, 2nd Series.)

many of the reported cases of intraosseous liposarcoma were actually malignant mesenchymomas. Before diagnosing a primary liposarcoma of bone, the possibility of metastatic liposarcoma should be considered and excluded by clinicoradiographic means. The signet ring cells in some liposarcomas may lead to confusion with adenocarcinomas, which are distinguished by their epithelial mucin positivity, as well as positive staining for epithelial markers such as cytokeratin and epithelial membrane antigen.

Treatment and Prognosis. Follow-up and method of treatment for the small number of reported cases have been variable. About half of the

patients developed metastases after amputation (7). There are too few cases to correlate biologic behavior with the subtype of liposarcoma.

LEIOMYOSARCOMA

Definition. A malignant, predominantly spindle cell neoplasm exhibiting smooth muscle differentiation.

Clinical Features. Fewer than 50 skeletal leiomyosarcomas have been reported (excluding the gnathic bones). Patients range from 9 to 80 years of age. The tumor is uncommon before 20 years of age and then has a fairly even distribution in each decade thereafter. Males are affected about twice as often as females. The usual complaint is pain that may be from several weeks' to 3 years' duration.

Sites. The most common site is the distal femur, followed closely by the proximal tibia. These two bones account for slightly more than 50 percent of reported cases. The humerus, pelvis, clavicle, ribs, and mandible are also affected.

Radiographic Appearance. The typical radiographic appearance is that of a nonspecific but malignant-appearing lytic defect located in the metaphyseal portion of the bone, often with extension into the diaphysis or the epiphysis. The tumor has ill-defined margins and ranges from 2 to 12 cm in greatest dimension. The cortex is frequently destroyed and periosteal reaction is seen in about half of cases (12).

Gross Findings. The cut surface is gray, white, or tan with focal areas of necrosis. Most intraosseous leiomyosarcomas exhibit soft tissue extension.

Microscopic Findings. The spectrum of microscopic appearances is almost identical to that of soft tissue leiomyosarcoma. Typically, there are interweaving fascicles of spindle cells having prominent eosinophilic, fibrillary cytoplasm. A nonspecific storiform pattern may be present, and the background stroma is variably collagenized. Occasionally, the neoplastic cells are more rounded, with pale to clear cytoplasm (15). Mitotic figures range from 1 to 35 per 10 high-power fields. Unlike soft tissue leiomyosarcoma, osteoclast-like giant cells are common, interspersed in the neoplastic stroma.

Ultrastructurally, the cytoplasm contains thin, actin-sized filaments with dense bodies arranged in bundles parallel to the longitudinal axis of the cell. Pinocytotic vesicles are prominent. These findings are characteristic of smooth muscle differentiation (13,16). Immunohistochemically, the cells stain with antibodies directed against muscle specific actin and, less often, desmin. As with soft tissue leiomyosarcomas, positivity for cytokeratin varies from widely scattered cells to more extensive staining (15).

Differential Diagnosis. The main consideration is distinguishing metastatic leiomyosarcoma from a primary intraosseous lesion. In a review of the literature, Fornasier and Paley (14) found only 10 reported cases of metastatic leiomyosarcoma, mostly from the uterus, initially presenting as a skeletal metastasis. The metastases were often to osseous sites that are uncommon for primary leiomyosarcoma such as the skull, spine, and scapula.

Some well-documented skeletal leiomyosarcomas were initially diagnosed as fibrosarcomas or malignant fibrous histiocytomas (15). Fibrosarcomas have a more distinct fascicular pattern with sharply delimited fascicles resulting in a herring-bone arrangement. Leiomyosarcoma shares with malignant fibrous histiocytoma foci of storiform architecture, as well as scattered giant cells. Immunostaining for muscle specific actin or desmin distinguishes leiomyosarcoma from fibrosarcoma and malignant fibrous histiocytoma. Spindle cell carcinomas are also separated on immunohistochemical grounds, as discussed in the section on metastatic neoplasms. The presence of occasional cytokeratin positivity in leiomyosarcomas mandates the use of a panel of immunohistochemical markers. In the event of equivocal immunohistochemical stains, electron microscopy will aid in differentiating epithelial cells from smooth muscle.

Treatment and Prognosis. About 50 percent of patients with skeletal leiomyosarcoma die of tumor, mainly due to pulmonary metastases. Widespread metastases, including cutaneous involvement, also have been reported (12). Amputation is the mainstay of therapy. Radiation may relieve pain at metastatic sites, but the role of chemotherapy is currently undetermined (15).

SCHWANNOMA OF BONE

Definition. A benign neoplasm of Schwann cell differentiation characterized, microscopically, by an orderly cellular pattern (Antoni A) and a loose, disorderly myxoid component (Antoni B). The term *neurilemmoma* is also used for these neoplasms.

General Features. Bone contains an abundant nerve supply that accompanies branches of the nutrient artery (25). Presumably, the associated Schwann cells give rise to these neoplasms. Fewer than 75 histologically documented intraosseous schwannomas of conventional type have been reported. The association between conventional schwannoma of bone and von Recklinghausen disease is not entirely clear. Patients with the latter condition may develop lytic bone lesions, but these are more commonly nonossifying fibromas of bone. In addition to conventional schwannomas, skeletal melanotic (psammomatous) schwannomas have on occasion been described in patients who have a heritable syndrome that includes cardiac myxoma and Cushing syndrome (18).

Clinical Features. Conventional intraosseous schwannomas equally affect males and females. Patients range in age from 2 to 65 years. Most of the tumors occur in the fourth decade of life. Patients present with pain or swelling over the affected bone, and, occasionally, a pathologic fracture. A few patients have been symptomatic for up to 15 years. Vertebral lesions may result in nerve deficits (24). Sacral lesions are often gigantic and may have a considerable anterior soft tissue extension (17).

Sites. The majority of intraosseous schwannomas have been located in the mandible, followed by the sacrum. Other sites include the vertebra, ulna, humerus, femur, tibia, patella, scapula, rib, and small bones of the hands (20). Some reported sacral schwannomas are an intraosseous extension of a lesion originating in the spinal canal or from the posterior nerve roots of the spinal cord.

Radiographic Appearance. Schwannomas are lytic, sharply demarcated defects that often expand the involved bone. Perilesional sclerosis may surround the area of central lucency. Periosteal reaction does not occur even when cortical erosion has taken place.

Gross Findings. The tissue may be gray, yellow, or hemorrhagic. If a block excision is performed, a thin sclerotic reaction may be seen in the bone with a suggestion of a fibrous capsule.

Microscopic Findings. Intraosseous schwannomas consist predominantly of Antoni A tissue with closely packed, spindle cells. The nuclei may orient in palisades, forming so-called Verocay bodies. Antoni type B tissue is loose and hypocellular in comparison, with randomly oriented spindle cells in a more edematous stroma. Secondary changes such as lipid- or hemosiderin-laden macrophages are common in the type B regions. As with their soft tissue counterparts, thick-walled blood vessels are also frequent in intraosseous schwannoma. Scattered, large, pleomorphic nuclei with densely staining, smudged chromatin may be present. These appear to represent a degenerative change also encountered in soft tissue schwannomas. In the absence of more clear-cut features of malignancy, such as increased mitotic rate and increased cellularity, they do not indicate more aggressive behavior.

Ultrastructurally, the broad, amorphous bands of basal lamina and the presence of long-spacing collagen are identical to soft tissue schwannomas (19). Immunohistochemically, schwannomas of the conventional type are almost always positive for S-100 protein, and about three fourths stain with Leu-7 (CD57) (21,26). Staining for glial fibrillary acidic protein has been variably reported as either present in about one third of cases (22) or completely absent (21). Staining for vimentin is invariably positive, and is only of value to confirm the antigenic viability of the tissue.

The rare melanotic schwannomas have pigmented spindle cells plus laminated calcific concretions (psammoma bodies) that may be radiographically detectable. Immunohistochemical staining with HMB-45 and for S-100 protein is strongly positive. Schwann cell differentiation, as well as melanogenesis has been confirmed ultrastructurally (23).

Differential Diagnosis. The cellular areas of Antoni type A tissue may be mistaken for spindle cell sarcoma if large, hyperchromatic nuclei are present. It should be noted that examples of primary neurofibrosarcoma of bone have not been well documented. The presence of Antoni type B tissue should prevent confusion. Benign fibrous histiocytomas and nonossifying fibromas may have spindle cells and lipid-filled cells, but these lesions tend to be more cellular, composed of multiple cell types, and they lack the thick-walled blood vessels and palisaded Antoni A areas of schwannoma. Desmoplastic fibroma is more densely collagenized than schwannoma and lacks the myxoid, edematous stroma of the Antoni B areas, as well as the palisading pattern in Antoni A regions. Immunohistochemical staining for S-100 protein or with Leu-7 may be of value in documenting Schwann cell differentiation in selected cases.

Treatment and Prognosis. En bloc excision is curative. Curettage and replacement with bone chips is also effective. Soft tissue melanotic schwannomas sometimes metastasize, but this has not been reported with the rare skeletal tumors.

MALIGNANT MESENCHYMOMA OF BONE

Definition. A sarcoma consisting of two or more differentiated mesenchymal elements other than fibrosarcoma. Many lesions previously interpreted as fibrosarcomas are currently considered to be malignant fibrous

LESIONS OF HEMATOPOIETIC, LYMPHOID, AND HISTIOCYTIC ELEMENTS

EOSINOPHILIC GRANULOMA

Definition. A proliferation of Langerhans cells usually accompanied by eosinophils, histiocytes, lymphocytes, neutrophils, and scattered plasma cells. The terms *histiocytosis X*, *Langerhans cell histiocytosis*, and *Langerhans granulomatosis* are synonymous.

General Features. In 1868, Paul Langerhans, a medical student, used a gold chloride stain to observe a population of dendritic cells in the human epidermis. The structure and function of these cells was essentially ignored until Birbeck et al. (1) discovered through electron microscopy that they contained a unique cytoplasmic "granule." Langerhans cells appear to have a variety of immunologic functions, although these have not been precisely defined. Langerhans resemble histiocytes cells on hematoxylin and eosin stained sections, but Langerhans cells stain, immunohistochemically, for S-100 protein and CD1 (OKT-6) antigen. In addition, they exhibit cell surface membrane and perinuclear staining with peanut agglutinin (13). This contrasts with the cell surface staining pattern of lymphoid cells and the diffuse or globular cytoplasmic pattern of staining seen in histiocytes. A number of other glycoproteins have been identified on the cell membrane of Langerhans cells, but their diagnostic utility is not yet clear (10). Ultrastructurally, Langerhans cells have variably shaped granules (Birbeck granules) that appear to form from complex invaginations of cell membranes, a feature not seen in histiocytes (7). Birbeck granules have been identified in mitotically active cells (4).

Eosinophilic granuloma is viewed by many as a reactive process or a disorder of immune regulation, rather than a neoplasm. All organ systems can be affected, and, rarely, it can be confined to extraosseous sites such as the intestinal tract, skin, or thyroid. Much of the confusion surrounding the prognosis of eosinophilic granuloma stems from differences in the extent of disease. The major clinical categories of involvement include: solitary bone lesions, multiple bone lesions, visceral lesions, and combinations of bone and visceral disease. Children with multiple bone lesions are also apt to have visceral involvement that may prove fatal. This is especially likely if the child has signs of visceral impairment such as liver failure, decreased bone marrow function, or symptomatic pulmonary disease. Approximately 50 to 60 percent of poor risk patients, usually children less than 2 years old, die of their disease (8,12). The subsequent discussion, however, is confined to eosinophilic granuloma limited to bones or presenting initially as osseous disease.

The clinical triad of diabetes insipidus, exophthalmos, and multiple lytic bone lesions has been referred to as *Hand-Schüller-Christian disease*. This is not a specific entity, however, as other destructive lesions centered in the anterior fossa can produce these clinical features. *Letterer-Siwe disease* is generally considered a variant of eosinophilic granuloma that occurs in infants, results in multiple visceral and cutaneous lesions, and, frequently, has a rapidly progressive, fatal course. Although these clinical features occur in some patients with eosinophilic granuloma, other diseases such as malignant histiocytosis, histiocytic lymphoma of childhood, and immunologic deficiencies may also share these features. Therefore, Hand-Schüller-Christian "disease" and Letterer-Siwe "disease" are perhaps better considered as clinical syndromes rather than specific entities.

Clinical Features. Patients with osseous eosinophilic granuloma range from 1 month to 71 years of age. About 85 percent of cases occur in the first three decades of life, with 60 percent in the first decade. Males are afflicted approximately twice as often as females. About 90 percent of patients complain of pain, and the remainder have a soft tissue swelling that may or may not be painful. Temporal bone disease presents with signs and symptoms indistinguishable from otitis media or mastoiditis. Some lesions are incidental findings on radiographs taken for other purposes or are separate asymptomatic lesions discovered after the identification of the initial symptomatic lesion. Mild peripheral eosinophilia is present in about 5 to 10 percent of patients.

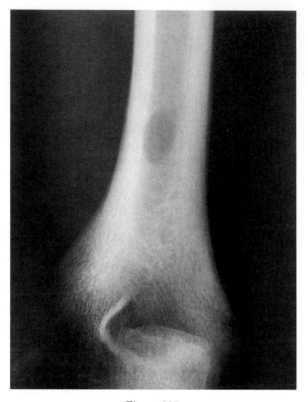

Figure 235
EOSINOPHILIC GRANULOMA
Sharply punched out lesion in the humerus of a 16-year-old boy complaining of pain in the elbow.

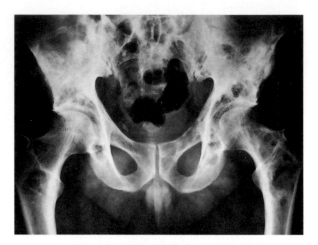

Figure 236
EOSINOPHILIC GRANULOMA
A 42-year-old man with a 3 year history of progressive involvement with polyostotic eosinophilic granuloma. Some lesions are sharply demarcated and others have irregular margins with sclerosis. The sclerotic foci may be regressing.

Patients with solitary lesions outnumber those with multiple lesions from 2 to 1 to more than 5 to 1 in published series. Because most reported series come from large institutions, it is likely that they are weighted by patients with multiple lesions who have severe clinical disease. Patients with solitary lesions undoubtedly outnumber those with polyostotic lesions by far more than 5 to 1.

Sites. Almost any bone can be involved. The calvarium is the single most common site, with the femur, pelvis, ribs, and mandible as other frequent sites. The small bones of the hands and feet are rarely affected. In one series confined to adults, the rib was the most frequent location (15). In the long bones, eosinophilic granuloma is typically diaphyseal or metaphyseal; epiphyseal lesions are rare.

Radiographic Appearance. Eosinophilic granuloma is a lytic process, usually centered in the medullary cavity, but occasionally localized to the cortex. There is often a "punched out"

appearance with no osseous reaction, or a thin or thick sclerotic rim of reactive bone. Punched out lesions usually are between 1 and 2 cm in size (fig. 235) (1). Occasionally, there is an expanded cortical shell that may be perforated and accompanied by a soft tissue mass. Long bone lesions often measure up to 4 to 6 cm in length and lack well-defined margins. Lesions in the skull often have a "beveled" appearance, due to an angled erosion of the cortical bone. Involvement of the ribs and clavicles may produce a permeative, highly aggressive-appearing radiographic pattern (11). Multiple lesions in the same individual can have a variety of appearances including punched out, ill-defined, and focally sclerotic defects (fig. 236). This variation in appearance suggests that the lesions have arisen, progressed, become static, or begun to resolve at differing times.

Gross Findings. The gross appearance is not distinctive. Depending on the mixture of cells, it may be yellow, gray, or brown. Older, regressing lesions may be yellow, due to the accumulation of lipid in histiocytes and Langerhans cells. Intralesional hemorrhage is common.

Microscopic Findings. Although eosinophilic granuloma contains a variety of cell types, only the Langerhans cell is diagnostic. The ratio of diagnostic Langerhans cells to inflammatory

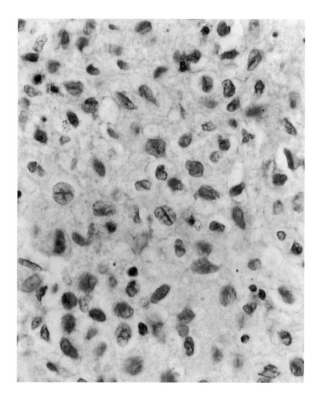

Figure 237
EOSINOPHILIC GRANULOMA
Langerhans cells may have discrete cell margins or they may be ill defined as in this field. Note the clear nuclei, some of which have clefts.

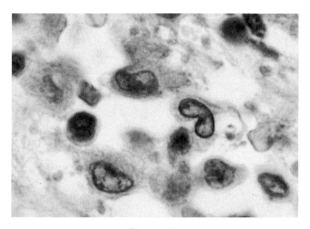

Figure 238
EOSINOPHILIC GRANULOMA
The Langerhans cells have a well-defined nuclear membrane and delicate chromatin, much of which is condensed along the nuclear membrane. Some nuclei are conspicuously reniform. (Fig. 13-3 from Fechner RE, Spjut HJ, Haggitt RC. Diseases of bones and joints. Based on the proceedings of the 51st Annual Anatomic Pathology Slide Seminar of the American Society of Clinical Pathologists. American Society of Clinical Pathologists Press, 1985:67.)

cells may vary greatly from field to field in a single lesion, as well as from case to case. Langerhans cells may be difficult to find or may be present in large numbers, producing a focally monotypic infiltrate, resembling a neoplasm. Langerhans cells contain highly variable amounts of cytoplasm and assume a variety of nuclear shapes. They may have well-demarcated cell borders or the nuclei may appear to be in a syncytium of cytoplasm (fig. 237). The prototypical cells have abundant, powdery, eosinophilic cytoplasm coupled with characteristic nuclear features. The diagnostic nuclei are bean shaped or reniform with convoluted nuclear grooves and indentations which are best seen by focusing up and down through the nucleus. The nuclear chromatin is either delicately dispersed or condensed along the prominent nuclear membrane (fig. 238). Multinucleated giant cells may have the same nuclear features as the mononuclear Langerhans cells (14). Mitotic figures vary in number and, occasionally, fewer than 5 per 10

high-power fields are present. Atypical Langerhans cells are distinguished by their hyperchromatic nuclei, increased nuclear to cytoplasmic ratio, and medium-sized nucleoli.

Eosinophilic granuloma contains variable numbers of ordinary histiocytes. These may often be recognized by their phagocytic activity, manifest by intracytoplasmic nuclear debris, hemosiderin, or Charcot-Leyden crystals from degenerating eosinophils. Lipid-laden histiocytes or "foam cells" are sometimes seen, and occasionally are numerous, especially in longstanding lesions. Langerhans cells are also capable of lipid accumulation, and it may be impossible to distinguish these cells from foamy histiocytes on hematoxylin and eosin stained sections.

Nondiagnostic eosinophils, neutrophils, lymphocytes, and plasma cells are common secondary components of eosinophilic granuloma. Eosinophils may predominate in some areas, forming diffuse sheets to the virtual exclusion of Langerhans cells. Occasionally, eosinophils form necrotic aggregates (eosinophilic abscesses), surrounded by histiocytes and Langerhans cells. Conversely, about 8 percent of cases have virtually no eosinophils (14). Lymphocytes and plasma cells also may predominate (fig. 239), leading to potential confusion with chronic osteomyelitis.

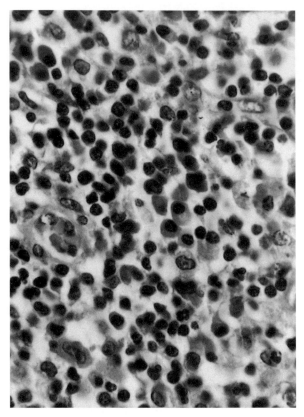

Figure 239
EOSINOPHILIC GRANULOMA
Lymphocytes and plasma cells predominate. The cells with lightly stained nuclei may be Langerhans cells or histiocytes. An S-100 stain would distinguish these two. (Figure 13-4 from Fechner RE, Spjut HJ, Haggitt RC. Diseases of bones and joints. Based on the proceedings of the 51st Annual Anatomic Pathology Slide Seminar of the American Society of Clinical Pathologists. American Society of Clinical Pathologists Press, 1985:68.)

In an intact eosinophilic granuloma, bony trabeculae are usually absent and bone at the periphery of the lesion often shows marked osteoclastic resorption. Prostaglandin production by Langerhans cells has been documented; these compounds are known to be strong stimulators of bone resorption (6). The presence of well-formed bony trabeculae within a presumed eosinophilic granuloma may indicate healing or secondary fracture; their absence should suggest the possibility that the lesion in question is not an eosinophilic granuloma.

Individual lesions may undergo partial or complete spontaneous resolution. Microscopically, resolving lesions become increasingly fibrotic with the progressive disappearance of Langerhans cells. Foamy histiocytes may persist in the proliferating fibrous tissue (14), creating an image reminiscent of nonossifying fibroma.

Differential Diagnosis. The differential diagnosis includes granulomatous inflammation, osteomyelitis, and Hodgkin disease. Osteomyelitis may be radiographically identical to eosinophilic granuloma, although destruction of the epiphyseal cartilage, loss of a vertebral disc space, or swollen joints are more consistent with osteomyelitis. In contrast to eosinophilic granuloma, osteomyelitis is rare in the skull. Microscopically, osteomyelitis is dominated by inflammatory cells other than eosinophils. Necrotic trabeculae are common in osteomyelitis, whereas bony trabeculae (either viable appearing or necrotic) are rare in eosinophilic granuloma. Xanthogranulomatous osteomyelitis, a lesion with large numbers of foamy histiocytes, neutrophils, and plasma cells has been described recently (3). Again, the absence of Langerhans cells and the dominance of neutrophils over eosinophils are helpful for differentiation.

Granulomatous inflammation may be confused with eosinophilic granuloma if the granulomas are ill defined or poorly developed. The presence of discrete granulomas, with or without necrosis, strongly suggests an infectious disease such as tuberculosis or fungal infection. Eosinophils are usually absent.

Hodgkin disease can present as a solitary osseous defect with a mixed inflammatory infiltrate. Radiographically apparent lesions tend to be larger than those of eosinophilic granuloma and often have a mixed osteoblastic-osteolytic appearance. Patients are typically over 20 years of age. The identification of Reed-Sternberg cells and the absence of Langerhans cells distinguishes the two. Immunohistochemical stains using antibodies directed against CD15 (Leu-M1) and CD30 (Ki-1) will aid in the recognition of Reed-Sternberg cells and may be of value when these cells are widely dispersed in a nondiagnostic inflammatory infiltrate.

Treatment and Prognosis. Solitary intraosseous eosinophilic granuloma is usually cured by simple curettage or intralesional injection with steroids. Low dose radiation may be of value for inaccessible lesions. With these forms of therapy, complete healing takes an average of about 1 year (9). Some radiographic lesions compatible with eosinophilic granuloma have completely disappeared ("healed") over time without therapy. Occasionally, an ill-defined lytic lesion develops a well-defined sclerotic margin and no further change takes place, presumably reflecting stable, partial healing (9). Recurrences following therapy are rare and develop from 3 months to 4 years after initial treatment (15).

Patients with solitary intraosseous eosinophilic granuloma are at risk for developing additional lesions, usually within 6 months to 1 year after initial diagnosis, but occasionally up to 2 years later (2,5). Cheyne (2) described one patient who developed further bone lesions after the presenting lesion had healed, but this is unusual. In one study, 5 of 36 patients presenting with solitary lesions developed polyostotic disease (9). Twenty-four of these patients had skeletal surveys that initially confirmed only one identifiable lesion. Six out of seven patients who presented with polyostotic eosinophilic granuloma developed additional bone lesions.

Adult patients with more than three osseous lesions are apt to have visceral involvement as well (15). Some studies have found that death due to eosinophilic granuloma is rare in adults, regardless of the extent of disease (15). Other studies, however, have found that the progression of multiple bone lesions in patients over 50 years of age is often accompanied by pulmonary disease and a high mortality rate (9).

MULTIPLE (PLASMA CELL) MYELOMA

Definition. Intraosseous plasma cell neoplasms may manifest as solitary lesions or involve many bones. The latter, disseminated form of disease is often referred to as multiple myeloma. Solitary myeloma is discussed separately, following this section.

General Features. Multiple myeloma is the most common primary neoplasm of bone and comprised about 45 percent of surgically diagnosed malignant bone tumors at the Mayo Clinic (18). About 85 percent were diagnosed by marrow aspirate. Surgical biopsies of myeloma were often done during repair of pathologic fractures or to relieve spinal cord compression, in addition to obtaining tissue for diagnostic purposes.

Clinical Features. Multiple myeloma is rare before the age of 40 years, and only a few cases

have been reported in patients in their second or third decades of life (18). The majority of patients are between the ages of 50 and 80 years. Most series report a slight male predominance.

Patients may present with diverse signs or symptoms including bone pain, anemia, pathologic fracture, neurologic complaints, fever, hypercalcemia, renal failure, or proteinuria. A small percentage of patients with multiple or solitary myeloma present with an extramedullary plasma cell tumor (plasmacytoma) that is frequently located in the upper respiratory tract. Some of these patients are found to have disseminated disease on further examination, but in others there may be an interval of months or years before multiple myeloma becomes manifest.

In 99 percent of patients with multiple myeloma, electrophoresis discloses increased levels of monoclonal immunoglobulin in the serum or light chains in the urine (Bence Jones protein). Serum protein IgG is seen in about 55 percent of patients, IgA in 25 percent, and, rarely, IgM, IgD, or IgE. In the remaining 20 percent of patients, Bence Jones proteinuria alone, without elevated serum immunoglobulins, is present. It should be noted that Bence Jones proteins are present in the urine along with elevated monoclonal immunoglobulins in 60 to 70 percent of all myeloma patients (24).

A few patients with multiple myeloma have an unusual constellation of laboratory and clinical features including polyneuropathy, organomegaly, endocrinopathy, serum protein abnormalities (so-called M-protein), and skin changes. The acronym POEMS has been given to this clinical syndrome (16). POEMS patients usually have sclerotic skeletal lesions, but bone pain is rare.

Radiographic Appearance. Distinctive but nondiagnostic radiographic abnormalities are seen in about 80 percent of patients (23). The earliest and most extensive changes, found in the vertebrae, pelvis, ribs, and skull, are sharply "punched out" areas of bone destruction, usually between 1 and 5 cm in diameter, without a surrounding zone of sclerosis (fig. 240). The cortex may be eroded (fig. 241). The ribs are especially likely to be expanded. In about 2 percent of cases, including patients with POEMS syndrome, there is increased density of the bones (osteosclerotic myelomas) (18,21). Bone scans are typically negative in multiple myeloma.

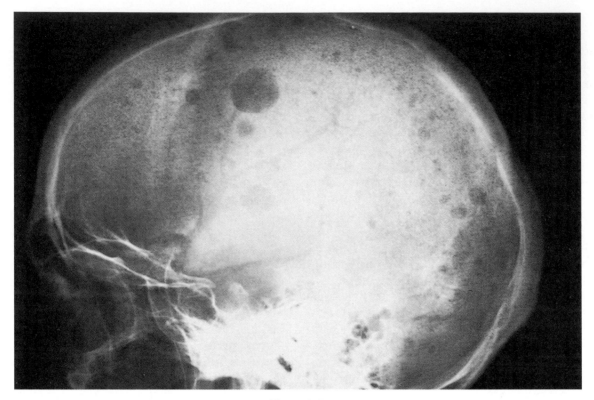

Figure 240
PLASMA CELL MYELOMA
The skull of a woman with disseminated multiple myeloma has "punched out," radiolucent defects of varying sizes. (Fig. 220 from Fascicle 5, Second Series.)

Gross Findings. Material usually in the form of curettings or a small biopsy specimen consists of red, gray, or mottled red-gray soft tissue. At autopsy, intact foci of tumor are either well-circumscribed or confluent nodules of red to gray soft tumor replacing the cancellous bone (fig. 242).

Microscopic Findings. Myeloma consists of sheets of closely packed plasma cells that vary from mature to blast-like in appearance. The background stroma is usually devoid of more than an occasional capillary and generally lacks prominent fibrosis. Amyloid is occasionally present, and, on rare occasion, may be so abundant as to obscure the neoplastic cells.

The most mature neoplastic cells resemble normal plasma cells and have an eccentric nucleus with abundant cytoplasm and a prominent Golgi area seen as a pale eosinophilic perinuclear halo. However, even well-differentiated myelomas usually have cells that deviate from normal. The perinuclear halo is absent in some cells, the chromatin pattern is more irregularly dispersed than in normal plasma cells, and the shape of the cell may be more polygonal (fig. 243). Occasional binucleated or trinucleated cells can be seen. Poorly differentiated lesions have conspicuous nuclear pleomorphism with coarse, irregular chromatin clumping and huge nucleoli (fig. 244). Regardless of the degree of differentiation, mitotic figures are uncommon.

Nuclear and cytoplasmic inclusions are sometimes evident in myeloma cells. The cytoplasmic inclusions are membrane bound, crystalline or globular, and usually located within rough endoplasmic reticulum. There does not appear to be a consistent association between morphologic appearances (including inclusions) and specific immunoglobulin abnormalities. The one exception appears in IgA myeloma where the plasma cells often contain amorphous, pale nuclear inclusions that may be as large as one third the diameter of the nucleus (26).

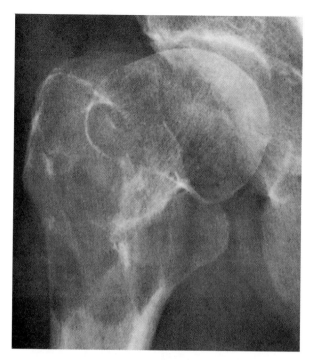

Figure 241
PLASMA CELL MYELOMA
A 64-year-old man with a pathologic fracture of the right femur. This destructive lesion exhibits cortical erosion, as well as loss of medullary bone. Multiple lesions were present in other bones. (Fig. 222 from Fascicle 5, 2nd Series.)

Differential Diagnosis. Chronic osteomyelitis is the main lesion in the differential diagnosis of myeloma. Osteomyelitis contrasts with most cases of myeloma by having prominent fibrous tissue, a mixed inflammatory infiltrate that includes lymphocytes and neutrophils in addition to plasma cells, and a well-vascularized stroma. If plasma cells are numerous, stains for kappa and lambda light chains are useful. If the ratio of one or the other is greater than 16 to 1, the diagnosis of myeloma is, in effect, assured (25). Lesser ratios probably indicate a polyclonal proliferation characteristic of reactive plasma cells. The more bizarre forms of myeloma may raise the question of carcinoma. Plasma cells do not contain cytokeratins but may stain with epithelial membrane antigen, negating its diagnostic value.

Distinguishing some lymphomas, particularly B-cell immunoblastic lymphoma (immunoblastic sarcoma) from poorly differentiated myeloma may be difficult on purely morphologic grounds.

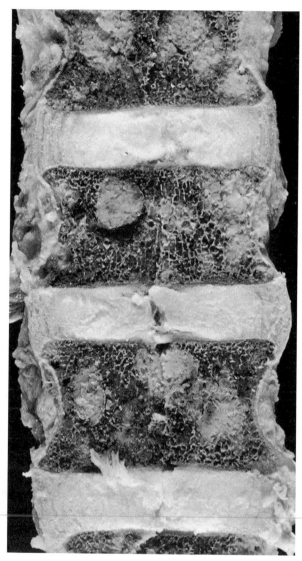

Figure 242
PLASMA CELL MYELOMA
This sagittal section of vertebrae from a 54-year-old woman shows nodular replacement of cancellous bone by multiple myeloma. The vertebrae are not collapsed and the discs are intact. (Fig. 223 from Fascicle 5, 2nd Series.)

Immunoblastic lymphomas usually involve lymph nodes, in contrast to myeloma. It has been suggested that there are immunohistochemical differences between myelomas and immunoblastic lymphomas, including the less common expression of leukocyte common antigen by the former neoplasms (27). However, because of overlapping immunophenotypes, these stains are of limited value in individual cases.

217

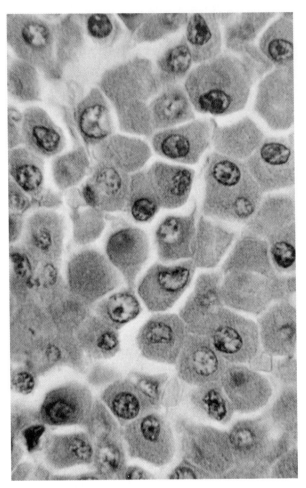

Figure 243
PLASMA CELL MYELOMA
The plasma cells are well differentiated, but abnormal in that the paranuclear halo is absent, the chromatin pattern is irregularly clumped, and some of the cells are polygonal. (Fig. 225 from Fascicle 5, 2nd Series.)

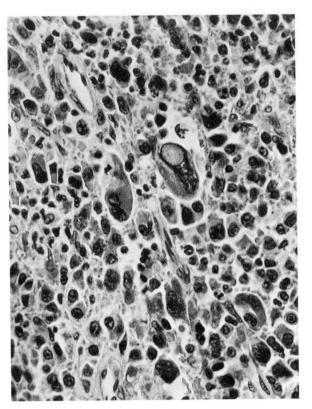

Figure 244
PLASMA CELL MYELOMA
This poorly differentiated myeloma in a 52-year-old man has many bizarre cells, as well as others that are only mildly atypical. (Fig. 227 from Fascicle 5, 2nd Series.) (Figures 244 and 245 are from the same patient.)

Treatment and Prognosis. The prognosis depends primarily on the stage of disease at the time of diagnosis (19), and, to a lesser extent, on the degree of differentiation (17,20). Patients with extensive lytic bone lesions rarely survive more than 6 to 12 months without therapy. Chemotherapy, usually in the form of alkylating agents, induces remission in approximately 50 to 70 percent of patients, but the median survival is still only 2 to 3 years. Radiation therapy is effective for individual lesions (fig. 245) and usually results in sclerosis of a given lesion, especially in the vertebrae. Most patients with myeloma die of infections or renal failure. The cause of the latter

is multifactorial, probably relating to proteinuria and, possibly, a direct toxicity to tubular epithelial cells. Patients with POEMS syndrome tend to have a prolonged course.

A rare clinical variant of myeloma, lacking radiographic osseous lesions but having more than 10 percent of the hematopoietic bone marrow consisting of normal plasma cells, has been termed *smoldering myeloma*. This variant shows little or no progression of disease for 5 years or more without treatment (22).

SOLITARY (PLASMA CELL) MYELOMA

Definition. A neoplasm of plasma cells that produces a single osseous lesion. Synonyms include *solitary myeloma* and *solitary plasmacytoma of bone*. For the sake of brevity, we will use the term solitary myeloma.

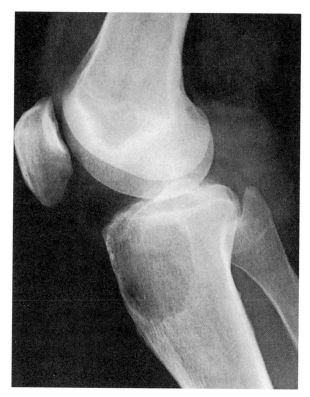

Figure 245
PLASMA CELL MYELOMA
This radiograph illustrates a destructive lesion in the proximal portion of the tibia. The tibial lesion was irradiated after biopsy and then curetted and packed with bone chips. Thorough study of the curetted material revealed no residual myeloma. The patient was living 8 years later with no evidence of further disease. (Fig. 226 from Fascicle 5, 2nd Series.)

General Features. In a series reported from the Mayo Clinic, solitary myeloma comprised 24 percent of the cases of plasma cell myeloma that were diagnosed surgically (28). Since bone scans are usually negative in patients with multiple myeloma, the diagnosis of solitary myeloma is warranted only after a radiographic skeletal survey fails to show additional lesions, and bone marrow aspirates do not have increased plasma cells (>10 percent).

Clinical Features. Patients range from 16 to 83 years of age, but the majority are over 50 years. About 80 percent present with pain, 10 percent have neurologic findings, and 10 percent are asymptomatic (29). A thoracic vertebra is the most common site followed by the lumbar vertebrae, ribs, scapula, pelvic bones, skull, mandible, and long bones. Serum or urine protein abnormalities are found in 50 to 77 percent of patients (29,31).

Radiographic Appearance. The vertebral lesions are lytic, but often show cortical ridging resulting in a "corduroy cloth" appearance. There may be destruction of the cortex, with or without extension into the soft tissues. Lesions in other bones may be lytic, and are sometimes expansile with a "bubbly" appearance (fig. 246).

Gross Findings, Microscopic Findings, and Differential Diagnosis. These are the same as for multiple myeloma.

Treatment and Prognosis. Most patients are treated with radiation to the tumor, often in conjunction with chemotherapy. Usually, there is resolution of the lesion, which may be accompanied by a decrease in serum protein abnormalities, if these were initially present. The persistence of serum protein abnormalities is not a poor prognostic sign (29). About 10 percent of solitary myelomas do not respond to therapy and these may be fatal if the vertebrae are involved.

Between 36 and 54 percent of patients with solitary myeloma develop multiple myeloma from a few months to more than 10 years after the original diagnosis. There are no consistent features that correlate with the risk of developing disseminated disease. Protein abnormalities, soft tissue extension, and site (whether vertebra or peripheral bone), are not associated with an increased risk (31). The only trend that seems to correlate with a high risk of subsequent multiple myeloma is a poorly differentiated tumor (30,31).

OSSEOUS LESIONS IN LEUKEMIAS

Definition. Disseminated bone marrow involvement is a defining feature of virtually all leukemias. This involvement may be asymptomatic or produce localized clinical and radiographic abnormalities.

General and Clinical Features. In spite of the diffuse bone marrow disease typical of almost all forms of leukemia, clinical and radiographic signs are less common and typically occur in young children with an acute form of the disease. In some studies, about 50 percent of patients with acute leukemia have had osseous symptoms, and a somewhat smaller percentage have had accompanying radiographic changes (32,35,36,38). Early studies of more advanced disease reported radiographic changes in up to two thirds of children

219

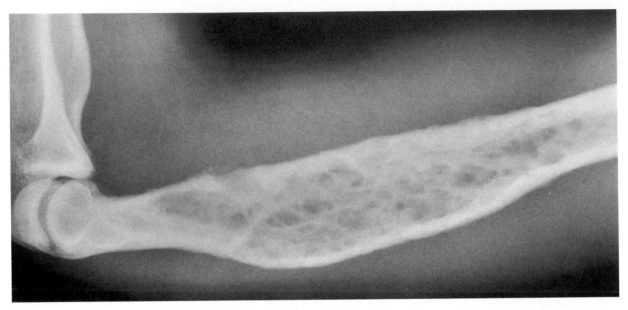

Figure 246
SOLITARY PLASMA CELL MYELOMA
A 26-year-old man had reduced range of movement of the elbow. This radiograph shows diffuse expansion of the humeral diaphysis with the cortex maintaining a normal thickness. A coarse, "bubbly" pattern is present. There were no other lesions. (Courtesy of Dr. T.W. Westgaard. Sandefjord, Norway.)

with leukemia (39). These changes are typically of little or no clinical significance.

In children, leukemic bone pain tends to be sharp, localized, and recurrent (38). In some instances, the pain may be associated with a joint effusion. These findings may lead to a misdiagnosis of osteomyelitis or septic arthritis with an associated delay in correct diagnosis. In adults, the pain is often more diffuse. The development of osseous lesions in patients with previously diagnosed chronic myelogenous leukemia may herald a blastic transformation (33).

Sites. In children, leukemic lesions most often involve the long bones of the extremities (38); in adults the axial skeleton is often involved. Involvement of the short tubular bones of the hands and feet is rare in all ages (37). These patterns of disease probably reflect the age-related localization of hematopoietic marrow.

Radiographic Appearance. Routine radiographic surveys are no longer recommended for patients with leukemia (37), although symptomatic lesions may be radiographed to determine if pathologic fracture has occurred or is likely. Osseous radiographic lesions due to leukemic infiltrates may assume several differing appearances, including radiolucent metaphyseal bands, generalized osteoporosis, osteolytic defects, diffuse or localized osteosclerosis, and periosteal reactions (fig. 247) (32,35,39).

Radiolucent, transverse metaphyseal bands may also extend into the epiphysis or diaphysis, and are a common finding in acute childhood leukemias. The bands apparently correspond to a disruption of normal endochondral ossification due to leukemic infiltration. Although a typical feature of acute leukemia, the bands are not diagnostic and may occasionally be seen in patients with chronic, severe illnesses such as scurvy (32,34,39). Generalized osteoporotic bone disease may be seen with both chronic and acute leukemias in children and adults (33,37). Osteolytic defects may occur in any bone, and are common in adults in the pelvis and vertebral bodies (32). Periosteal reactions have been reported in association with 36 percent of leukemias occurring in infancy, but are less common in adults. Typically, these are in the form of a single parallel line. Osteosclerotic changes were reported in 2 to 9 percent of infantile cases (36,37). Osteosclerosis may also be seen in adults, secondary to chronic myelogenous leukemia with myelofibrosis.

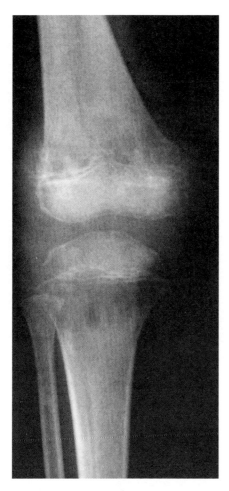

Figure 247
LEUKEMIA
This 4-year-old boy with acute leukemia had severe bone pain. Radiographic changes include osteolytic lesions, radiolucent bands with growth arrest lines, and periosteal reaction. (Modified from fig. 429, Fascicle 5, 2nd Series.)

The incidence of skeletal involvement is higher at relapse, than at the time of initial presentation (37). Up to 65 percent of children dying of leukemia have radiographic bone lesions.

Gross Findings. If properly diagnosed by clinical and radiographic means, these lesions are not biopsied. Occasionally, however, bone pain and an apparently solitary radiographic defect may be the mode of presentation, accompanied by peripheral blood changes that are nondiagnostic (aleukemic phase). Leukemic bone lesions have also been studied at autopsy. Grossly, there is a hyperemic or hemorrhagic marrow with destruction of bony trabeculae or,

conversely, osteosclerosis. Areas of bone infarction may be obvious grossly.

Microscopic Findings. The microscopic appearance is dependent on the form of leukemia. The typical childhood acute lymphoblastic leukemias appear microscopically as patternless sheets of small, blue cells.

Differential Diagnosis. Microscopically, the small, blue cells of an acute leukemia may be confused with other small cell tumors including Ewing sarcoma, metastatic neuroblastoma, or matrix-free areas of small cell osteosarcoma or mesenchymal chondrosarcoma. Confusion with chronic osteomyelitis is also possible. Distinction is typically straightforward if appropriate clinical and hematologic information is available. Wright stained touch preparations of tumor cells may be of value in identifying the typical chromatin patterns of leukemic "blasts." In problematic cases, fresh tissue should be snap-frozen for appropriate immunohistochemical or DNA studies.

Treatment and Prognosis. The general treatment for leukemia is chemotherapy based and varies with the form of disease. The presence of localized pain or a radiographic lesion at the time of diagnosis does not appear to alter the prognosis. As noted above, however, patients with chronic myelogenous leukemia who develop bone lesions later in their course may be undergoing "blast transformation" (33).

NON-HODGKIN LYMPHOMA OF BONE

Definition. Primary osseous lymphoma has been arbitrarily defined as a lymphoma arising within the medullary cavity of a single bone, without concurrent regional lymph node or visceral involvement for at least 6 months following diagnosis (41,54). The vast majority are of non-Hodgkin type, and most are large cell lymphomas (54).

General Features. Secondary, clinically occult, osseous involvement by lymphomas arising in extraosseous sites is quite common, particularly with malignant lymphomas of small cleaved cell type. A much smaller number of patients with lymphoma present with signs, symptoms, and radiographic evidence of bone involvement. Approximately half of these patients (the percentage varies markedly from series to series) have involvement of regional lymph nodes, but the remainder have primary osseous lymphomas.

In 1939, Parker and Jackson (53) first clearly distinguished primary "reticulum cell sarcoma" of bone from Ewing sarcoma and noted that the former tumor had a much better prognosis. Thirteen of their 17 patients were alive from 6 months to 14 years after initial diagnosis. Their study was followed by a series of publications defining "reticulum cell sarcoma" as a distinct entity (41,47,49–51). Intraosseous lymphoma is now well recognized, accounting for 3.1 percent of primary malignant osseous tumors in the large Mayo Clinic series of bone neoplasms (43).

In the United States, the great majority of intraosseous lymphomas are B-cell proliferations (46,54). Specifically, many are multilobated B-cell lymphomas, a group of lesions noted for a high percentage of extranodal presentations involving the skin and subcutaneous tissues, as well as bone (54). The background population of small lymphocytes commonly seen in osseous lymphomas is a reactive, predominantly T-cell proliferation (46,54). In Japan, where T-cell lymphomas, in general, are far more common, about 10 percent of osseous lymphomas are of the T-cell type (55).

Flow cytometric studies of osseous lymphomas have shown no significant differences when compared to non-Hodgkin lymphomas of lymph node origin (56).

Clinical Features. Primary osseous lymphomas have a broad age distribution, but they most often occur after the second decade of life and are rare in children. There is a definite male predilection of approximately 1.5 to 1 (43).

Patients usually present with localized dull or aching pain. Some have a palpable mass. About 50 percent have symptoms for longer than 1 year, and a few may have been symptomatic for several years. Generalized symptomatology is usually absent, and the apparent good health of the patient often contrasts markedly with the extensive destruction seen radiographically. Despite often massive osseous destruction, pathologic fractures are seen in only about 25 percent of cases (43). A few patients have joint pain with effusion, but direct extension into the joint space is extremely rare.

Sites. Any bone may be involved, but there is a predilection for the lower extremity (30 percent), and the femur is the single most common site (25 percent) (fig. 248). Pelvic bones are also frequently involved (19 percent). Osseous lymphomas are

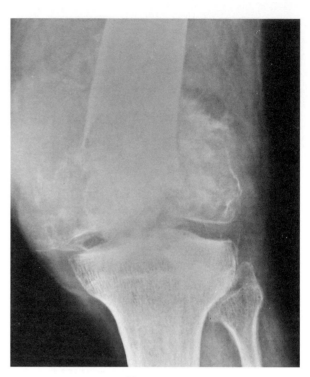

Figure 248
LYMPHOMA
A 70-year-old man noticed progressive swelling and intermittent pain in his knee. The radiograph shows sclerosis of the medullary portion of the distal femur, erosion of the cortex, and extensive periosteal reaction. A compression fracture of the more proximal femur through the lytic area abuts the articular cartilage. (Figures 248 and 249 are from the same patient.)

rare in the distal upper extremity but, in contrast, are common in the distal lower extremity. Primary osseous lymphoma is more common in the appendicular versus axial skeleton by a factor of 2–3 to 1 (48). In contrast, secondary involvement with disseminated lymphoma has the reverse distribution, favoring the axial skeleton. In the Mayo Clinic series of osseous lymphomas without extraosseous disease, 29 percent had multiple foci of intraosseous involvement (43). Although the latter tumors are traditionally considered as disseminated disease, their associated prognosis is similar to that of patients having solitary osseous lesions (43,52).

Radiographic Appearance. Lesions almost always appear malignant but the images are quite variable. The appearance may be predominantly blastic, predominantly lytic, or mixed lytic and blastic (42). Other than the often extensive nature of the lesion, which commonly involves 25

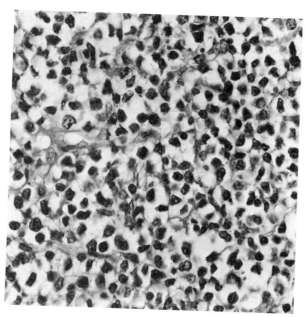

Figure 249
LYMPHOMA

Biopsy of the lesion seen in figure 248 disclosed a lymphoma with a mixture of lymphocytes having dense nuclei and "histiocyte-like" cells with larger, irregular, vesicular nuclei.

to 50 percent or more of the affected bone, there are no characteristic features that strongly suggest the diagnosis. The earliest change is a destruction, often multifocal, of medullary bone, giving it a mottled or patchy appearance. These early changes often begin in the diaphysis. With time, separate areas of bone erosion coalesce into larger fields and the permeative growth pattern gives the bone a "moth-eaten" appearance. The edges of the lesion usually blend imperceptibly with normal bone. Conventional radiographs often grossly underestimate the extent of disease. When the lesion penetrates the cortex, a periosteal reaction is typically present (fig. 248). This may be associated with soft tissue calcifications (43). There may eventually be complete destruction of the bone with loss of the cortical outline and a large soft tissue mass. Osseous lymphomas with marked intralesional sclerosis may be confused with metastatic carcinoma, osteosarcoma, chronic osteomyelitis, or Paget disease.

Gross Findings. Most lesions are not excised if properly diagnosed by biopsy. In excised lesions, the main intraosseous mass and the extraosseous extension are often centered in the metaphyseal region. The diffuse infiltrative nature of the tumor is obvious, the margins are indistinct, and the intraosseous component often contains a mixture of bone spicules and marrow fat. The extraosseous tissue has a tan or white appearance and resembles lymphomatous lymph nodes.

Microscopic Findings. The cytologic appearances of osseous large cell lymphoma are identical to those of their far more common nodal counterparts. There is invariably a diffuse growth pattern (40,43), typically with a mixture of small lymphocytic cells, as well as a larger "histiocytic" component (fig. 249). Nuclei exhibit marked variation in shape, with the predominant cells often having grooved or folded vesicular nuclei and prominent nucleoli. Cytoplasmic glycogen is absent and a complex reticulin framework is typically present in the intercellular background. The latter is somewhat variable, however, and may be lacking in some cases. Intraosseous lymphomas often have a prominent fibroblastic component, which may be associated with spindling of the neoplastic lymphoid cells. The resultant image may be confused with a spindle cell sarcoma, particularly in suboptimal sections, but application of immunohistochemical stains for lymphoid markers such as leukocyte common antigen should allow distinction. Ostrowski and colleagues (52) noted other diagnostic pitfalls which included cells with clear cytoplasm and signet ring cells mimicking adenocarcinoma, as well as clustering of neoplastic cells in a pattern resembling carcinoma.

Differential Diagnosis. *Ewing Sarcoma.* The distinguishing features of Ewing sarcoma and intraosseous lymphoma are discussed in the chapter dealing with the former lesion. Immunohistochemical stains for lymphoid cell markers have made this once problematic distinction straightforward.

Chronic Osteomyelitis. Distinguishing between malignant lymphoma and chronic osteomyelitis may be extremely difficult in poorly processed, distorted specimens. The often prominent sclerosis and common background population of small reactive lymphocytes may obscure the larger, neoplastic cells. Recognition of the larger neoplastic component is essential for the diagnosis and, conversely, the reactive small lymphocytes are of value in suggesting a lymphoid malignancy, as a prominent lymphoid background is uncommon in nonlymphoid osseous neoplasms (54).

Tu

no
di
m
of
te
or
al

w
s
d
o
u
c
i
ı
l

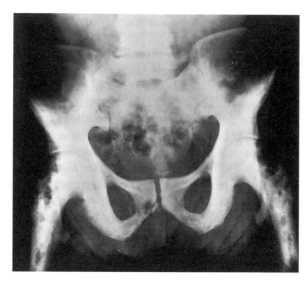

Figure 251
SYSTEMIC MASTOCYTOSIS
Radiograph shows extensive osteolytic and osteoblastic lesions of the femurs and pelvic bones in a patient with systemic mastocytosis. (Fig. 1 from Brunning RD, McKenna RW, Rosai J, et al. Systemic mastocytosis. Extracutaneous manifestations. Am J Surg Pathol 1983;7:425–38.)

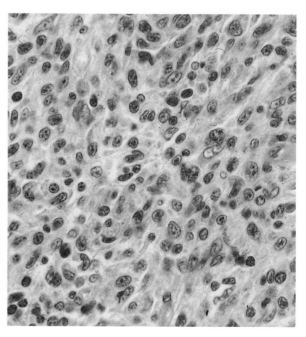

Figure 252
SYSTEMIC MASTOCYTOSIS
Mast cells with predominantly ovoid nuclei have eosinophilic cytoplasm and indistinct cell boundaries. A few lymphocytes are intermixed. (Courtesy of Dr. R.W. McKenna, Dallas, TX.)

Microscopic Findings. Mast cells are highly variable in appearance (figs. 252, 253). They may be round, irregular, or spindle shaped, with round, oval, indented, or elongated nuclei. Cell borders may be distinct or blurred. The cytoplasm ranges from pale to slightly eosinophilic. Mast cell granules are best visualized by their metachromatic staining with toluidine blue. Toluidine blue stains decalcified, paraffin-embedded tissue, and may be applied to decolorized hematoxylin and eosin stained sections (68). The chloroacetate esterase stain, which reacts with mast cells and neutrophils, can be used to identify mast cells in nondecalcified formalin-fixed specimens.

The bone marrow may be diffusely infiltrated (fig. 254), but more commonly has focal lesions that are perivascular, paratrabecular, or isolated in the fat. The focal lesions can be broadly classified into monomorphic or polymorphic types. The monomorphic type is composed mainly of mast cells with only a few lymphocytes or eosinophils interspersed. The polymorphic type contains, in addition to mast cells, many lymphocytes, neutrophils, eosinophils, histiocytes, and fibroblasts in varying proportions. Sometimes,

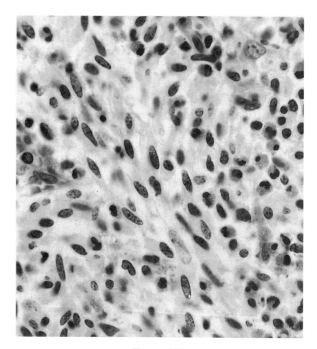

Figure 253
SYSTEMIC MASTOCYTOSIS
Mast cells are predominantly spindle shaped. A few eosinophils and lymphocytes are intermixed. (Courtesy of Dr. R.W. McKenna, Dallas, TX.)

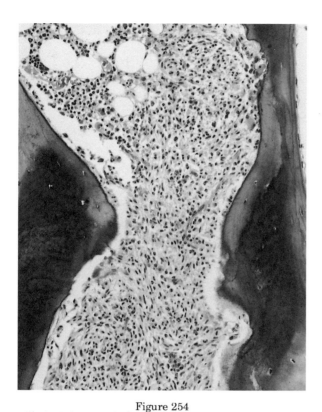

Figure 254
SYSTEMIC MASTOCYTOSIS
A bone marrow trephine biopsy shows diffuse involvement. (Courtesy of Dr. R.W. McKenna, Dallas, TX.)

lymphocytes form the center of the lesion with the mast cells around the periphery. The eosinophils that are scattered among the mast cells also may have their greatest concentration at the periphery of the lesion (68).

Differential Diagnosis. The differential diagnosis includes myelofibrosis, metastatic carcinoma, and large cell lymphoma. The differentiation from these other conditions relies on identifying the mast cells, which may require toluidine blue or chloroacetate esterase staining.

SINUS HISTIOCYTOSIS WITH MASSIVE LYMPHADENOPATHY (ROSAI-DORFMAN DISEASE)

Definition. Also known as Rosai-Dorfman disease (80), this is a rare, usually self-limited, non-neoplastic histiocytic proliferation which is distinct from eosinophilic granuloma. Although cervical lymphadenopathy is most common, a variety of organs, including bone may be affected. Osseous lesions occasionally occur without lymphadenopathy.

General Features. The cause of sinus histiocytosis with massive lymphadenopathy (SHML) is unknown, although the disease is thought to represent a defect in immune regulation, perhaps in response to an unknown pathogen. A registry of SHML has been established and currently includes over 420 cases. About 40 percent have extranodal disease and over 30 cases (8 percent) have osseous involvement. Nine of the 30 did not have associated lymphadenopathy (74). In several instances, SHML has presented as a solitary osseous lesion with no demonstrable extraosseous disease (75,77,79,82).

Clinical Features. In a review of all published cases of SHML, Foucar et al. (74) noted that the condition has occurred both congenitally and in a 74-year-old patient. The mean age is about 20 years, however, and most patients are in their second or third decades of life. Of patients in the SHML registry, 43.6 percent are black, 43.6 percent are white, 4.6 percent are oriental, and 8.2 percent are mixed or belong to other racial groups. Males predominate 58 to 42 percent. Two sets of identical twins and two sets of siblings with SHML have been reported, suggesting the possibility of a genetic predisposition or familial transmission of an unknown pathogen (74). Typically, SHML produces a group of clinical findings including painless, often massive cervical lymphadenopathy, fever, elevated sedimentation rate, leukocytosis, polyclonal hypergammaglobulinemia, and hypochromic or normochromic anemia (78).

Sites. Osseous lesions are often multiple and may involve virtually any bone. Involvement of the skull, facial bones, vertebrae, sacrum, long bones, phalanges, and ribs is common. Long bone lesions may be metaphyseal, diaphyseal, or epiphyseal, often with multiple lesions in the same bone. Some osseous involvement, especially in the region of the paranasal sinuses, appears to represent intraosseous extension from a primarily soft tissue mass.

Radiographic Appearance. Lytic lesions predominate, but blastic and mixed blastic/lytic examples have been described (81). Involvement is usually within the medullary cavity, with cortical defects occasionally occurring (81,83). The margins of the lytic defects have been described as somewhat fuzzy and lacking a sclerotic rim of

227

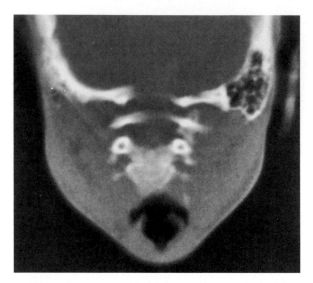

Figure 255
SINUS HISTIOCYTOSIS
A 19-year-old woman had a 3-cm mass palpable in the occipital region. A CT scan demonstrates an expansile, partly lytic lesion in the skull. (Courtesy of Dr. J.T. Wolfe III, Jacksonville, FL.) (Figures 255 and 256 are from the same patient.)

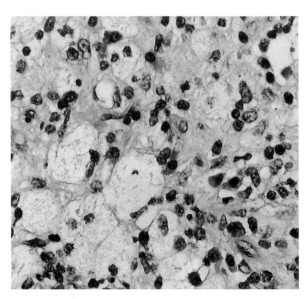

Figure 256
SINUS HISTIOCYTOSIS
Large, foamy histiocytes are intermixed with lymphocytes. The patient never developed lymphadenopathy and remains well 5 years later. (Courtesy of Dr. J.T. Wolfe III, Jacksonville, FL.)

reactive bone (fig. 255). Periosteal reaction and intralesional calcification have not been reported (83). Serial radiographs may document spontaneous, progressive decrease in the size of the defect with eventual complete resolution (83).

Gross Findings. Lewin et al. (77) described a "ray" amputation for SHML involving the distal metaphysis and epiphysis of the fifth metacarpal. Grossly, the medullary cavity was filled with a soft, yellow to white tumor mass. The cortical bone was thinned and partially destroyed, in association with a pathologic fracture. There were no areas of hemorrhage or necrosis, and a periosteal reaction was not described. Hamels et al. (75) described the curettage fragments from a patient with SHML as being "soft, fungoid fragments of a greyish colour."

Microscopic Findings. The findings on hematoxylin and eosin stained sections are usually diagnostic. The intertrabecular spaces are filled with a cellular, polymorphous infiltrate consisting of large histiocytes, lymphocytes, and plasma cells. The diagnostic histiocytes have vesicular, round to oval nuclei with smooth contours and distinct, small nucleoli (fig. 256). The cytoplasm is abundant and varies from eosinophilic to finely vacuolated and foamy. Phagocytosed lympho-

cytes, plasma cells, red blood cells, and neutrophils may be seen within the cell cytoplasm. This feature, particularly the phagocytosis of lymphocytes, is important diagnostically. Binucleate or multinucleate histiocytes may also be present, including some with the appearance of Touton giant cells. Mitotic figures in the histiocytic cells are extremely rare. Other cell types present include mature plasma cells, often with scattered Russell bodies, and neutrophils which tend to aggregate in small clumps; eosinophils are rare or absent.

The intralesional tissue typically contains sparse bony trabeculae, some of which may show osteoblastic rimming. The background stroma of SHML may exhibit a prominent fibroblastic component with storiform growth pattern. In such areas, the entrapped histiocytic cells assume a spindled configuration.

Ultrastructurally, the histiocytic cells contain complex cytoplasmic filopodia, lipid vacuoles, lysosomes, and phagocytosed cells and cell debris (74). They specifically lack the characteristic Birbeck or Langerhans cell granules typical of eosinophilic granuloma. Immunohistochemical stains, performed on paraffin-embedded tissue, demonstrate that the cells of SHML strongly express S-100 protein, strongly label with the macrophage marker Mac-387, and express other histiocytic markers, including lysozyme, alpha-1-antitrypsin, and alpha-1-antichymotrypsin (73,75, 79). Leu-22, a lymphoid marker, is also present in the majority of cases (73). T-cell and B-cell markers, seemingly expressed by the histiocytic cells, may represent phagocytosed lymphocytes.

Differential Diagnosis. The radiographic appearance of SHML may be easily confused with that of eosinophilic granuloma (histiocytosis X, Langerhans cell histiocytosis). However, the former lesion typically has more blurred radiographic margins and more commonly involves the bones of the hands and feet. The histiocytic cells of SHML lack the irregular nuclear contours, grooves, and indentations of Langerhans cells. Both cell types strongly express S-100 protein, but the cells of SHML also contain lysozyme, alpha-1-antitrypsin, alpha-1-antichymotrypsin, and stain with Mac-387 and Leu-22, markers which are lacking in eosinophilic granuloma (73).

Treatment and Prognosis. Of the 33 patients with osseous SHML reviewed by Foucar et al. (74), 3 died of disease, invariably secondary to involvement of multiple, nonosseous sites.

Most of the remainder were free of disease at last follow-up. Most patients require no therapy because the disease is usually self-limited and characterized by spontaneous regression (76). The course may be protracted, however. About 17 percent of patients have persistent symptoms after 5 to 10 years, and the longest described clinical course was said to be 30 years (78).

Occasionally, SHML will produce severe, multisystem disease that requires intervention. An ideal treatment regimen has not been identified. The best chemotherapy results, achieved with the combination of a vinca alkaloid, an alkalating agent, and corticosteroids, gives only about a 50 percent full or partial response rate (76). This is less than the chemotherapeutic response of malignant lymphomas or eosinophilic granuloma. Radiation therapy, at varying doses, gives a partial or complete response in only 33 percent of patients (76). Again, the responses, even at higher doses, are less than those expected of malignant lymphomas. Many of these "responses" may represent spontaneous regressions in patients receiving therapy. Surgical intervention is usually reserved for life-threatening obstruction of vital structures.

REFERENCES

Eosinophilic Granuloma

1. Birbeck MS, Breathnach AS, Everall JD. An electron microscopic study of basal melanocytes and high-level clear cell (Langerhans cell) in vitiligo. J Invest Dermatol 1961;37:51–64.
2. Cheyne C. Histiocytosis X. J Bone Joint Surg [Br] 1971;53:366–82.
3. Cozzuto C. Xanthogranulomatous osteomyelitis. Arch Pathol Lab Med 1984;108:973–6.
4. Favara BE, McCarthy RC, Mierau GW. Histiocytosis X. Hum Pathol 1983;14:663–76.
5. Fowles JV, Bobechko WP. Solitary eosinophilic granuloma in bone. J Bone Joint Surg [Br] 1970;52:238–43.
6. Gonzalez-Crussi F, Hsueh W, Wiederhold MD. Prostaglandins in histiocytosis-X. PG synthesis by histiocytosis-X cells. Am J Clin Pathol 1981;75:243–53.
7. Hammar S. Langerhans cells. Pathol Annu 1988;23(Pt 2):293–328.
8. Komp DM, Herson J, Starling KA, Vietti TJ, Hvizdala E. A staging system for histiocytosis X: a Southwest Oncology Group study. Cancer 1981;47:798–800.
9. McCullough CJ. Eosinophilic granuloma of bone. Acta Orthop Scand 1980;51:389–98.
10. Murphy GF. Cell membrane glycoproteins and Langerhans cells. Hum Pathol 1985;16:103–12.
11. Nauert C, Zornoza J, Ayala A, Harle TS. Eosinophilic granuloma of bone: diagnosis and management. Skeletal Radiol 1983;10:227–35.
12. Raney RB Jr, D'Angio GJ. Langerhans' cell histiocytosis (histiocytosis X): experience at the Children's Hospital of Philadelphia, 1970–1984. Med Pediatr Oncol 1989;17:20–8.
13. Ree HJ, Kadin ME. Peanut agglutinin. A useful marker for histiocytosis X and interdigitating reticulum cells. Cancer 1986;57:282–7.
14. Risdall RJ, Dehner LP, Duray P, Kobrinsky N, Robinson L, Nesbit ME Jr. Histiocytosis X (Langerhans' cell histiocytosis). Prognostic role of histopathology. Arch Pathol Lab Med 1983;107:59–63.
15. Wester SM, Beabout JW, Unni KK, Dahlin DC. Langerhans' cell granulomatosis (histiocytosis X) of bone in adults. Am J Surg Pathol 1982;6:413–26.

Multiple (Plasma Cell) Myeloma

16. Bardwick PA, Zvaifler NJ, Gill GN, Newman D, Greenway GD, Resnick DL. Plasma cell dyscrasia with polyneuropathy, organomegaly, endocrinopathy, M protein and skin changes: the POEMS syndrome. Report on two cases and a review of the literature. Medicine (Baltimore) 1980;59:311–22.
17. Bartl R, Frisch B, Fateh-Moghadam A, Kettner G, Jaeger K, Sommerfeld W. Histologic classification and staging of multiple myeloma: a retrospective and prospective study of 674 cases. Am J Clin Pathol 1987;87:342–55.
18. Dahlin DC, Unni KK. Bone tumors. General aspects and data on 8,542 cases. 4th ed. Springfield, Ill: Charles C. Thomas, 1986:194.
19. Gassmann W, Pralle H, Haferlach T, et al. Staging systems for multiple myeloma: a comparison. Br J Haematol 1985;59:703–11.
20. Greipp PR, Raymond NM, Kyle RA, O'Fallon WM. Multiple myeloma: significance of plasmablastic subtype in morphological classification. Blood 1985;65:305–10.
21. Hall FM, Gore SM. Osteosclerotic myeloma variants. Skeletal Radiol 1988;17:101–5.
22. Kyle RA. Multiple myeloma: review of 869 cases. Mayo Clin Proc 1975;50:29–40.
23. _____, Greipp PR. Smoldering multiple myeloma. N Engl J Med 1980;302:1347–9.
24. Osserman EF, Merlini G, Butler VP Jr. Multiple myeloma and related plasma cell dyscrasias. JAMA 1987;258:2930–7.
25. Peterson LC, Brown BA, Crosson JT, Mladenovic J. Application of the immunoperoxidase technic to bone marrow trephine biopsies in the classification of patients with monoclonal gammopathies. Am J Clin Pathol 1986; 85:688–93.
26. Reed M, McKenna RW, Bridges R, Parkin J, Frizzera G, Brunning RD. Morphologic manifestations of monoclonal gammopathies. Am J Clin Pathol 1981;76:8–23.
27. Strickler JG, Audeh MW, Copenhaver CM, Warnke RA. Immunophenotypic differences between plasmacytoma/multiple myeloma and immunoblastic lymphoma. Cancer 1988;61:1782–6.

Solitary (Plasma Cell) Myeloma

28. Dahlin DC, Unni KK. Bone tumors: general aspects and data on 8,542 cases. 4th ed. Springfield, Ill: Charles C. Thomas, 1986.
29. Frassica DA, Frassica FJ, Schray MF, Sim FH, Kyle RA. Solitary plasmacytoma of bone: Mayo Clinic experience. Int J Radiation Oncol Biol Phys 1989;16:43–8.
30. Greenberg P, Parker RG, Fu YS, Abemayor E. The treatment of solitary plasmacytoma of bone and extramedullary plasmacytoma. Am J Clin Oncol 1987;10:199–204.
31. Meis JM, Butler JJ, Osborne BM, Ordóñez NG. Solitary plasmacytomas of bone and extramedullary plasmacytomas. A clinicopathologic and immunohistochemical study. Cancer 1987;59:1475–85.

Osseous Lesions in Leukemias

32. Brünner S, Gudbjerg CE, Iversen T. Skeletal lesions in leukemia in children. Acta Radiol 1958;49:419–24.
33. Chabner BA, Haskell CM, Canellos GP. Destructive bone lesions in chronic granulocytic leukemia. Medicine (Baltimore) 1969;48:401–10.
34. Jaffe HL. Skeletal manifestations of leukemia and malignant lymphoma. Bull Hosp Joint Dis 1952;13:217–38.
35. Marsh WL Jr, Bylund DJ, Heath VC, Anderson MJ. Osteoarticular and pulmonary manifestations of acute leukemia. Case report and review of the literature. Cancer 1986;57:385–90.
36. Nixon GW, Gwinn JL. The roentgen manifestations of leukemia in infancy. Radiology 1973;107:603–9.
37. Parker BR, Marglin S, Castellino RA. Skeletal manifestations of leukemia, Hodgkin disease, and non-Hodgkin lymphoma. Semin Roentgenol 1980;15:302–15.
38. Thomas LB, Forkner CE Jr, Frei E III, Besse BE Jr, Stabenau JR. The skeletal lesions of acute leukemia. Cancer 1961;14:608–21.
39. Willson JK. The bone lesions of childhood leukemia: a survey of 140 cases. Radiology 1959;72:672–81.

Non-Hodgkin Lymphoma of Bone

40. Bacci G, Jaffe N, Emiliani E, et al. Therapy for primary non-Hodgkin's lymphoma of bone and a comparison of results with Ewing's sarcoma. Ten years' experience at the Istituto Ortopedico Rizzoli. Cancer 1986;57:1468–72.
41. Boston HC Jr, Dahlin DC, Ivins JC, Cupps RE. Malignant lymphoma (so-called reticulum cell sarcoma) of bone. Cancer 1974;34:1131-7.
42. Clayton F, Butler JJ, Ayala AG, Ro JY, Zornoza J. Non-Hodgkin's lymphoma in bone. Pathologic and radiologic features with clinical correlates. Cancer 1987;60:2494–501.
43. Dahlin DC, Unni KK. Bone tumors: general aspects and data on 8,542 cases. 4th ed. Springfield, Ill: Charles C. Thomas, 1986:208–26.
44. Dosoretz DE, Murphy GF, Raymond AK, et al. Radiation therapy for primary lymphoma of bone. Cancer 1983; 51:44–6.
45. _____, Raymond AK, Murphy GF, et al. Primary lymphoma of bone: the relationship of morphologic diversity to clinical behavior. Cancer 1982;50:1009–14.
46. Fiche M, Le Tourneau A, Audouin J, Touzard RC, Diebold J. A case of primary osseous malignant immunoblastic B-cell lymphoma with intracytoplasmic mu lambda immunoglobulin inclusions. Histopathology 1990;16:167–72.
47. Francis KC, Higinbotham NL, Coley BL. Primary reticulum cell sarcoma of bone. Report of 44 cases. Surg Gynecol Obstet 1954;99:142–6.
48. Huvos AG. Bone tumors: diagnosis, treatment, and prognosis. 2nd ed. Philadelphia: WB Saunders, 1991:625–37.
49. Ivins JC, Dahlin DC. Malignant lymphoma (reticulum cell sarcoma) of bone. Mayo Clin Proc 1963;38:375–85.
50. _____, Dahlin DC. Reticulum-cell sarcoma of bone. J Bone Joint Surg [Am] 1953;35:835–42.

51. McCormack LJ, Ivins JC, Dahlin DC, Johnson EW Jr. Primary reticulum-cell sarcoma of bone. Cancer 1952;5:1182–92.
52. Ostrowski ML, Unni KK, Banks PM, et al. Malignant lymphoma of bone. Cancer 1986;58:2646–55.
53. Parker F Jr, Jackson H Jr. Primary reticulum cell sarcoma of bone. Surg Gynecol Obstet 1939;68:45–53.
54. Pettit CK, Zukerberg LR, Gray MH, et al. Primary lymphoma of bone. A B-cell neoplasm with a high frequency of multilobated cells. Am J Surg Pathol 1990; 14:329–34.
55. Ueda T, Aozasa K, Ohsawa M, et al. Malignant lymphomas of bone in Japan. Cancer 1989;64:2387–92.
56. Vassallo J, Mellin W, Pill C, Roessner A, Grundmann E. Flow cytometric DNA analysis of malignant lymphomas with primary bone manifestation. J Cancer Res Clin Oncol 1987;113:249–52.
57. Wang CC, Fleischli DJ. Primary reticulum cell sarcoma of bone. With emphasis on radiation therapy. Cancer 1968;22:994–8.

Osseous Involvement by Hodgkin Disease

58. Beckstead JH, Wood GS, Turner RR. Histiocytosis X cells and Langerhans cells: enzyme histochemical and immunologic similarities. Hum Pathol 1984;15:826–33.
59. Frierson HF Jr, Innes DJ Jr. Sensitivity of anti-Leu-M1 as a marker in Hodgkin's disease. Arch Pathol Lab Med 1985;109:1024–8.
60. Gold RH, Mirra JM. Case report 101. Primary Hodgkin disease of humerus. Skeletal Radiol 1979;4:233–5.
61. Granger W, Whitaker R. Hodgkin's disease in bone, with special reference to periosteal reaction. Br J Radiol 1967;40:939–48.
62. Kaplan HS. Hodgkin's disease. 2nd ed. Cambridge: Harvard University Press, 1980:220–2.
63. Mills SE, Sloop FB Jr, Thiele AL, Miller CW, Zazakos CP Jr. Case report 251. Hodgkin disease, nodular sclerosing variant, primary form. Skeletal Radiol 1983;10:287–9.
64. Newcomer LN, Silverstein MB, Cadman EC, Farber LR, Bertino JR, Prosnitz LR. Bone involvement in Hodgkin's disease. Cancer 1982;49:338–42.
65. Pinkus GS, Thomas P, Said JW. Leu-M1—a marker for Reed-Sternberg cells in Hodgkin's disease. An immunoperoxidase study of paraffin-embedded tissues. Am J Pathol 1985;119:244–52.
66. Zukerberg LR, Collins AB, Ferry JA, Harris NL. Coexpression of CD15 and CD20 by Reed-Sternberg cells in Hodgkin's disease. Am J Pathol 1991;139:475–83.

Systemic Mastocytosis

67. Brinkley AB Jr, O'Brien MW. Case report 320. Localized eosinophilic fibrohistiocytic lesion of bone (tibia)—a localized form of mastocytosis. Skeletal Radiol 1985;14:68–72.
68. Brunning RD, McKenna RW, Rosai J, Parkin JL, Risdall R. Systemic mastocytosis. Extracutaneous manifestations. Am J Surg Pathol 1983;7:425–38.
69. Fallon MD, Whyte MP, Teitelbaum SL. Systemic mastocytosis associated with generalized osteopenia. Histopathological characterization of the skeletal lesion using uncalcified bone from two patients. Hum Pathol 1981;12:813–20.
70. Rafii M, Firooznia H, Golimbu C, Balthazar E. Pathologic fracture in systemic mastocytosis. Radiographic spectrum and review of the literature. Clin Orthop 1983;180:260–7.
71. Rosenbaum RC, Frieri M, Metcalfe DD. Patterns of skeletal scintigraphy and their relationship to plasma and urinary histamine levels in systemic mastocytosis. J Nucl Med 1984;25:859–64.
72. Webb TA, Li CY, Yam LT. Systemic mast cell disease: a clinical and hematopathologic study of 26 cases. Cancer 1982;49:927–38.

Sinus Histiocytosis with Massive Lymphadenopathy (Rosai-Dorfman Disease)

73. Eisen RN, Buckley PJ, Rosai J. Immunophenotypic characterization of sinus histiocytosis with massive lymphadenopathy (Rosai-Dorfman disease). Semin Diagn Pathol 1990;7:74–82.
74. Foucar E, Rosai J, Dorfman RF. Sinus histiocytosis with massive lymphadenopathy (Rosai-Dorfman disease): review of the entity. Semin Diagn Pathol 1990;7:19–73.
75. Hamels J, Fiasse L, Thiery J. Atypical lymphohistiocytic bone tumour (osseous variant of Rosai-Dorfman disease?). Virchows Arch [A] 1985;408:183–9.
76. Komp DM. The treatment of sinus histiocytosis with massive lymphadenopathy (Rosai-Dorfman disease). Semin Diagn Pathol 1990;7:83–6.
77. Lewin JR, Das SK, Blumenthal BI, D'Cruz C, Patel RB, Howell GE. Osseous pseudotumor. The sole manifestation of sinus histiocytosis with massive lymphadenopathy. Am J Clin Pathol 1985;84:547–50.
78. McAlister WH, Herman T, Dehner LP. Sinus histiocytosis with massive lymphadenopathy (Rosai-Dorfman disease). Pediatr Radiol 1990;20:425–32.
79. Nawroz IM, Wilson-Storey D. Sinus histiocytosis with massive lymphadenopathy (Rosai-Dorfman disease). Histopathology 1989;14:91–9.
80. Rosai J, Dorfman RF. Sinus histiocytosis with massive lymphadenopathy. A newly recognized benign clinicopathological entity. Arch Pathol 1969;87:63–70.
81. Sartoris DJ, Resnick D. Osseous involvement in sinus histiocytosis with massive lymphadenopathy (Rosai-Dorfman disease) [Letter]. Eur J Pediatr 1986;145:238–40.
82. Unni KK. Case report 457. Sinus histiocytosis with massive lymphadenopathy (Rosai-Dorfman disease) presenting as a lesion in the sacrum. Skeletal Radiol 1988;17:129–32.
83. Walker PD, Rosai J, Dorfman RF. The osseous manifestations of sinus histiocytosis with massive lymphadenopathy. Am J Clin Pathol 1981;75:131–9.

EXTRAGNATHIC ADAMANTINOMA

Definition. A primary intraosseous epithelial neoplasm of low-grade malignancy which shows a marked predilection for the tibia and is often associated with osteofibrous dysplasia.

General Features. In the second series Fascicle on bone tumors, adamantinoma was listed as a tumor of uncertain differentiation, although it was noted that ultrastructural studies had suggested epithelial features (13). Subsequent electron microscopic and immunohistochemical studies have firmly established extragnathic adamantinoma as an intraosseous epithelial neoplasm (6,8,12,14). More than 200 cases have been reported (11). Even before its epithelial nature was confirmed, the microscopic resemblance of this tumor to gnathic adamantinoma (ameloblastoma) was noted, giving rise to its name. Although the pathogenesis of extragnathic adamantinoma is uncertain, it seems clear that it is unrelated to its gnathic counterpart. Adamantinomas of the gnathic bones presumably arise from the odontogenic epithelial apparatus, epithelium that is lacking in the tibia or other extragnathic bones.

Pretibial soft tissue adamantinomas without an osseous component have been reported (2,7,10). Mills and Rosai (10) suggested that some intraosseous adamantinomas may begin as pretibial soft tissue neoplasms that subsequently erode the underlying bone. Other studies have noted morphologic, ultrastructural, histochemical, and immunohistochemical similarities between extragnathic adamantinoma and cutaneous eccrine carcinoma (3,6).

The association of adamantinoma with an intraosseous fibro-osseous proliferation has been recognized for half a century. Although this component was often called fibrous dysplasia, it is now clear that it more closely resembles osteofibrous dysplasia, both microscopically and radiographically. In fact, Czerniak et al. (5) postulate that osteofibrous dysplasia is a secondary reparative process that overgrows regressing adamantinomas. It is possible that osteofibrous dysplasia is the end result of the total elimination of an adamantinoma, although some cases of osteofibrous dysplasia may arise de novo, unrelated to an epithelial neoplasm.

It now seems reasonable to divide adamantinoma into two categories: *classic* and *differentiated*. The classic tumors usually present in older patients, grow beyond the cortex, and sometimes metastasize. The differentiated adamantinomas occur at an earlier age, are confined to the cortex, and do not metastasize. The subsequent discussion does not distinguish between the two forms, because published reports rarely have made a distinction.

Clinical Features. Patients range from 3 to 72 years of age, although occurrence in the first decade of life is distinctly uncommon. About 50 percent of tumors present in the second or third decade, and the remainder are fairly evenly distributed in the remaining decades. Most studies indicate that males and females are affected equally, although some have reported a male predominance. Patients complain of pain and swelling, painless swelling, or pain alone. A few present with pathologic fracture. A history of localized trauma can be elicited in up to 50 percent of cases, but the role, if any, of trauma in the development of this lesion remains unclear. The duration of symptoms ranges from a few weeks to 50 years (7). Approximately one third have symptoms of from 1 to 4 years' duration and another third have symptoms for longer than 5 years.

Sites. There is a striking predilection for the tibia, which accounts for almost 90 percent of cases. The diaphyseal portion of the bone is favored; involvement of the metaphyses is less common. A small number of patients have an ipsilateral fibular tumor, in addition to their tibial lesion. Purported adamantinomas also have been described in the femur, ulna, humerus, radius, fibula, ischium, and small bones of the hands and feet.

Radiographic Appearance. Extragnathic adamantinoma typically produces an eccentric, sharply defined osteolytic defect, often with a lobulated, multicystic, or "soap bubble" configuration (fig. 257). There may be considerable perilesional sclerosis. Although most lesions are centered in the midshaft, larger examples often

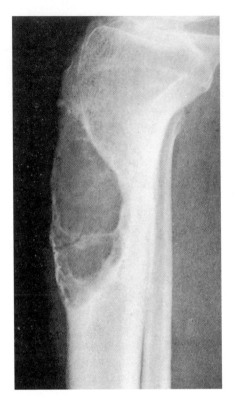

Figure 257
ADAMANTINOMA
Lateral view of a tibia in a 44-year-old man shows an expanding destructive lesion with sharply defined margins. The tumor had been curetted and packed with bone chips; however, it persisted and was still expanding 14 years later. (Fig. 344B from Fascicle 5, 2nd Series.) (Figures 257 and 260 are from the same patient.)

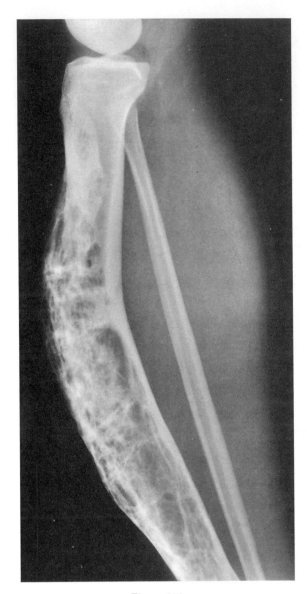

Figure 258
ADAMANTINOMA AND
OSTEOFIBROUS DYSPLASIA
Most of the tibia in this 19-year-old woman is involved with a lytic and sclerotic lesion causing anterior bowing. Biopsy specimens obtained at 2 years of age and again at 19 years of age were microscopically identical. The patient has had no therapy and is asymptomatic at the age of 21 years. (Courtesy of Dr. J.A. Richman, Cooperstown, NY.) (Figures 258 and 259 are from the same patient.)

extend to the metaphysis; occasionally they arise in the metaphyseal region. Lesions arising in the medullary cavity often asymmetrically expand the overlying cortex, which remains intact in most cases. In tibial lesions, the expansion is often along the anterior surface of the bone (fig. 258). Approximately 15 percent of extragnathic adamantinomas penetrate the cortex and have an associated soft tissue component. About 90 percent of all cases involve both the cortical and medullary portions of the bone; only about 10 percent are confined to the cortex (7). Occasional extragnathic adamantinomas appear to arise in a juxtacortical location with an extensive soft tissue component and erosion of the outer cortex.

Gross Findings. The sharp demarcation of the lesion seen radiographically is also a gross feature. Often a distinctly lobulated configuration can be seen as well. Solid areas are soft to firm, gray or white, and granular or fibrous in consistency. Cystic spaces and areas of intralesional hemorrhage are common. More than 80 percent of the tumors are at least 5 cm in length, and some involve the entire shaft (7).

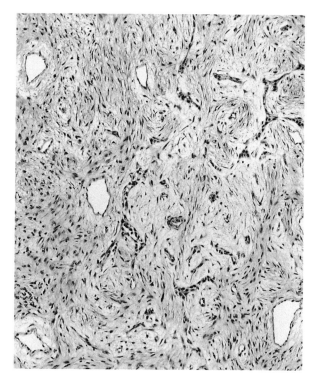

Figure 259
ADAMANTINOMA

Small, irregular strands of plump cells with hyperchromatic nuclei are surrounded by haphazardly arranged spindle cells in a fibrous stroma. The strands of cells, as well as scattered stromal spindle cells, were keratin positive. (Courtesy of Dr. H.D. Alpern, Cooperstown, NY.)

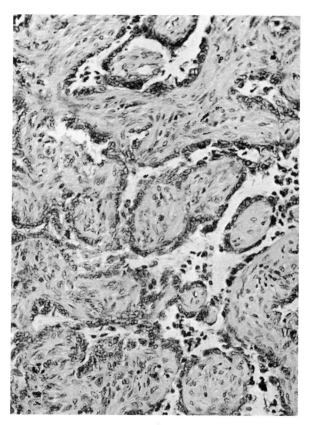

Figure 260
ADAMANTINOMA

Anastomosing, epithelial-lined spaces impart a pseudovascular appearance. The intervening stroma has plump cells that are probably neoplastic. (Fig. 345 from Fascicle 5, 2nd Series.)

Microscopic Findings. There is an enormous diversity of the epithelial elements. Four basic histologic patterns have been described: spindled, basaloid, tubular, and squamoid (4,16). The most difficult pattern to recognize is a spindle cell proliferation with a storiform, "herringbone" or fascicular appearance. The plump spindle cells are situated in a loose fibrous tissue background and may be virtually indistinguishable from reactive fibroblasts. The spindle cells may gradually assume an outline around small tubule-like empty spaces.

The more clearly defined epithelial elements are situated in a loose or dense fibrous stroma and may assume many low-power configurations. They may form tubular structures lined by one or two cells, which sometimes branch and anastomose (fig. 259). In cross section, they appear as small, vascular-like tubules with well-formed lumens (fig. 260). The basaloid pattern has a peripheral layer of cuboidal cells more or less oriented at right angles to the inner cell masses. The central cells may form solid nests or have irregular lumens and a papillary pattern.

Extragnathic adamantinomas may have areas of squamous differentiation (fig. 261). These can range from immature, basaloid squamous cells with scant cytoplasm arranged in whorls to more mature-appearing squamous epithelium, occasionally with overt keratinization. The squamous cells may be present as nests, cords, or larger, solid, circumscribed, or stellate arrangements.

Regardless of the low-power pattern of extragnathic adamantinoma or its cytologic appearance, the nuclei are usually bland. Nuclear atypia is present in only about 15 percent of tumors and the degree of atypia is minimal (7). Mitotic figures are usually absent, but may be as numerous as 10 per 10 high-power fields (4).

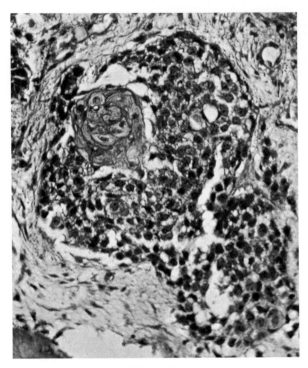

Figure 261
ADAMANTINOMA
This basaloid nest of adamantinoma contains an aggregate of larger, squamous cells. (Fig. 348 from Fascicle 5, 2nd Series.)

When osteofibrous dysplasia accompanies adamantinoma, the osteofibrous areas may predominate with only rare epithelial structures (5). If the epithelium is a simple tubule cut in cross section, it may be indistinguishable from blood vessels and require immunohistochemical staining for cytokeratin or other epithelial markers to confirm its epithelial nature. The zonation seen in pure osteofibrous dysplasia is maintained in osteofibrous dysplasia associated with adamantinoma (1).

Differential Diagnosis. As discussed above, extragnathic adamantinomas may contain osteofibrous dysplasia–like areas. In some cases, this component may dominate, and the epithelial elements, particularly if of the spindle cell pattern, may be overlooked. Immunohistochemical stains for epithelial markers may be of value for identifying the epithelial component. It should be noted, however, that isolated cytokeratin-positive cells are a common finding in otherwise typical osteofibrous dysplasia (15).

Extragnathic adamantinoma may be confused, microscopically, with metastatic carcinoma, although the diverse epithelial pattern present in most adamantinomas, as well as their bland cytologic appearance, would be quite unusual for a metastatic carcinoma. The radiograph provides important clues for distinction. The soap bubble appearance of adamantinoma would rarely be duplicated by metastatic carcinoma.

The tubular pattern of adamantinoma may be misinterpreted as a vascular neoplasm, such as an epithelioid hemangioendothelioma. Often, other more obviously epithelial areas will be present, allowing ready distinction. Strong immunohistochemical staining for multiple epithelial markers and lack of staining for endothelial markers such as factor VIII–related antigen allows recognition of adamantinoma in cases not readily interpreted by light microscopic features alone.

The tubular pattern of extragnathic adamantinoma, in conjunction with a prominent stroma, leads to a biphasic appearance reminiscent of synovial sarcoma. Indeed, there are published reports of tibial adamantinoma under the rubric of "synovial sarcoma." In this instance, immunohistochemical positivity for epithelial markers is of no value, or may further the confusion, if adamantinoma has not been considered as a diagnostic possibility. The stroma of adamantinoma, however, lacks the marked cellularity and pleomorphism of synovial sarcoma.

Treatment and Prognosis. As many as 60 percent of patients treated with curettage have local recurrence, which can include implants in the soft tissue (7). Recurrences may develop from a few months to 26 years after initial therapy (9). Patients treated with wide excision have a lower rate of local recurrence.

The metastatic potential of adamantinoma is considerable. In one series, 5 of 20 patients treated initially with amputation died of metastatic disease (7). The long interval between initial therapy and the occurrence of regional lymph node metastases or distant metastases requires lifelong follow-up. Lymph node metastases can appear up to 15 years after initial diagnosis (7). Pulmonary metastases can occur from 1 to 15 years after amputation. Metastases may involve bones, as well as lungs and lymph nodes.

There is considerable variation in reporting features associated with an increased risk of metastases. At the moment, there does not seem to be a constant association with age, duration of symptoms, or histologic features. Some lesions with virtually no mitotic activity in the original material may have an increased mitotic rate (6 mitotic figures per 50 high-power fields) in metastases (16). The metastases usually duplicate the histologic spectrum of appearances seen in the primary tumor. Occasionally, however, different patterns are seen, such as a squamoid element that was not present in the primary tumor (16). Others have described a sarcomatous appearance in the metastases (11).

REFERENCES

1. Alguacil-Garcia A, Alonso A, Pettigrew NM. Osteofibrous dysplasia (ossifying fibroma) of the tibia and fibula and adamantinoma. A case report. Am J Clin Pathol 1984;82:470–4.

2. Bambirra EA, Noguerira AM, Miranda D. Adamantinoma of the soft tissue of the leg [Letter]. Arch Pathol Lab Med 1983;107:500–1.

3. Brandt H, Albores-Saavedra J, Mora-Tiscareño A. Eccrine sweat gland carcinoma. Its microscopic and ultrastructural similarity to adamantinoma of long bones. Patologia 1977;15:33–43.

4. Campanacci M, Giunti A, Bertoni F, Laus M, Gitelis S. Adamantinoma of the long bones. The experience at the Istituto Ortopedico Rizzoli. Am J Surg Pathol 1981; 5:533–42.

5. Czerniak B, Rojas-Corona RR, Dorfman HD. Morphologic diversity of long bone adamantinoma. The concept of differentiated (regressing) adamantinoma and its relationship to osteofibrous dysplasia. Cancer 1989;64:2319–34.

6. Eisenstein W, Pitcock JA. Adamantinoma of the tibia. An eccrine carcinoma. Arch Pathol Lab Med 1984;108:246–50.

7. Keeney GL, Unni K, Beabout JW, Pritchard DJ. Adamantinoma of long bones. A clinicopathologic study of 85 cases. Cancer 1989;64:730–7.

8. Knapp RH, Wick MR, Scheithauer BW, Unni KK. Adamantinoma of bone. An electron microscopic and immunohistochemical study. Virchows Arch [A] 1982;398:75–86.

9. Markel SF. Ossifying fibroma of long bone: its distinction from fibrous dysplasia and its association with adamantinoma of long bone. Am J Clin Pathol 1978;69:91–7.

10. Mills SE, Rosai J. Adamantinoma of the pretibial soft tissue. Clinicopathologic features, differential diagnosis, and possible relationship to intraosseous disease. Am J Clin Pathol 1985;83:108–14.

11. Moon NF, Mori H. Adamantinoma of the appendicular skeleton—updated. Clin Orthop 1986;204:215–37.

12. Perez-Atayde AR, Kozakewich HP, Vawter GF. Adamantinoma of the tibia. An ultrastructural and immunohistochemical study. Cancer 1985;55:1015–23.

13. Rosai J. Adamantinoma of the tibia. Electron microscopic evidence of its epithelial origin. Am J Clin Pathol 1969;51:786–92.

14. _____, Pinkus GS. Immunohistochemical demonstration of epithelial differentiation in adamantinoma of the tibia. Am J Surg Pathol 1982;6:427–34.

15. Sweet DE, Vinh TN, Devaney K. Cortical osteofibrous dysplasia of long bone and its relationship to adamantinoma. A clinicopathologic study of 30 cases. Am J Surg Pathol 1992;16:282–90.

16. Weiss SW, Dorfman HD. Adamantinoma of long bone. An analysis of nine new cases with emphasis on metastasizing lesions and fibrous dysplasia-like changes. Hum Pathol 1977;8:141–53.

❖❖❖

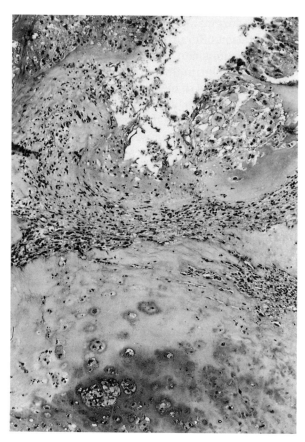

Figure 264
CHONDROID CHORDOMA
In addition to conventional elements of chordoma (top), areas of cartilaginous differentiation are present (bottom). (Fig. 8-12 from Mills SE, Fechner RE. Tumors and tumorlike lesions of the craniofacial bones and cervical vertebrae. In: Gnepp DR, ed. Pathology of the head and neck. New York: Churchill Livingstone, 1988:359–401.)

lacunae separated by a stroma of hyaline cartilage. The chondrocytes may be minimally atypical, as in an enchondroma, or moderately pleomorphic, simulating a low-grade chondrosarcoma. The proportion of cartilaginous tissue ranges from scant to predominant. Even a single microscopic focus of clear-cut cartilaginous differentiation appears to be sufficient to place the neoplasm in this prognostically more favorable subgroup.

Differential Diagnosis. There are two potential pitfalls associated with these tumors, depending on the amount of chondroid material present. If the chondroid component is a minor element, it may be missed on limited sampling or overlooked on cursory microscopic examination.

Alternately, if the majority of the tumor is cartilaginous, the chordoma element may be overlooked, leading to a misdiagnosis of chondroma, osteochondroma, or low-grade chondrosarcoma. To avoid these problems, all chordomas and cartilage-containing lesions arising in the spheno-occipital region should be completely sectioned and carefully examined microscopically.

Treatment and Prognosis. Local recurrences almost invariably develop and account for the very high long-term mortality. Unlike conventional chordoma, however, survival is markedly prolonged. The mean survival in the series by Heffelfinger et al. (15) was 15.8 years, as compared to 4.1 years for conventional chordomas.

"DEDIFFERENTIATED" CHORDOMA

Definition. A biphasic, clinically distinctive neoplasm consisting, in part, of conventional chordoma or, rarely, a chondroid chordoma with a secondary component of high-grade sarcoma. The latter most commonly resembles malignant fibrous histiocytoma.

General Features. Conventional chordomas may display considerable pleomorphism that is of no apparent prognostic importance. Occasionally, however, there may be zones of overt sarcoma, or a sarcoma may arise at the site of a previously excised chordoma (2,6,10,18,19,22,25,27–29). This was first described by Debernardi in 1913 (10), and several cases have been documented. Because of the analogy between this phenomenon and similar transformations in low-grade cartilaginous and lipogenic tumors, these neoplasms have been viewed as "dedifferentiated" chordomas. We realize, as have others (19), that this term is probably incorrect mechanistically, because the sarcoma more likely represents a "failure of differentiation" by primitive, mitotically active cells, rather than a "dedifferentiation" of end-stage chordoma cells. Nonetheless, the term adequately conveys the resultant transformation and has gained acceptance.

Clinical Features. It is uncommon for the sarcoma to be present within a chordoma at the time of initial diagnosis. Typically, there is a history of multiple recurrences over many years before a sarcoma is identified. Some of these patients had received radiation therapy, and it may be argued that the transformation was radiation

242

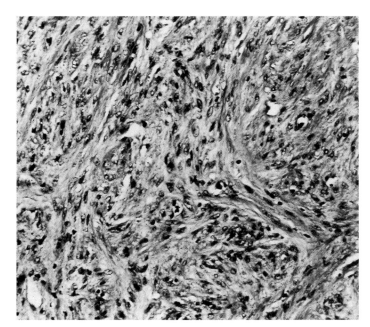

Figure 265
DEDIFFERENTIATED CHORDOMA
This tumor with the appearance of malignant fibrous histiocytoma occurred in the site of a previously typical chordoma. (Fig. 8-13 from Mills SE, Fechner RE. Tumors and tumorlike lesions of the craniofacial bones and cervical vertebrae. In: Gnepp DR, ed. Pathology of the head and neck. New York: Churchill Livingstone, 1988:359–401.)

induced, but in other instances only surgical excision was employed.

Sites. Dedifferentiation appears to be more common in sacrococcygeal chordomas, than in vertebral or spheno-occipital tumors. However, in their study of chordomas from the skull base, Heffelfinger et al. (15) identified two conventional chordomas that had high-grade sarcomatous components in their recurrences.

Microscopic Findings. Usually, the sarcomas resemble a malignant fibrous histiocytoma (fig. 265) (2,25,27–29), but elements of so-called fibrosarcoma, osteosarcoma, and high-grade chondrosarcoma have also been described (6,15, 18,27). It is somewhat surprising that chordoma, a tumor with predominantly epithelial features both ultrastructurally and immunohistochem-

ically, should give rise to a sarcomatous component, but this has been observed in multiple instances, and the sarcomatous elements have predominantly mesenchymal features, immunohistochemically and ultrastructurally (19,29). Interestingly, the notochord from which these tumors appear to arise has been postulated to have a dual ectodermal and mesenchymal origin (19).

Treatment and Prognosis. Once a high-grade sarcoma has developed, the prognosis worsens considerably, and hematogenous metastases composed solely of the sarcomatous elements typically occur. Because of their marked effect on prognosis, all chordomas, but particularly recurrent lesions, should be sectioned carefully to exclude the possibility of a high-grade sarcomatous component.

REFERENCES

1. Abenoza P, Sibley RK. Chordoma: an immunohistologic study. Hum Pathol 1986;17:744–7.
2. Belza MG, Urich H. Chordoma and malignant fibrous histiocytoma. Evidence for transformation. Cancer 1986; 598:1082–7.
3. Berdal P, Myhre E. Cranial chordomas involving the paranasal sinuses. J Laryngol Otol 1964;78:906–19.
4. Bottles K, Beckstead JH. Enzyme histochemical characterization of chordomas. Am J Surg Pathol 1984;8:443–7.
5. Brooks JJ, LiVolsi VA, Trojanowski JQ. Does chondroid chordoma exist? Acta Neuropathol (Berl) 1987;72:229–35.
6. Chambers PW, Schwinn CP. Chordoma. A clinicopathologic study of metastasis. Am J Clin Pathol 1979; 72:765–76.
7. Chu TA. Chondroid chordoma of the sacrococcygeal region. Arch Pathol Lab Med 1987;111:861–4.
8. Dahlin DC, MacCarty CS. Chordoma. A study of fifty-nine cases. Cancer 1952;5:1170–8.

9. _____, Unni KK. Bone tumors: general aspects and data on 8,542 cases. Springfield, Ill: Charles C. Thomas, 1986;379–93.

10. Debernardi L. Cordoma sarcomatose del sacro contributo alla conoscenza istologica e clinica dei tumori di origine cordale. Arch Sci Med [Torino] 1913;37:404–42.

11. de Vries J, Oldhoff J, Hadders HN. Cryosurgical treatment of sacrococcygeal chordoma. Report of four cases. Cancer 1986;58:2348–54.

12. Ericksson B, Gunterberg B, Kindblom LG. Chordoma. A clinicopathologic and prognostic study of a Swedish national series. Acta Orthop Scand 1981;52:49–58.

13. Falconer MA, Bailey IC, Duchen LW. Surgical treatment of chordoma and chondroma of the skull base. J Neurosurg 1968;29:261–75.

14. Friedmann I, Harrison DF, Bird ES. The fine structure of chordoma with particular reference to the physaliphorous cell. J Clin Pathol 1962;15:116–25.

15. Heffelfinger MJ, Dahlin DC, MacCarty CS, Beabout JW. Chordomas and cartilaginous tumors at the skull base. Cancer 1973;32:410–20.

16. Higinbotham NL, Phillips RF, Farr HW, Hustu HO. Chordoma. Thirty-five-year study at Memorial Hospital. Cancer 1967;20:1841–50.

17. Hizawa K, Inaba H, Nakanishi S, Otsuka H, Izumi K. Subcutaneous pseudosarcomatous polyvinylpyrrolidone granuloma. Am J Surg Pathol 1984;8:393–8.

18. Hruban RH, May M, Marcove RC, Huvos AG. Lumbosacral chordoma with high-grade malignant cartilaginous and spindle cell components. Am J Surg Pathol 1990;14:384–9.

19. _____, Traganos F, Reuter VE, Huvos AG. Chordomas with malignant spindle cell components. A DNA flow cytometric and immunohistochemical study with histogenetic implications. Am J Pathol 1990;137:435–47.

20. Huvos AG. Bone tumors: diagnosis, treatment, and prognosis. 2nd ed. Philadelphia: WB Saunders, 1991:599–624.

21. Kaiser TE, Pritchard DJ, Unni KK. Clinicopathologic study of sacrococcygeal chordoma. Cancer 1984;53:2574–8.

22. Knechtges TC. Sacrococcygeal chordoma with sarcomatous features (spindle cell metaplasia). Am J Clin Pathol 1970;53:612–6.

23. Kuo TT, Hsueh S. Mucicarminophilic histiocytosis. A polyvinylpyrrolidone (PVP) storage disease simulating signet-ring adenocarcinoma. Am J Surg Pathol 1984;8:419–28.

24. Mabrey RE. Chordoma. A study of 150 cases. Am J Cancer 1935;25:501–17.

25. Makek M, Leu HJ. Malignant fibrous histiocytoma arising in a recurrent chordoma. Case report and electron microscopic findings. Virchows Arch [A] 1982;397:241–50.

26. Meis JM, Giraldo AA. Chordoma. An immunohistochemical study of 20 cases. Arch Pathol Lab Med 1988;112:553–6.

27. _____, Raymond AK, Evans HL, Charles RE, Giraldo AA. "Dedifferentiated" chordoma. A clinicopathologic and immunohistochemical study of three cases. Am J Surg Pathol 1987;11:516–25.

28. Miettinen M, Karaharju E, Järvinen H. Chordoma with a massive spindle-cell sarcomatous transformation. A light- and electron-microscopic and immunohistological study. Am J Surg Pathol 1987;11:563–70.

29. _____, Lehto VP, Virtanen I. Malignant fibrous histiocytoma within a recurrent chordoma. A light microscopic, electron microscopic, and immunohistochemical study. Am J Clin Pathol 1984;82:738–43.

30. Murad TM, Murthy MS. Ultrastructure of chordoma. Cancer 1970;25:1204–15.

31. Pardo-Mindan FJ, Guillen FJ, Villas C, Vazquez JJ. A comparative ultrastructural study of chondrosarcoma, chordoid sarcoma, and chordoma. Cancer 1981;47:2611–9.

32. Pena CE, Horvat BL, Fisher ER. The ultrastructure of chordoma. Am J Clin Pathol 1970;53:544–51.

33. Perzin KH, Pushparaj N. Nonepithelial tumors of the nasal cavity, paranasal sinuses, and nasopharynx. A clinicopathologic study. XIV: Chordomas. Cancer 1986;57:784–96.

34. Rich TA, Schiller A, Suit HD, Mankin HJ. Clinical and pathologic review of 48 cases of chordoma. Cancer 1985;56:182–7.

35. Rutherfoord GS, Davies AG. Chordomas—ultrastructure and immunohistochemistry: a report based on the examination of six cases. Histopathology 1987;11:775–87.

36. Salisbury JR, Isaacson PG. Demonstration of cytokeratins and an epithelial membrane antigen in chordomas and human fetal notochord. Am J Surg Pathol 1985;9:791–7.

37. _____, Isaacson PG. Distinguishing chordoma from chondrosarcoma by immunohistochemical techniques [Letter]. J Pathol 1986;148:251–2.

38. Spjut HJ, Luse SA. Chordoma: an electron microscopic study. Cancer 1964;17:643–56.

39. Valderrama E, Kahn LB, Lipper S, Marc J. Chondroid chordoma. Electron-microscopic study of two cases. Am J Surg Pathol 1983;7:625–32.

40. Volpe R, Mazabraud A. A clinicopathologic review of 25 cases of chordoma (a pleomorphic and metastasizing neoplasm). Am J Surg Pathol 1983;7:161–70.

41. Walker WP, Landas SK, Bromley CM, Sturm MT. Immunohistochemical distinction of classic and chondroid chondromas. Mod Pathol 1991;4:661–6.

42. Weiss SW. Ultrastructure of the so-called "chordoid sarcoma." Evidence supporting cartilaginous differentiation. Cancer 1976;37:300–6.

43. Wick MR, Burgess JH, Manivel JC. A reassessment of "chordoid sarcoma." Ultrastructural and immunohistochemical comparison with chordoma and skeletal myxoid chondrosarcoma. Mod Pathol 1988;1:433–43.

✧✧✧

METASTATIC TUMORS INVOLVING BONE

Definition. A secondary osseous neoplasm that arises from detached, transported cells of a primary tumor and grows separately from it.

General Features. Virtually every malignant neoplasm has been reported to have metastasized to bone, including such rarely metastasizing tumors as paraganglioma (26) and basal cell carcinoma (2). In most patients with osseous metastases, the lesions are multiple, there is a known primary tumor, and the skeletal involvement is not biopsied. However, some patients with occult visceral tumors present with osseous metastases. If the osseous lesions are multiple, they are often assumed to be metastases, but unless a primary site can be found, a bone biopsy must be performed to firmly establish the diagnosis. If the osseous metastasis is solitary, it is often clinically confused with a primary bone tumor, and may be biopsied without a thorough evaluation for an undetected primary neoplasm. Patients with multiple primary tumors often require biopsy of osseous metastases to determine which form of neoplasia has metastasized. In one series of 319 patients with skeletal metastases due to carcinoma of the breast, 22 (7 percent) had a concomitant second malignancy (20).

In a series of 1,000 consecutive autopsies of patients who died of carcinoma, metastases to bone were found in 27 percent (1). If extensive sampling directed at detecting metastases is carried out, skeletal metastases occur in at least 70 percent of patients (14). For the most common carcinomas (breast, lung, prostate, kidney, and thyroid), the frequency of skeletal metastasis is approximately 85 percent (14). One cannot rely on clinical radiographs for the identification of metastatic sites. Radiographs of the spine removed at autopsy failed to show tumor in 13 of 30 patients with grossly visible metastases (39). Specimen radiographs of 4 mm slices of vertebrae were more sensitive, but still failed to detect many different kinds of metastatic cancer (8).

Metastatic tumor cells primarily reach the bones via the venous and arterial vascular systems. The vertebral plexus of veins (Batson plexus) lacks venous valves to control blood flow. Therefore, when pressure is increased in the

chest or abdomen, such as during exhalation, blood may bypass the caval systems and flow into the vertebral plexus. The latter is in continuity with the veins of the vertebrae, shoulder girdle, and skull. It is likely that this is the major pathway for skeletal metastases from carcinomas of the kidney, urinary bladder, prostate, gastrointestinal tract, and breast (3).

Metastases to the hands and feet (acrometastases) are uncommon, but can be the initial presentation of an occult carcinoma (12). These are arterially borne metastases, most often from the lung. Pulmonary carcinomas readily invade pulmonary veins and, unlike other venous metastases, the tumor cells rapidly enter the arterial circulation without being filtered by pulmonary capillaries. Libson et al. (18) have suggested that some metastases to the bones of the feet may be due to retrograde venous flow. They point out that there are communications between the Batson plexus in the lumbar region and the iliofemoral venous system. In patients with venous valvular incompetence, tumor emboli might descend on a gravitational basis. This could explain the relatively high percentage of intra-abdominal neoplasms, especially colorectal carcinomas, that metastasize to the bones of the feet.

Lymphatics, another potential conduit for metastases, are present in the periosteum and accompany the nutrient vessels. Although difficult or impossible to detect in normal bones, intraosseous lymphatics have been demonstrated in patients with lymphedema (37).

The interaction between metastatic tumor and bone almost always involves both osteoblastic and osteoclastic activity. It is the balance between these factors that determines whether a metastasis has a radiographically lytic or blastic appearance (9). Diffusible activating factors are probably produced by tumor cells, because activation of osteoblasts and osteoclasts at a distance of several hundred microns from the nearest tumor cell has been demonstrated (6). Furthermore, carcinomas adjacent to, but not directly involving, ribs have been shown to stimulate osteoclasts and osteoblasts in the underlying cortical and cancellous bone (6).

Malignant cells secrete many factors that stimulate osteoclasts including several growth factors, prostaglandins, cytokines, transforming growth factors alpha and beta, and platelet-derived growth factor (23). The release of these substances from metastatic cells probably accounts for the increased numbers and activity of osteoclasts, inducing bone resorption. The cells of squamous carcinoma have been shown in one in vitro study to produce interleukin-1, one of the most potent stimulators of bone resorption (32). Macrophages, another source of osteoclast activating factors, can account for up to 20 to 30 percent of the cells in a tumor mass (19). Preliminary studies have indicated that the cells of malignant melanoma can produce a factor that stimulates macrophages to release interleukin-1 and tumor necrosis factor in vitro (31). Direct osteolysis at the point of contact between tumor cells and bone has been clearly demonstrated in vitro using cultures of human breast cancer cells (7). Nonetheless, it is now generally thought that in vivo bone resorption is due to osteoclasts, rather than as a direct effect of malignant cells (23), despite the fact that malignant cells occasionally are seen in resorption bays on bone surfaces.

The increased bone in osteoblastic metastases has two patterns, usually seen in conjunction with one another. The production of new osteoid on the surface of existing cancellous bone results in trabeculae that are thicker than normal. In addition, there is stimulation for osteoblasts to form new trabeculae in the marrow spaces between preexisting medullary bone. In tissue culture, cells from a prostate cancer have been shown to produce osteoblast-stimulating factor (13).

Clinical Features. Pain, swelling, or tenderness are the most common symptoms of metastatic disease. The pain is usually insidious in onset, increases in intensity over weeks or months, and often antedates any changes in conventional radiographs (12). Abrupt onset of severe pain is usually due to fracture. In one study of 45 patients with surgically repaired pathologic fractures of major long bones, 11 had the fracture as the first symptom of malignant disease (17).

In a review of 46 patients with skeletal metastases of unknown origin, a diagnostic sequence consisting of medical history, physical examination, chest radiograph, intravenous pyelogram, and computerized tomography in selected patients identified the primary tumor in only 16 patients (34). Seven of the primary tumors were in the lung, 6 were in the kidney, 2 were carcinomas of the breast, and 1 was a prostatic carcinoma. The patients without an identifiable primary had adenocarcinomas, clear cell carcinomas, undifferentiated carcinomas, and, in one instance, squamous carcinoma. Six of 10 patients who were autopsied had a previously diagnosed primary site confirmed. In one case, no primary site was identified. A primary tumor was found for the first time in the kidney, pancreas, and lung (one case each). Two of these tumors were less than 2 cm in size.

Sites. Although any bone may be involved with metastatic disease, the most common skeletal sites are those bones of the axial and proximal appendicular skeleton with active, hematopoietic marrow. The rich sinusoidal vascular system in hematopoietic marrow, as opposed to fatty marrow, may be a factor in promoting the development of metastases. The sites most commonly affected include vertebrae, pelvis, rib, skull, sternum, and proximal femur. Metastases to the fatty marrow distal to the elbows or knees are unusual in adults, as are metastases to the mandible.

Occasionally, metastases are bilateral and symmetrical (fig. 266). In addition to the case illustrated in figure 266, similar cases have been reported: carcinoma of the breast metastatic to each thumb and carcinoma of the lung metastatic to both humeri (27,28).

There may be variations in the osseous distribution of metastases from different cancers. As discussed above, metastases to the bones of the hands or feet, although rare, usually originate in the lung (18), whereas symptomatic pathologic fractures of the femur are usually due to carcinoma of the breast, and only rarely due to carcinoma of the lung (29).

Radiographic Findings. Conventional radiographs are not highly sensitive for detecting metastatic disease. Borak (5) drilled holes 1 cm in diameter through dried vertebrae but radiographs of the vertebrae failed to show defects in the cancellous bone even though the cortical defects were visible. Radioisotopic scanning of bone is much more sensitive, and this technique can identify metastases at least 4 months before they become radiographically apparent (15).

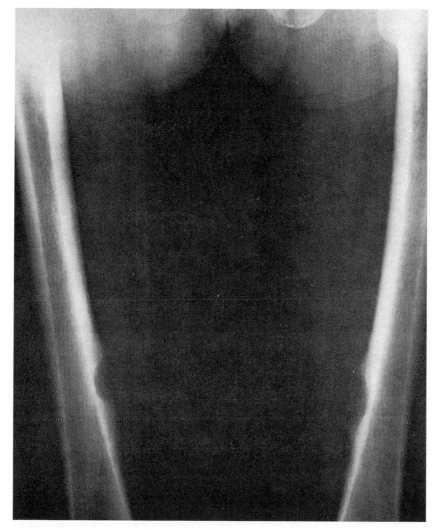

Figure 266
METASTATIC CARCINOMA
FROM LUNG
The femoral shafts of a 58-year-old man have bilateral, symmetrical cortical metastases. He had complained of pain in both thighs for a year, and biopsy of one of the lesions demonstrated a metastatic squamous cell carcinoma. (Fig. 410 from Fascicle 5, 2nd Series.)

However, scans may not detect multiple myeloma or metastatic renal cell carcinoma, neoplasms that cause bone destruction without significant osteoblastic response (33).

Skeletal metastases are generally subdivided into *osteolytic*, *osteoblastic*, or *mixed lesions*. As the names suggest, osteolytic metastases destroy bone, whereas osteoblastic metastases stimulate more than the normal quantity of bone. The majority of metastatic lesions are osteolytic. Tumors that almost always cause osteolytic metastases include carcinomas of the kidney, thyroid, lung, and gastrointestinal tract. Carcinoma of the breast usually results in osteolytic metastases but may produce osteoblastic metastases or mixed lesions. Carcinoma of the prostate, carcinoid tumors, and medulloblastoma almost al-

ways result in osteoblastic metastases (fig. 267) (30,36). Painless osteoblastic metastases may be mistaken for osteopoikilosis (10).

Osseous metastases can markedly expand the affected bone (figs. 268, 269). This is most commonly seen in patients with renal cell or thyroid carcinoma. However, it may occur in metastases from carcinoma of the breast and lung, and malignant melanoma (21). Periosteal reaction is generally said to be uncommon in metastases, but there are widely conflicting data regarding this, due perhaps to varying interpretations of what constitutes periosteal reaction. In an analysis of 35 patients with solitary metastatic lesions, Norman and Ulin (25) found a periosteal reaction in 37 percent. These included a lamellated reaction (onion peel), a perpendicular

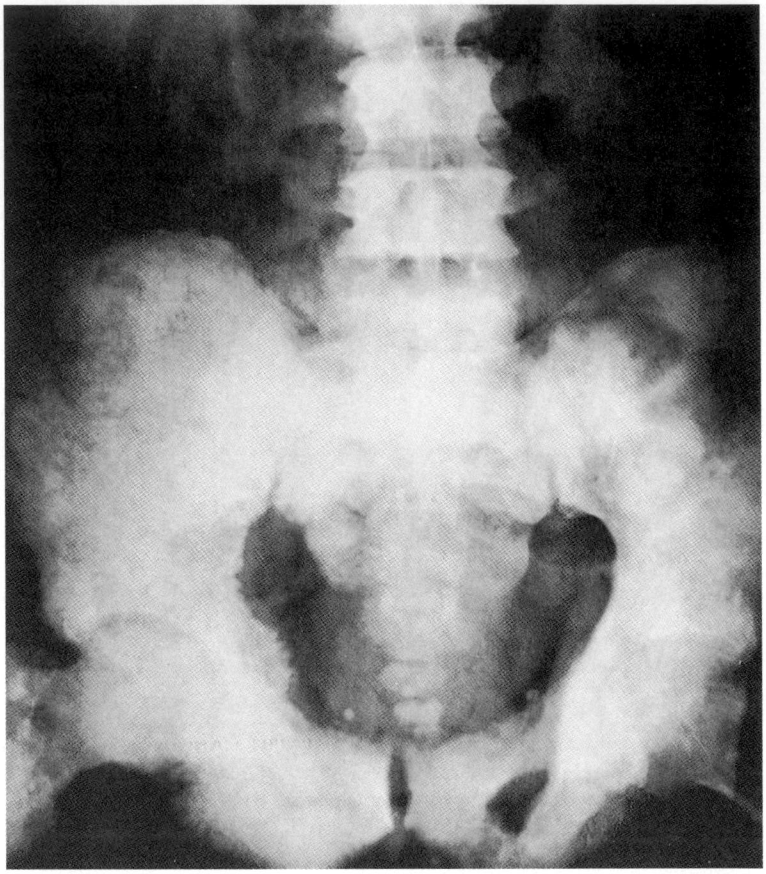

Figure 267
OSTEOBLASTIC METASTATIC
CARCINOMA FROM PROSTATE
Extreme sclerotic changes are present in the pelvic bones, femoral heads, sacrum, and vertebrae. (Fig. 414 from Fascicle 5, 2nd Series.)

or spiculated (sunburst) appearance, a dense periosteal reaction difficult to differentiate from thickened cortex and often associated with osteoblastic metastases, and a reactive triangle at the margin of a lesion (Codman triangle). In another report, the periosteal sunburst reaction was found in a disproportionate number of metastases distal to the elbow or knee and in patients with osteoblastic metastases due to carcinoma of the prostate (4). Exuberant reactive bone formation also can occur in response to a pathologic fracture due to metastatic carcinoma and, if biopsied, this formation may lead to diagnostic confusion with osteosarcoma (16).

Gross Findings. There are no specific gross features of metastatic neoplasms that allow their distinction from primary tumors. When metastases are osteolytic, they are usually sharply demarcated from the surrounding bone. Osteoblastic metastases result in a firm, less sharply demarcated mass with a sclerotic consistency, and a slightly mottled gross appearance.

Metastatic renal cell and thyroid carcinomas are noted for their highly vascular appearance, both grossly and microscopically.

Microscopic Findings. In most instances, a metastatic neoplasm is easily diagnosed, and sometimes it is possible to identify or strongly suggest the primary site (e.g., clear cell adenocarcinoma of the kidney or follicular carcinoma of the thyroid). Adenocarcinomas of the prostate, although lacking a highly specific pattern, may be identified by demonstrating prostate specific antigen or prostate specific acid phosphatase by immunohistochemistry. The osteoblastic response to a metastasis results in a proliferation of small trabeculae that use the normal bone as a scaffolding (fig. 270) and may be so pronounced that the neoplasm is present only as individual cells or small aggregates that may be easily overlooked. Immunohistochemical stains for cytokeratin or epithelial membrane antigen may be helpful for identifying these widely separated epithelial cells.

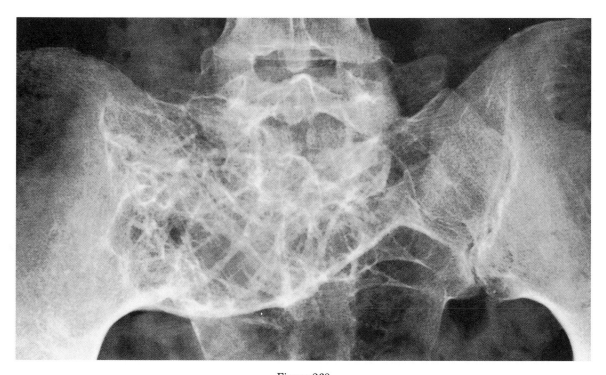

Figure 268
METASTATIC CARCINOMA FROM THYROID
A large expansile sacral lesion was originally interpreted as giant cell tumor. (Fig. 411 from Fascicle 5, 2nd Series.)
(Figures 268 and 269 are from the same patient.)

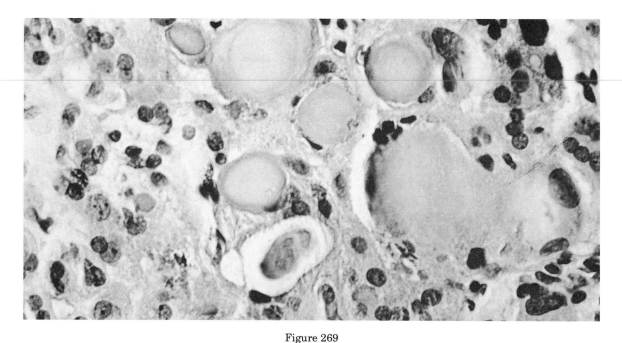

Figure 269
METASTATIC CARCINOMA FROM THYROID
Biopsy of the lesion shown in figure 268 discloses a poorly differentiated follicular carcinoma metastatic from the thyroid of a 41-year-old woman. (Fig. 412 from Fascicle 5, 2nd Series.)

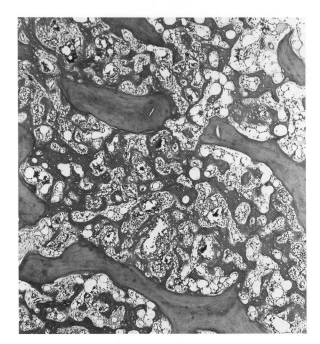

Figure 270
METASTATIC CARCINOMA FROM PROSTATE
Proliferating small trabeculae of bone replace the marrow. Only a few tumor cells are evident.

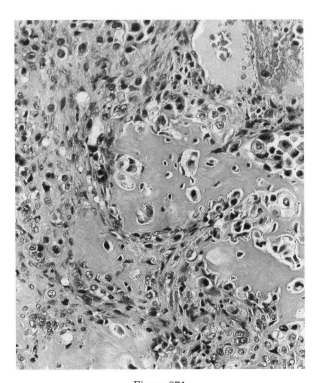

Figure 271
METASTATIC CARCINOMA FROM LUNG
A 53-year-old woman presented with a solitary vertebral mass. Large tumor cells are surrounded by osteoid and lie between the trabeculae. The pattern is indistinguishable from osteosarcoma. (Figures 271 and 272 are from the same patient.)

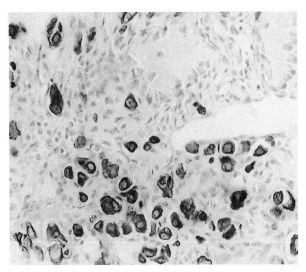

Figure 272
METASTATIC CARCINOMA FROM LUNG
Many cells seen in figure 271 stained for cytokeratin, BER-EP4, and epithelial membrane antigen (shown). Ten months after this biopsy was obtained, a nodule was identified in the lung and proved to be a large cell undifferentiated carcinoma cytologically identical to the osseous metastasis.

Differential Diagnosis. A metastatic neuroblastoma to bone may be potentially confused with Ewing sarcoma although this is rarely a problem since the distinction can usually be made on clinical grounds. Differentiating clinical and microscopic features are discussed under Ewing sarcoma.

Osteoblastic metastases sometimes have metastatic cells surrounded by exuberant osteoid, in a pattern mimicking osteosarcoma (fig. 271). A careful study of the reactive bone, however, discloses that normal osteoblasts are forming the osteoid. Immunohistochemical staining for cytokeratin or other epithelial markers distinguishes the neoplastic epithelial cells from reactive osteoblasts (fig. 272).

Osseous metastases composed of spindle cells, with or without epithelioid-like neoplastic cells, can pose tremendous diagnostic difficulty. The differential diagnosis includes a variety of primary osseous sarcomas such as malignant fibrous histiocytoma, leiomyosarcoma, and fibrosarcoma. Spindle cell (sarcomatoid) carcinomas have been reported to arise in the skin,

Table 10

PANEL OF IMMUNOHISTOCHEMICAL STAINS
FOR SPINDLE CELL NEOPLASMS

Tumor	Antigens				
	CK*	EMA**	S-100	Vimentin	MSA[+]
Spindle cell carcinoma	+	+	+/-	+/-	-
Malignant melanoma	-	-	+	+	-
Malignant fibrous histiocytoma	-	-	-	+	-
Leiomyosarcoma	+/-	-	-	+/-	+
Fibrosarcoma	-	-	-	+	-

*Cytokeratin
**Epithelial membrane antigen
[+]Muscle specific actin

upper aerodigestive tract, and virtually every visceral organ (38). In particular, osseous metastases from spindle cell (sarcomatoid) renal cell carcinomas commonly involve bone and may closely mimic malignant fibrous histiocytoma. Immunohistochemistry is of major importance in distinguishing between these two groups of lesions. Proper decalcification has not been shown to significantly alter the intensity or sensitivity of immunohistochemical staining (22). It must be remembered, however, that some antigens are shared by both carcinomas and sarcomas. Vimentin, almost invariably present in sarcomas, may be synthesized by carcinomas and malignant melanoma. Cytokeratin, present in most carcinomas, has been reported to occur in skeletal leiomyosarcoma (24) and other mesenchymal neoplasms. A useful diagnostic immunohistochemical panel for spindle cell lesions includes cytokeratin, epithelial membrane antigen, S-100, vimentin, desmin, and muscle specific actin. The presence of epithelial membrane antigen or keratin strongly suggests the diagnosis of metastatic carcinoma. Diffuse S-100 positivity suggests a malignant melanoma, given the appropriate light microscopic appearance, and this can be confirmed by staining with the melanocytic marker, HMB-45.

If the cytokeratin, epithelial membrane antigen, and S-100 stains are negative, the differential diagnosis then lies among different primary sarcomas. Vimentin stains some cells in malignant fibrous histiocytoma and fibrosarcoma, and may be present in leiomyosarcoma. The latter, however, strongly stains with muscle specific actin, desmin, and smooth muscle actin (Table 10).

Treatment and Prognosis. About half of patients presenting with skeletal metastases die within 8 months, and most of the remainder do so within 24 months. There are rare long-term survivors of up to 6 years after initial diagnosis (34), many of whom have metastatic follicular thyroid carcinoma, a tumor known for its often indolent clinical course. Identification of the primary tumor site is often important because of variations in chemotherapy applied to different tumors. For example, hormonal therapy is an important component in the treatment of metastatic carcinoma of the breast or prostate gland. Different regimens of chemotherapy have been developed for various forms of carcinoma. If solitary, symptomatic, or in danger of fracture, radiation therapy is often used for local control of metastases. Radiation brings complete local response in about 50 percent of patients and partial relief in an additional 35 percent (35). Surgery may be beneficial for relief of pain in patients who have slowly growing cancers with a protracted clinical course (e.g., carcinoma of breast or prostate). Major surgical procedures may be justified for solitary lesions, including resection and replacement of the hip joint (11).

GENERAL REFERENCES

Rubens RD, Fogelman I, eds. Bone metastases: diagnosis and treatment. London: Springer-Verlag, 1991.

Sim FH. Diagnosis and management of metastatic bone disease: a multidisciplinary approach. New York: Raven Press, 1987.

REFERENCES

1. Abrams HL, Spiro R, Goldstein N. Metastases in carcinoma. Analysis of 1000 autopsied cases. Cancer 1950;3:74–85.
2. Assor D. Basal cell carcinoma with metastasis to bone. Report of two cases. Cancer 1967;20:2125–32.
3. Berrettoni BA, Carter JR. Mechanisms of cancer metastasis to bone. J Bone Joint Surg [Am] 1986;68:308–12.
4. Bloom RA, Libson E, Husband JE, Stoker DJ. The periosteal sunburst reaction to bone metastases. A literature review and report of 20 additional cases. Skeletal Radiol 1987;16:629–34.
5. Borak J. Relationship between the clinical and roentgenological findings in bone metastases. Surg Gynecol Obstet 1942;75:599–604.
6. Cramer SF, Fried L, Carter KJ. The cellular basis of metastatic bone disease in patients with lung cancer. Cancer 1981;48:2649–60.
7. Eilon G, Mundy GR. Direct resorption of bone by human breast cancer cells in vitro. Nature 1978;276:726–8.
8. Fornasier VL, Horne JG. Metastases to the vertebral column. Cancer 1975;36:590–4.
9. Galasko CS. Mechanisms of lytic and blastic metastatic disease of bone. Clin Orthop 1982;20–7.
10. Ghandur-Mnaymneh L, Broder LE, Mnaymneh WA. Lobular carcinoma of the breast metastatic to bone with unusual clinical, radiologic, and pathologic features mimicking osteopoikilosis. Cancer 1984;53:1801–3.
11. Harrington KD. The management of acetabular insufficiency secondary to metastatic malignant disease. J Bone Joint Surg [Am] 1981;63:653–64.
12. Healey JH, Turnbull ADM, Miedema B, Lane JM. Acrometastases. A study of twenty-nine patients with osseous involvement of hands and feet. J Bone Joint Surg [Am] 1986;68:743–6.
13. Jacobs SC, Pikna D, Lawson RK. Prostatic osteoblastic factor. Invest Urol 1979;17:195–8.
14. Jaffe HL. Tumors and tumorous conditions of the bones and joints. Philadelphia: Lea & Febiger, 1958:600.
15. Joo KG, Parthasarathy KL, Bakshi SP, Rosner D. Bone scintigrams: their clinical usefulness in patients with breast carcinoma. Oncology 1979;36:94–8.
16. Kahn LB, Wood FW, Ackerman LV. Fracture callus associated with benign and malignant bone lesions and mimicking osteosarcoma. Am J Clin Pathol 1969;52:14–24.
17. Koskinen EV, Nieminen RA. Surgical treatment of metastatic pathological fracture of major long bones. Acta Orthop Scand 1973;44:539–49.
18. Libson E, Bloom RA, Husband JE, Stoker DJ. Metastatic tumors of the bones of the hand and foot. A comparative review and report of 43 additional cases. Skeletal Radiol 1987;16:387–92.
19. McBride WH. Phenotype and functions of intratumoral macrophages. Biochem Biophys Acta 1986;865:27–41.
20. Miller F, Whitehill R. Carcinoma of the breast metastatic to the skeleton. Clin Orthop 1984;184:121–7.
21. Mootoosamy IM, Anchor SC, Dacie JE. Expanding osteolytic bone metastases from carcinoma of the breast: an unusual appearance. Skeletal Radiol 1985;14:188–90.
22. Mukai K, Yoshimura S, Anzai M. Effects of decalcification on immunoperoxidase staining. Am J Surg Pathol 1986;10:413–9.
23. Mundy GR. Hypercalcemia of malignancy revisited. J Clin Invest 1988;82:1–6.
24. Myers JL, Arocho J, Bernreuter W, Dunham W, Mazur MT. Leiomyosarcoma of bone. A clinicopathologic, immunohistochemical, and ultrastructural study of five cases. Cancer 1991;67:1051–6.
25. Norman A, Ulin R. A comparative study of periosteal new-bone response in metastatic bone tumors (solitary) and primary sarcomas. Radiology 1969;92:705–8.
26. North CA, Zinreich ES, Cristensen WN, North RB. Multiple spinal metastases from paraganglioma. Cancer 1990;66:2224–8.
27. Ozarda AT. Bilateral symmetrical metastatic osseous lesions. Am Surg 1965;31:56–7.
28. Panebianco AC, Kaupp HA. Bilateral thumb metastasis from breast carcinoma. Arch Surg 1968;96:216–8.
29. Poigenfurst J, Marcove RC, Miller TR. Surgical treatment of fractures through metastases in the proximal femur. J Bone Joint Surg [Br] 1968;50:743–56.
30. Powell JM. Metastatic carcinoid of bone. Report of two cases and review of the literature. Clin Orthop 1988;230:266–72.
31. Sabatini M, Chavez J, Mundy GR, Bonewald LF. Stimulation of tumor necrosis factor release from monocytic cells by the A375 human melanoma via granulocyte-macrophage colony-stimulating factor. Cancer Res 1990;50:2673–8.
32. Sato K, Mimura H, Han DC, et al. Production of bone-resorbing activity and colony-stimulating activity in vivo and in vitro by a human squamous cell carcinoma associated with hypercalcemia and leukocytosis. J Clin Invest 1986;78:145–54.
33. Sim FH, Frassica FJ. Metastatic bone disease. In: Unni KK, ed. Bone tumors. New York: Churchill Livingstone, 1988:226.
34. Simon MA, Bartucci EJ. The search for the primary tumor in patients with skeletal metastases of unknown origin. Cancer 1986;58:1088–95.
35. Tong D, Gillick L, Hendrickson FR. The palliation of symptomatic osseous metastases: final results of the study by the Radiation Therapy Oncology Group. Cancer 1982;50:893–9.
36. Vieco PT, Azouz EM, Hoeffel JC. Metastases to bone in medulloblastoma. A report of five cases. Skeletal Radiol 1989;18:445–9.
37. Wallace S. Dynamics of normal and abnormal lymphatic systems as studies with contrast media. Cancer Chemother Rep 1968;52:31–58.
38. Wick MR, Brown BA, Young RH, Mills SE. Spindle-cell proliferations of the urinary tract. An immunohistochemical study. Am J Surg Pathol 1988;12:379–89.
39. Young JM, Funk FJ Jr. Incidence of tumor metastasis to the lumbar spine. A comparative study of roentgenographic changes and gross lesions. J Bone Joint Surg [Am] 1953;35:55–64.

NON-NEOPLASTIC LESIONS THAT MIMIC NEOPLASMS

ANEURYSMAL BONE CYST

Definition. A benign but often rapidly expansile, and locally destructive, multicystic lesion. The cysts are blood-filled with walls composed of spindle cells, osteoid, and multinucleated giant cells.

General Features. Although aneurysmal bone cysts are not true neoplasms, they represent one of the most rapidly growing and destructive bone lesions. They account for about 2 percent of primary biopsied bone tumors and are half as common as giant cell tumor (7). The pathogenesis of aneurysmal bone cyst is not certain, but there is evidence that these cysts represent a reactive change secondary to a localized arteriovenous malformation (4,5). Gross arteriovenous malformations have been found in completely excised specimens (14), and manometric studies have documented that the cyst contents, in some cases, are under arteriolar pressure, suggesting a malformation at that level (4). The rapid growth of aneurysmal bone cysts, their documented association with trauma or fracture, and their tendency to recur after curettage are all consistent with a vascular etiology.

Between 32 and 50 percent of aneurysmal bone cysts are associated with other pathologic entities including giant cell tumor, giant cell reparative granuloma, nonossifying fibroma, fibrous dysplasia, chondromyxoid fibroma, chondroblastoma, osteoblastoma, osteosarcoma, unicameral bone cyst, hemangioma, and infantile hamartoma of the rib (4,10,12,13). By convention, the diagnosis is that of the primary entity and the cystic areas are viewed as a secondary change. Conditions with secondary aneurysmal bone cyst have approximately the same rate of postcurettage recurrence as primary aneurysmal bone cysts. When secondary aneurysmal bone cysts recur, about 86 percent contain both the primary process and the secondary cystic component. Some authors have suggested that virtually all aneurysmal bone cysts are, in fact, secondary, reactive lesions but that in many instances the precursor lesion has been destroyed. This hypothesis is, of course, impossible to prove. The important point is to examine all tissue carefully to exclude an associated process. Epiphyseal aneurysmal bone cysts have an identifiable primary lesion in up to 70 percent of cases, and cysts in this location should be examined particularly carefully (4).

Clinical Features. These cysts may occur at any age. Between 70 to 85 percent of patients are 20 years of age or younger, although occurrence prior to 5 years of age is uncommon (18). Some series show a slight female predominance (4,18). Pain that varies in duration from weeks to a few years is the most common complaint. About half of patients are symptomatic for 3 months or less (18). Swelling is also frequent, often with a history of rapid increase in size. Throbbing pain and pressure tenderness are less common, and rare lesions may be visibly pulsatile.

Sites. Almost any single bone may be involved, but multibone disease, outside the vertebral column, is rare. The metaphyseal region of the long bones and the vertebrae together account for 70 to 80 percent of lesions (14,18), with the distal femur and proximal tibia the most common sites. Secondary aneurysmal bone cysts follow the sites of predilection of their precursor lesions. Most vertebral lesions involve the posterior arch and spinous processes. The vertebral body may be involved by extension, but confinement to the body is unusual. Aneurysmal bone cyst has the uncommon ability to involve adjacent bones. This is particularly true with vertebral lesions, where up to 50 percent affect multiple spinous processes (18).

Radiographic Appearance. Aneurysmal bone cyst, particularly of the tubular bones, has been subdivided according to the pattern of involvement and the phase of progression (14,17). There are three patterns of involvement: eccentric, parosteal, and central. Eccentric involvement is most common in the large tubular bones, including the femur and tibia; parosteal lesions are the least common and form a predominantly soft tissue mass with only minimal erosion or saucerization of the cortex (6).

The radiographic appearance varies with the phase of development (6,14). In the *initial* or *incipient phase*, there is a small, often eccentric, lytic lesion that does not grossly expand the bone but may have an alarming, permeative growth

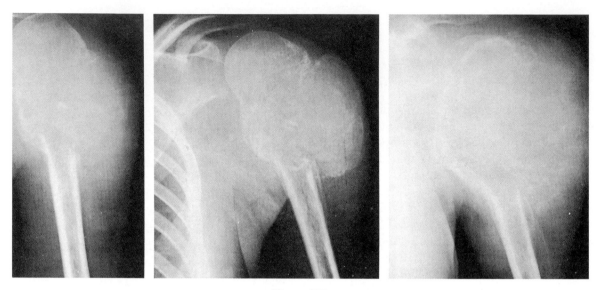

Figure 273
ANEURYSMAL BONE CYST

These three radiographs demonstrate progression of an aneurysmal bone cyst of the humerus in a 13-year-old girl. The radiographs (from left to right) were taken on December 19, 1959; January 2, 1960; and February 22, 1960. The lesion was locally resected and a prosthesis inserted. (Fig. 401 from Fascicle 5, 2nd Series.)

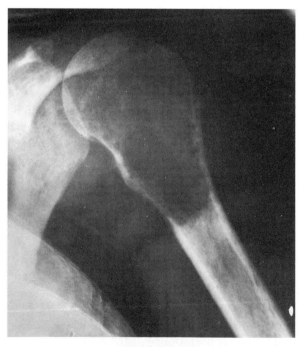

Figure 274
ANEURYSMAL BONE CYST

This radiograph from an 18-year-old woman shows a destructive lesion in the proximal humerus with cortical erosion and only slight expansion of bone. (Figures 274–280 are from the same patient.)

pattern. In the *growth phase* there is rapid, destructive growth characterized by massive lysis of bone and cortical destruction (figs. 273, 274). Codman triangles may be prominent. The lesion grows so rapidly that the periosteal bone cannot encompass it, and there is little or no bony circumscription. These naked margins may lead to confusion with malignancy but the "blowout" appearance is characteristic, and the intramedullary component usually has a well-circumscribed margin. In the *stable phase*, the radiograph has the classic appearance of aneurysmal bone cyst with expanded, grossly distorted bone and a distinct bony shell surrounding a lesion that contains numerous internal trabeculations. Finally, in the *healing phase*, there is progressive ossification of the bony trabeculae to form an irregular, coarsely trabeculated, bony mass.

Gross Findings. Aneurysmal bone cysts are seldom removed intact. Rare intact lesions have a thin osseous shell surrounding honeycombed, cavernous vascular spaces that are usually filled with unclotted blood (6). The size of the vascular spaces and the thickness of the trabecular walls are variable (figs. 275, 276). Some cysts, especially from older lesions, may be filled with serous

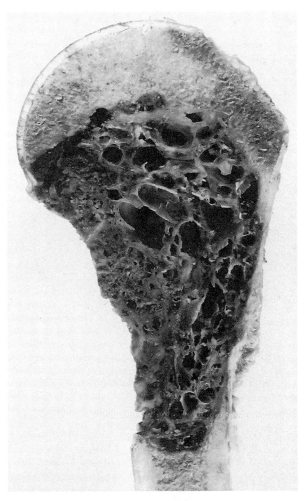

Figure 275
ANEURYSMAL BONE CYST
Because of the size of the lesion, and its extension into the subchondral portion of the joint, an excision was performed with insertion of a prosthesis. On cut section, there is complete loss of cortex on left. Vascular spaces are small in semisolid foci (left) with larger cavernous spaces elsewhere.

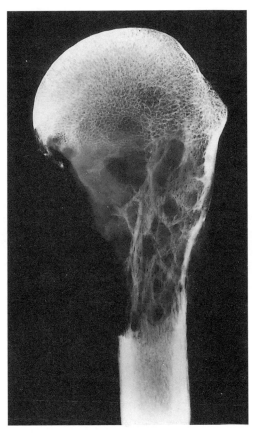

Figure 276
ANEURYSMAL BONE CYST
Specimen radiograph of the lesion demonstrates the cortical erosion and variable sized spaces to good advantage. The trabeculae of bone are remaining remnants of cortical bone that have not been completely destroyed.

or serosanguinous fluid rather than freely circulating blood. A careful search should be made for more solid areas that may contain an associated precursor lesion. The so-called solid variant, discussed below, is a noncystic, focally hemorrhagic, firm to soft, grey-white lesion (16).

Microscopic Findings. The microscopic appearance is variable. The essential histologic feature is the presence of many cavernous spaces that are filled with blood but lack the smooth muscle walls and endothelial lining of normal vessels (figs. 277, 278) (4,6,18). The absence of an

endothelial lining, at least in large part, has been confirmed with immunohistochemical and ultrastructural studies (1–3). The mental reconstruction of these spaces from curetted fragments is often difficult. The vascular spaces are separated by fibrous walls that may contain osteoid, chondroid, giant cells, and inflammation. In completely resected specimens, the cysts may be seen permeating between adjacent trabeculae of normal bone at the periphery of the lesion (18). If the cortex has been completely destroyed, lesional tissue abuts the adjacent soft tissue (fig. 279).

The areas of osteoid formation are occasionally surrounded by a primitive chondroid matrix or, more commonly, the osteoid appears to arise in a "metaplastic" fashion analogous to that seen in fibrous dysplasia. The osteoid in aneurysmal

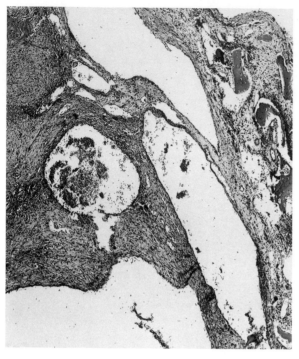

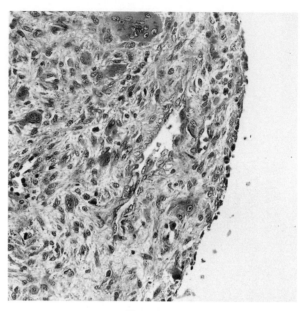

Figure 277
ANEURYSMAL BONE CYST
Vascular spaces vary widely in size and shape. The septa range from thin to broad. Well-formed bone is focally present.

Figure 278
ANEURYSMAL BONE CYST
The septum contains fibroblasts, mononuclear histiocyte-like cells, and multinucleated giant cells, as well as capillaries. The lining of the large vascular spaces may be indistinct or consist of a single layer of attenuated stromal cells as seen here.

bone cyst often has a trabecular pattern similar to osteoblastoma. Osteoid is frequently laid down as long, linear depositions within the septa. The osteoid often has a crinkled appearance, presumably due to rearrangement of the architecture of the cyst (fig. 280).

The chondroid zones have a characteristic fibrillary, fibromyxoid quality, and usually lack the appearance of conventional hyaline cartilage (14,16,18). They may be present in large numbers in the trabecular regions, often line the vascular spaces, and may have a degenerating, focally calcified appearance. It has been suggested that these chondromyxoid foci are highly characteristic of aneurysmal bone cysts (14,16).

Mitotic figures may be numerous, particularly in the areas of osteoid formation, and the low-power pattern may be indistinguishable from that of telangiectatic osteosarcoma (see differential diagnosis). Although the mitotic rate is often high, the stromal cells lack features of anaplasia and atypical mitotic figures are not present.

Sanerkin and colleagues (16) described four noncystic intraosseous lesions with microscopic

features similar to those seen in the trabeculae of aneurysmal bone cyst. The seeming oxymoron of "the solid variant of aneurysmal bone cyst" was applied to these proliferations. Similar, if not identical, cases have been described in the pelvis under the designation of "giant cell containing fibrous lesion of the sacrum" (8). These proliferations contained collections of fibroblasts, fibrohistiocytic cells, giant cells, osteoblasts with osteoid, and occasional areas of calcifying fibromyxoid/chondroid tissue similar to that seen in the septa of typical aneurysmal bone cysts (18). In some areas, the osteoblastic component formed extensive and somewhat atypical islands of osteoid that could be confused with osteosarcoma or osteoblastoma (16). Most, but not all, cases contained at least small foci of dilated vascular sinusoids, more typical of conventional aneurysmal bone cyst. The solid variant lesions may, in many microscopic fields, be indistinguishable from giant cell reparative granuloma. Indeed, these two lesions appear to be close morphologic and, in some cases, pathogenetic relatives.

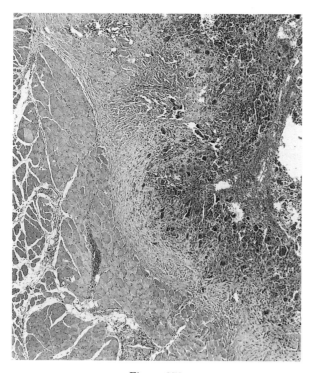

Figure 279
ANEURYSMAL BONE CYST
Where the cortex has been completely destroyed, the lesional tissue abuts striated muscle.

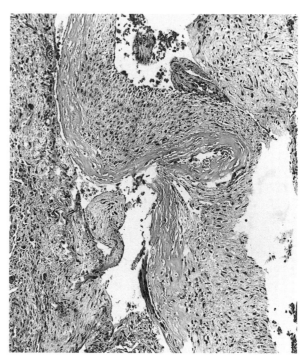

Figure 280
ANEURYSMAL BONE CYST
A fibrous septum contains a long strand of osteoid that appears to have "buckled" in the center.

Differential Diagnosis. The histologic diagnosis is one of exclusion. One must sample extensively to find or exclude a precursor lesion. Any solid area should be completely sectioned, especially if it is greater than 1 cm in size.

Telangiectatic Osteosarcoma. The confusion between aneurysmal bone cyst and telangiectatic osteosarcoma represents one of the most dangerous pitfalls in bone pathology. Misdiagnoses have been made in both directions. Telangiectatic osteosarcoma is much less common, and the diagnosis should be approached with caution. Occasionally, the radiographic appearance will be nonspecific, or worse, suggest the wrong diagnosis. More often aneurysmal bone cysts have a well-defined margin with cortical "blowout" and an eggshell rim. Telangiectatic osteosarcoma usually has a more ill-defined margin and looks malignant, radiographically. The distinction must ultimately be made histologically and rests on the finding of obviously anaplastic cells in the trabeculae of telangiectatic osteosarcoma. Atypical mitotic figures are frequently

present and the osteoid has a more irregular, closely-packed pattern.

Osteosarcoma with Areas of Aneurysmal Bone Cyst. Although this may sound initially like telangiectatic osteosarcoma, it is distinctly different. Conventional osteosarcomas may have areas of secondary aneurysmal bone cyst change, in which the stroma is benign and typical of that lesion, unlike the malignant fibrous septa of telangiectatic osteosarcoma. Elsewhere, however, the lesion has the appearance, at least in small foci, of high-grade osteosarcoma. If these small foci of malignancy are missed by the pathologist or, worse, not present in the biopsy tissue, only the radiographic appearance can suggest the underlying condition. Such rare cases emphasize the fact that aneurysmal bone cyst is a diagnosis of exclusion and should never be made without radiographic correlation. If other elements appear to be present radiographically, they must be searched for in the available tissue or a rebiopsy.

Giant Cell Tumor. Aneurysmal bone cyst may contain numerous giant cells and, adding to the confusion, true giant cell tumor may have a secondary aneurysmal bone cyst component. Giant cell tumor usually occurs in skeletally mature patients over the age of 20 years. In contrast, aneurysmal bone cyst usually occurs in younger patients with open epiphyses. Giant cell tumors are less polycystic and do not generally show the tremendous osseous distortion and periosteal "blowout" seen in aneurysmal bone cysts. Giant cell tumors arise in or at least involve the closed epiphysis. Aneurysmal bone cysts often occur before epiphyseal plate closure, and are typically metaphyseal or diaphyseal lesions. Epiphyseal aneurysmal bone cysts are usually secondary to chondroblastoma or other primary epiphyseal lesions.

Microscopically, giant cell tumors do not show the marked osteoblastic changes seen in the trabeculae of aneurysmal bone cysts. In our experience, the giant cells in aneurysmal bone cysts do not have the enormous numbers of nuclei seen in the multinucleated cells of giant cell tumor.

Ossifying Hematoma / Pseudotumor of Hemophilia. This is a subperiosteal hematoma secondary to trauma and often related to a bleeding diathesis. Radiographically, it mimics a parosteal aneurysmal bone cyst and produces considerable bony destruction with a surrounding rim of eggshell calcification. It usually lacks the trabeculations of an aneurysmal bone cyst and, microscopically, consists of an organizing hematoma with hemosiderin and new bone formation (6).

Unicameral Bone Cyst. Unicameral bone cysts are typically located centrally and cause little or no expansion of the involved bone (6). As the name implies, they differ from aneurysmal bone cysts by being unicystic lesions that contain clear serosanguinous fluid.

Treatment and Prognosis. Although aneurysmal bone cysts may produce extreme deformation of the involved bone, prognosis is good and 90 percent of patients eventually have cosmetically and functionally acceptable resolution of their lesion (5,18). A few cases followed radiographically without therapy became stationary, followed by lesional sclerosis (17). Most lesions, however, require therapeutic intervention. The most successful form of therapy is surgical excision with grafting of the defect. Unfortunately, this approach can produce major functional derangement. Radiation has been advocated by some and may be particu-

larly helpful with vertebral lesions in danger of producing cord compression. The dose should be as low as possible and should be reserved only for patients not amenable to other forms of therapy, as irradiated aneurysmal bone cysts are associated with a low but definite incidence of postradiation sarcoma (6,11,18).

Curettage leads to recurrences in 20 to 70 percent of patients (5,15,17,18). Some studies have documented a trend towards increasing recurrence rates in younger patients and patients with smaller lesions (4,18), but other studies have specifically noted no such association (5,15). It has also been suggested that vertebral lesions have a lower recurrence rate (18). Recurrences almost always develop less than 2 years after the initial therapy and usually within the first 6 months (18). Recurrence is manifest, radiologically, as increased destruction at the periphery of the lesion and resorption of bone chips (18).

Aneurysmal bone cysts also may be treated with cryotherapy. In contrast to the 20 to 70 percent recurrence rate for curettage alone, lesions that had liquid nitrogen instilled into the cavity after curettage had only an 8 percent recurrence rate in one series (4). The effect of cryotherapy on lesions near the growth plate in small children has not been adequately studied, however.

Kyriakos and Hardy (9) described a patient with an aneurysmal bone cyst who developed an osteosarcoma 50 months after the initial onset of symptoms and 28 months after her last curettage for the cyst. They found 13 cases of similar malignant transformation in the world literature, most of which were osteosarcomas, with a few fibrosarcomas. Many of these patients had had radiation therapy, unlike the case reported by Kyriakos and Hardy.

CORTICAL IRREGULARITY SYNDROME

Definition. A reactive fibrous or fibro-osseous proliferation associated with radiographic erosion of the cortex at the insertion of major muscles. *Distal metaphyseal femoral defect* and *distal femoral cortical defect* are synonymous. The terms *periosteal* or *cortical desmoid* have been used in the past.

General Features. The cortical irregularity syndrome is not a neoplastic or even aggressive

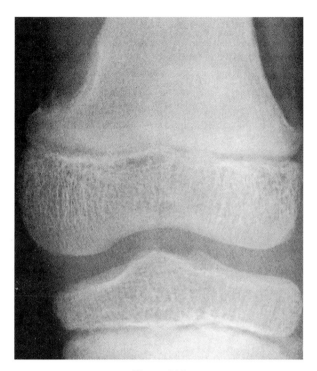

Figure 281
CORTICAL IRREGULARITY SYNDROME
This radiograph reveals a sharply demarcated cortical defect in the femoral metaphysis of an 8-year-old boy. Note the absence of periosteal new bone formation and the intact inner margin of the cortex. (Fig. 292 from Fascicle 5, 2nd Series.) (Figures 281 and 282 are from the same patient.)

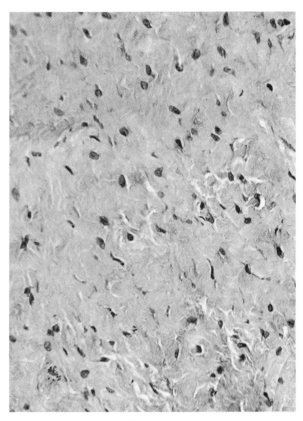

Figure 282
CORTICAL IRREGULARITY SYNDROME
The radiographic defect consists of well-differentiated tendon-like fibrous tissue with abundant stromal collagen. (Fig. 293 from Fascicle 5, 2nd Series.)

lesion. Its common presence in physically active adolescents supports a traumatic pathogenesis. Because these are not true neoplasms, the older terms of periosteal or cortical desmoid should be abandoned (21).

Clinical Features. Most lesions occur in young males 3 to 20 years of age. Many are incidental radiographic findings, but some patients complain of pain. About one third of lesions are bilateral (20).

Sites. The most common site is the posteromedial aspect of the distal femur, which is the site of insertion of the extensor portion of the adductor magnus muscle. Similar lesions have been described in the humerus at the insertion of the pectoralis major (19).

Radiographic Appearance. Cortical irregularities in the femur are radiolucent areas 1 to 3 cm in size (fig. 281). The margin may either be well defined or somewhat irregular (20). Periosteal new bone formation is sometimes present in

response to the lesion. MRI studies have been useful in some cases for showing sharp circumscription, indicative of a nonaggressive lesion (23).

Gross Findings. The tissue has a nonspecific, grossly fibrous appearance, often with a few spicules of bone intermixed.

Microscopic Findings. Much of the specimen typically consists of densely collagenized fibrous tissue that is microscopically identical to normal tendon (fig. 282). Reactive bone or cartilage may be interspersed. When the former is present, the trabeculae are evenly spaced, lined by normal osteoblasts, and appear similar to florid periostitis or callus.

Differential Diagnosis. If the biopsy material consists only of fibrous tissue, it may be indistinguishable from soft tissue desmoid tumor (aggressive fibromatosis) or desmoplastic fibroma of bone. However, desmoplastic fibroma has an intramedullary lytic epicenter on radiograph. The rare case of true periosteal desmoid involves a broad expanse of bone, and has a concave sclerotic margin, rather than the irregular appearance of cortical irregularity syndrome (21).

Treatment and Prognosis. There is no specific treatment for this non-neoplastic process and, indeed, the prognosis is excellent, even for untreated cases. There are no recurrences following biopsy. Untreated lesions may persist into adulthood (22).

SOLITARY BONE CYST

Definition. An almost invariably unilocular, intramedullary cavity filled with clear or sanguinous fluid. It is lined by a thin fibrovascular connective tissue membrane. The terms *unicameral bone cyst*, *simple cyst*, and *benign bone cyst* are also used.

General Features. Solitary bone cysts account for approximately 3 percent of primary bone lesions undergoing biopsy. The pathogenesis is unknown, but the lesions appear to be reactive or developmental rather than true neoplasms (29). Radiographic studies have reported an increased frequency of simple bone cysts in U.S. Navy divers, about one third of whom have small, asymptomatic cysts, predominantly in the humerus or femur (30). This suggests that some solitary bone cysts may be a reaction to a traumatic event such as a bone infarct, to which compressed gas divers are prone. Rarely, solitary bone cysts may occur at the site of a previous, nonpathologic fracture (33).

Clinical Features. In most series, there is a male sexual predilection of up to 3 to 1. Patients range from 2 to 69 years of age. About 65 percent occur in teenagers, and an additional 20 percent occur in the first decade of life (34). Symptoms include pain, swelling, or stiffness of the nearest joint. Approximately two thirds of patients have a sudden onset of pain due to fracture through a previously asymptomatic cyst.

Sites. Eighty to 90 percent of solitary bone cysts are in the proximal humerus, mid-humerus, or proximal femur. Occasional solitary bone cysts are found in the pelvis of adolescents (24). In patients older than 20 years of age, approximately half involve the ilium or calcaneus

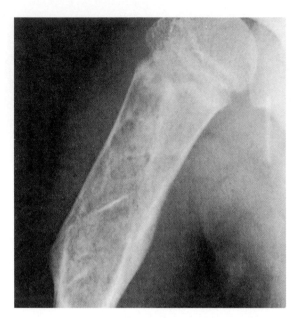

Figure 283
SOLITARY BONE CYST
This solitary bone cyst is in the humerus of a 7-year-old girl. The radiograph shows the close proximity of the cyst to the epiphysis and slight deformity in the area of a fracture. (Fig. 381 from Fascicle 5, 2nd Series.) (Figures 283 and 284 are from the same patient.)

(35). The pelvic lesions are often incidental radiographic findings.

Radiographic Appearance. The typical solitary bone cyst of long bones involves the metaphysis and is near or touching the epiphyseal plate (fig. 283). The overlying cortex is thin and may be slightly expanded, but is never penetrated. The cyst often arises in contact with the epiphyseal plate, but in skeletally immature individuals the growth of the cyst seems to be slower than normal bone growth, so that the cyst is "pushed" away from the growth plate as the bone lengthens (fig. 284). The total length of the cyst is variable, ranging from a few centimeters to involvement of almost the entire shaft. Cysts may appear trabeculated or multiloculated due to osseous ridges on the inner wall. A few contain calcified granules representing the calcospherites described below (fig. 285). Approximately 20 percent of cysts contain one or more "fallen fragments" of bone that have been dislodged from the cortex (35).

Gross Findings. Solitary bone cysts are rarely encountered by pathologists as intact specimens and are much more frequently seen

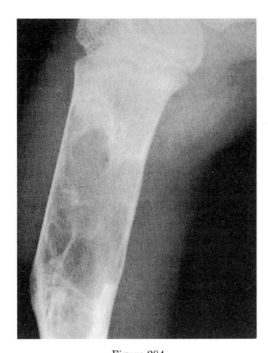

Figure 284
SOLITARY BONE CYST
This radiograph reveals the untreated fracture 4 months later. Note that the cyst has "moved" from the epiphysis due to normal bone growth. (Fig. 382 from Fascicle 5, 2nd Series.)

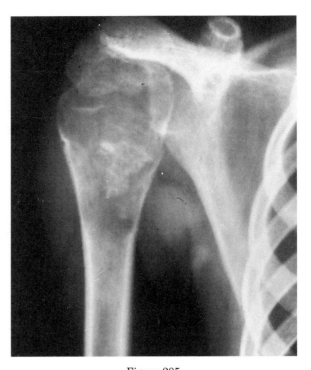

Figure 285
SOLITARY BONE CYST
This unicameral bone cyst from a 7-year-old boy contains calcified material. At surgery, a few small fragments of solid tissue lay within an otherwise typical bone cyst. (Figures 285 and 289 are from the same patient.)

as sparse, curetted fragments. They contain serous fluid, serosanguinous fluid, or, occasionally, appear to be gas filled. The wall of the cyst is white and shiny, and usually less than 1 mm in thickness, although rare cases have been described as having a wall up to 1 cm thick (26). At surgery, a few cysts have been found with "no bottom," communicating freely with a hollow humeral shaft (26). If fibrous septa are present, the lesion is converted into a truly multilocular cyst (fig. 286). These have been demonstrated by injection studies with radiopaque material (28).

Microscopic Findings. The pathologist receives little tissue from a curetted lesion because it consists only of a thin, twisted membrane. There are, therefore, no specific diagnostic features. The lining membrane varies from a few strands of collagen (fig. 287) with an occasional capillary, to a thicker fibrous wall with small arteries and veins. There may be new bone formation, even in the absence of fracture (fig. 288). Often there are hemosiderin deposits, granulation tissue, and a scattering of lymphocytes.

About 9 percent of solitary bone cysts contain approximately spherical, calcified structures in a loose fibrous stroma (fig. 288). Microscopically, these resemble cementum (fig. 289), but ultrastructurally they are seen as an unusual form of bone (32). Some of these calcospherites probably form by the biochemical process known as the Liesegang phenomenon. The resultant structures are known as Liesegang rings and result from alternating diffusion and precipitation of supersaturated solutions (31). Radiographically solid "bone cysts," a seeming contradiction in terms, may contain extensive calcified cementum-like substance. Adler (25) described four such cases in the proximal femurs of patients between the ages of 47 and 56 years. It seems highly possible that these were once solitary cysts that gradually filled in with this material.

Treatment and Prognosis. Traditionally, simple bone cysts have been curetted and packed with bone chips. This is followed by a recurrence rate of about 15 to 20 percent (figs. 290, 291).

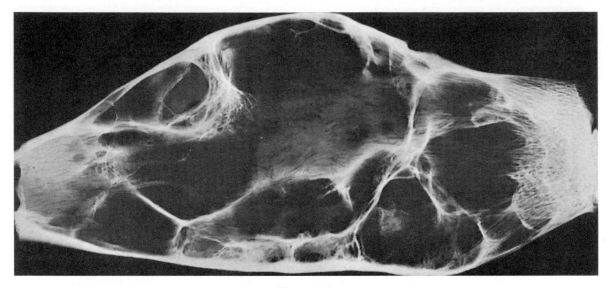

Figure 286
SOLITARY BONE CYST
This specimen radiograph of a resected cyst from the fibula of a 10-year-old girl shows thin ridges that incompletely divide the lesion. (Fig. 384 from Fascicle 5, 2nd Series.)

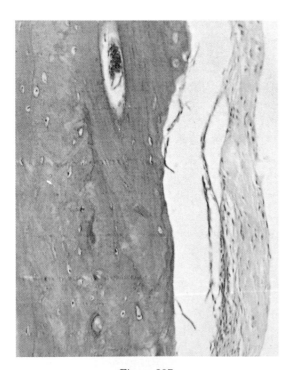

Figure 287
SOLITARY BONE CYST
The lining is a thin fibrous layer adjacent to cortical bone. (Fig. 386 from Fascicle 5, 2nd Series.)

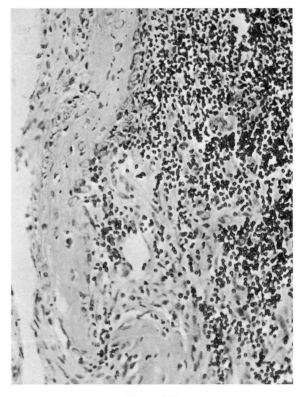

Figure 288
SOLITARY BONE CYST
This cyst lining has osteoid, a finding that may lead to misinterpretation as an aneurysmal bone cyst. Erythrocytes and inflammatory cells including lymphocytes are also present. (Fig. 387 from Fascicle 5, 2nd Series.)

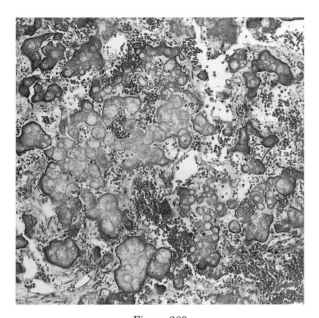

Figure 289
SOLITARY BONE CYST
Curetted material from the cyst shown in figure 285 has calcified spherules, most of which are coalescent.

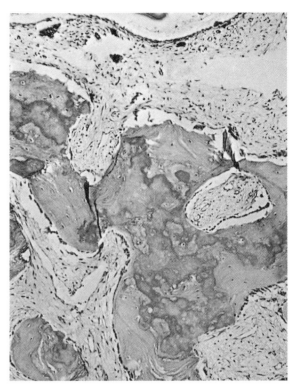

Figure 291
SOLITARY BONE CYST
This histologic section of the material from the second curettage shows a thin fibrous lining membrane of the cyst and remnants of the bone chips around which there is new appositional bone formation. (Fig. 390 from Fascicle 5, 2nd Series.)

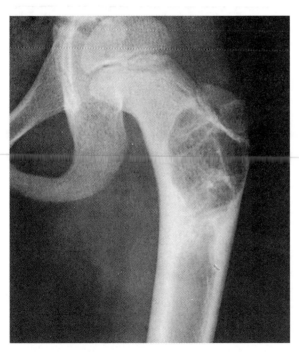

Figure 290
SOLITARY BONE CYST
This cyst abuts against the epiphysis of the greater trochanter. This 9-year-old boy had been treated 18 months previously by insertion of bone chips. Symptoms recurred and this radiograph is the recurrent bone cyst. (Fig. 389 from Fascicle 5, 2nd Series.) (Figures 290 and 291 are from the same patient.)

Large lesions and cysts in children less than 10 years of age have a greater likelihood of recurrence. Recently, aspiration of cyst fluid, followed by injection with cortisone has been used for treatment. The recurrence rate is comparable to that of surgical therapy (27). Rarely, sarcomas have arisen in the walls of unicameral bone cysts (29).

SUBCHONDRAL CYST

Definition. A sharply circumscribed epiphyseal cavity immediately adjacent to the articular cartilage and almost invariably associated with degenerative joint disease. The term *synovial cyst* has been used for subchondral cysts, but proof of synovial origin or differentiation is lacking.

General Features. Subchondral cysts occur in association with a variety of processes that result in degenerative articular changes, including osteoarthritis, rheumatoid arthritis, aseptic

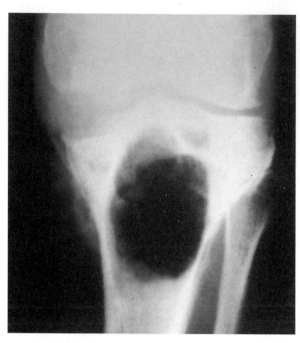

Figure 292
SUBCHONDRAL CYST
A 70-year-old man with degenerative arthritis had an unusually large subchondral cyst that raised concern for a neoplasm. At surgery the cyst contained gray, semi-liquid fluid. The defect was packed with bone chips.

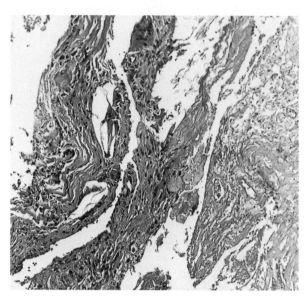

Figure 293
SUBCHONDRAL CYST
A 42-year-old man had severe degenerative arthritis secondary to trauma. Subchondral cysts were present in the subarticular bone. During repair, these were curetted. Most of the material was amorphic, basophilic debris (right). In addition, there were fragments of a fibrous cyst wall measuring 1 to 5 mm in thickness.

necrosis, and calcium pyrophosphate deposit disease. Bones surrounding a silicone rubber prosthesis may develop subchondral cysts that contain silicone (40). The pathogenesis is unknown and may differ from patient to patient. Landell (37) thought that the cysts were formed by synovial fluid entering through defects in cartilage and underlying bone destroyed by arthritis. Rahney and Lam (39) postulated that osteonecrosis preceded fracture of the subchondral bone plate with subsequent continuity of the joint space and underlying cyst.

Clinical Features. Because subchondral cysts are secondary lesions, they typically occur in older individuals where degenerative joint disease, regardless of cause, is more common. They are almost invariably asymptomatic. Attention is usually directed to the area of the primary arthritic changes, resulting in radiographs that show the secondary cyst formation.

Sites. The bones of the hip are most commonly involved, followed by the tibia (38).

Radiographic Appearance. Most subchondral cysts are sharply circumscribed, lytic

defects that vary in size from 0.5 to 1.5 cm and have a slightly sclerotic rim. Larger cysts occur (fig. 292), and they may expand and breach the cortex (36).

Gross Findings. The cyst is typically filled with gray or yellow fluid. Occasionally, the cyst contents may be gelatinous.

Microscopic Findings. A subchondral cyst is essentially a defect in subchondral bone. As such, it has few distinguishing features. The edge of the cyst often has no lining and abuts normal bone. In other areas, the periphery of the cyst may be demarcated by loosely arranged or dense collagen (fig. 293). No distinct lining is seen, although widely scattered, flattened cells resembling fibroblasts may lie along the periphery.

Differential Diagnosis. Radiographically, subchondral cysts may superficially mimic neoplasms that abut the articular cartilage, such as chondroblastoma or giant cell tumor. Recognition of the associated articular disease, the small size of most defects, and the older age of the patients should allow distinction. Even if these cysts contain a slightly myxoid material, they can be distinguished from intraosseous ganglia by their lack of a well-formed fibrous capsule and their association with degenerative joint disease. There may be rare examples in which the distinction is arbitrary.

Treatment and Prognosis. No therapy is required. Rare, larger lesions may be biopsied because the size of the cyst leads to concern about a possible neoplasm (36).

INTRAOSSEOUS GANGLION

Definition. An intramedullary, non-neoplastic, mucin-filled cyst lined by fibrous tissue. The World Health Organization uses the term *juxta-articular bone cyst* for this lesion.

General Features. The pathogenesis of intraosseous ganglion is not understood. Presumably, there is a reactive process in which an unknown stimulus causes fibroblast-like stromal cells to produce large quantities of mucin. Intraosseous ganglion may be caused by a localized vascular disturbance, although signs of associated avascular bone necrosis are not demonstrable. Some intraosseous lesions have been in continuity with soft tissue ganglia and are thought to be secondary to the soft tissue component (42). However, otherwise typical intraosseous ganglia only rarely communicate with an adjacent joint (43).

Clinical Features. Patients range in age from 14 to 86 years, but most are between 30 and 60 years of age (41,44). Males are affected slightly more often than females. Patients typically complain of tenderness and, sometimes, a mass. Pathologic fracture is rare.

Sites. About two thirds of the cases involve, in order of decreasing frequency, the distal tibia, proximal tibia, proximal femur, and ulna. Small bones of the hands and feet have also been involved. Multiple lesions, often bilateral and symmetrical, are occasionally seen (45).

Radiographic Appearance. Intraosseous ganglia always occupy the epiphysis and range from several millimeters to 6 cm in size. Most are 2 to 4 cm in greatest dimension. They are eccentric, lytic defects with sharply defined margins and slight perilesional sclerosis (fig. 294). The adjacent articular surface is usually normal, in contrast to the degenerative changes seen in association with subchondral cysts.

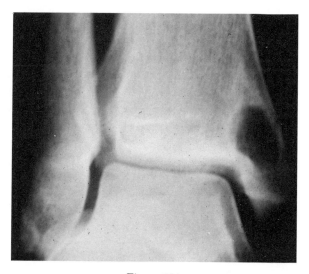

Figure 294
INTRAOSSEOUS GANGLION
The medial malleolus of a 44-year-old man has a well-demarcated, lytic lesion. Note the lack of arthritic changes.

Gross Findings. The cyst contents consist of strands of fibrous tissue intermixed with yellow, white, or gray gelatinous to mucoid material.

Microscopic Findings. Most of the tissue is myxoid stroma with variable numbers of intermixed, fibroblast-like cells (fig. 295). Fibrous tissue may be haphazardly dispersed in the lesion, or more organized to form septa. The cyst is surrounded by an outer fibrous wall or capsule which is heavily collagenized and contains only a few capillaries. A lining layer of attenuated fibroblast-like cells may be present on the inner aspect of the capsule. The outer portion of the capsule is often surrounded by reactive new bone formation.

Differential Diagnosis. Intraosseous ganglion may be confused with extragnathic fibromyxoma, chondromyxoid fibroma, or subchondral cysts. Distinction from extragnathic fibromyxoma is discussed under that tumor. Chondromyxoid fibroma may have mucinous areas, but also has more cellular fibrous septa and is lobulated, microscopically. Subchondral cysts contain small amounts of fluid or slightly myxoid material, and are associated with a variety of articular abnormalities.

Treatment and Prognosis. Curettage with bone graft, if necessary, is almost always curative, although a few patients have one or more recurrences (45).

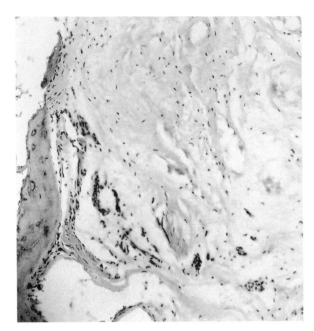

Figure 295
INTRAOSSEOUS GANGLION
This intraosseous ganglion consists of myxoid material with only a few interspersed, fibroblast-like cells. The myxoid material is separated from the peripheral rim of bone by an inconstant band of collagen. (Fig. 5 from Pope TL Jr, Fechner RE, Keats TE. Intra-osseous ganglion. Report of four cases and review of the literature. Skeletal Radiol 1989;18:185–7.)

FLORID REACTIVE PERIOSTITIS

Definition. A reactive fibrous, osteoblastic, and focally cartilaginous proliferation (52), primarily involving the fingers and toes, which has been known by a variety of terms including *parosteal fasciitis* (48,49), *fibro-osseous pseudotumor* (47), and *periostitis ossificans* (50).

Clinical Features. Patients vary in age from children to the elderly, with a mean age of approximately 25 to 30 years (46,47,50). There is a slight female predominance (1.5 to 1). A history of trauma can be elicited in about 40 percent of cases (47). The typical clinical presentation is a painful, often fusiform swelling of the affected bone.

Sites and Radiographic Appearance. A soft tissue swelling is always present radiographically (52), and a periosteal reaction, often laminated, is seen in about 30 percent of cases (fig. 296). Radiographic features of malignancy are invariably absent (52). Involvement of the digits favors hand (91 percent) over foot (9 per-

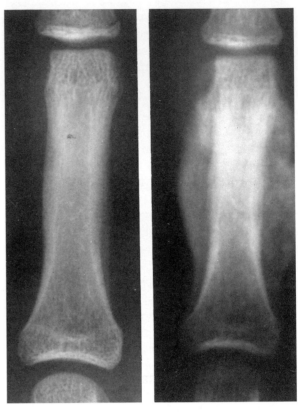

Figure 296
FLORID PERIOSTITIS
An 18-year-old man presented with a 6-month history of decreased range of motion and painless swelling in his finger. He had no recollection of trauma. A radiograph (left) showed minimal periosteal reaction and slight soft tissue swelling. The radiograph on the right was taken 1 month later. There is extensive soft tissue swelling and a conspicuous periosteal reaction encasing the proximal phalanx of the fourth finger. Because of the rapid increase in size and uncertainty regarding the diagnosis, an amputation was performed. (Courtesy of Dr. T.L. Pope, Jr., Winston-Salem, NC.) (Figures 296 and 298 are from the same patient.)

cent). The proximal phalanx is the most common site, followed by the middle/distal phalanges and the metacarpal/metatarsal bones. Virtually any bone may be involved, however (50).

Microscopic Findings. A haphazard, proliferating fibrous tissue background contains variable amounts of amorphous osteoid (fig. 297), mature bone (fig. 298), and, occasionally, immature to mature cartilage. Either the fibrous or osseous portions may dominate. The former consists of frequently nodular proliferations of large, spindled fibroblasts with prominent nucleoli and often numerous, normal-appearing

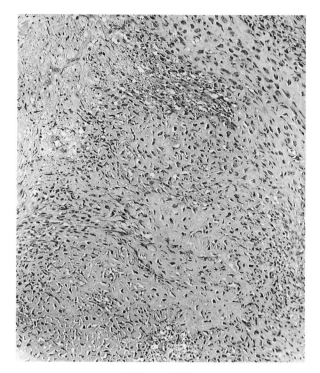

Figure 297
FLORID PERIOSTITIS
The tissue reaction can include amorphous osteoid in a haphazard, densely cellular stroma reminiscent of osteosarcoma.

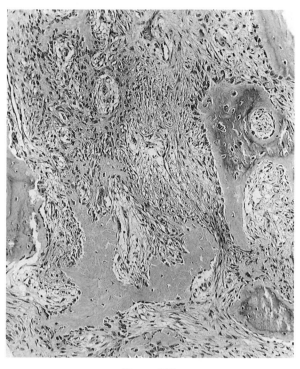

Figure 298
FLORID PERIOSTITIS
More "mature" areas consist of irregularly shaped trabeculae of bone in a cellular fibrous stroma. Osteoblast rimming is prominent.

mitotic figures. Although often highly cellular, nuclear pleomorphism is minimal and atypical mitotic figures are not seen. The osseous elements range from immature, tightly compacted or lace-like osteoid reminiscent of osteosarcoma to zones of more mature woven and even lamellar bone with intense osteoblastic rimming. There may be a "macrozonation phenomenon" in which completely excised lesions demonstrate central maturation. More commonly, there is "microzonation" in which fragments of tissue demonstrate a regional maturation from immature, cytologically alarming osteoid or cartilage to mature bone.

Differential Diagnosis. Myositis ossificans, a typically deep soft tissue lesion, is microscopically virtually identical to florid reactive periostitis. Radiographically, myositis ossificans is a circumscribed, large soft tissue mass. It lacks the parosteal involvement of florid reactive periostitis and seldom elicits a periosteal reaction. Fracture callus, another reactive fibro-osseous and cartilaginous proliferation, is also closely related, microscopically. The clinical history and radiographic features allow easy distinction. Bizarre parosteal osteochondromatous proliferation predilects the hand and favors the proximal phalanx (51). It has a number of features in common with florid reactive periostitis, and some have suggested that the two lesions are fundamentally the same process (53). Bizarre parosteal osteochondromatous proliferations are distinguished by several features. Radiographically, they are cartilage-capped exostoses that appear "stuck on" the cortical surface, an appearance distinct from florid reactive periostitis. Microscopically, the cartilage is more abundant and predominantly peripheral compared to florid reactive periostitis.

Treatment and Prognosis. Local excision is usually curative. About 10 percent of patients develop recurrences.

BIZARRE PAROSTEAL OSTEOCHONDROMATOUS PROLIFERATION

Definition. An exophytic outgrowth from the cortical surface that consists of a mixture of cartilage, bone, and fibrous tissue. There may be considerable nuclear atypia in the lesional cartilage and a callus-like appearance to the cartilage-bone interface.

General Features. Bizarre parosteal osteochondromatous proliferation is part of a spectrum of benign, but often microscopically disturbing proliferations of the hands and feet that include florid reactive periostitis, subungual exostosis, and chondromas of soft tissue. Prior to its description by Nora et al. (57), some of these lesions were undoubtedly included under more malignant diagnoses such as "early juxtacortical osteosarcoma" (56) or interpreted as unusual osteochondromas. Although seemingly related to typical osteochondroma, there are significant clinical, radiographic, and, most importantly, microscopic distinctions.

Clinical Features. Nora et al. (57) described 35 cases of bizarre parosteal osteochondromatous proliferation in 1983, and only a few additional case reports have appeared since that time (54,55). Patients range from 14 to 74 years of age, but most are between 20 and 35 years of age. Males and females are affected equally. Complaints of swelling, tenderness and, occasionally, rapid growth are typical. There is no association with trauma, including prior radiation.

Sites. Nearly all bizarre parosteal osteochondromatous proliferations arise from the tubular bones of the hands and feet, most commonly the proximal phalanges of the hand. The humerus or radius is rarely involved (56).

Radiographic Appearance. There is a calcified, rounded mass that arises directly from the surface of the bone and often has a well-defined pedicle. The underlying bone is otherwise normal. The flaring of the cortex seen in the pedicle of osteochondromas is absent. The contour of the mass is smooth and ranges from 0.4 to 3.0 cm in diameter (fig. 299).

Gross Findings. Most lesions grossly resemble osteochondromas by having an obvious cartilaginous cap. Occasionally, the mass is multilobulated.

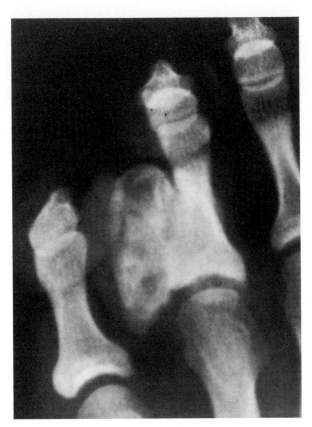

Figure 299
BIZARRE PAROSTEAL
OSTEOCHONDROMATOUS PROLIFERATION
A 20-year-old man had a hard mass develop approximately 6 months after injury to the foot. A well-defined osseous mass is attached in continuity with the cortex of the proximal phalanx. (Fig. 1 from deLange EE, Pope TL Jr, Fechner RE, Keats TE. Case report 428. Bizarre parosteal osteochondromatous proliferation (BPOP). Skeletal Radiol 1987;16:481–3.) (Figures 299 and 300 are from the same patient.)

Microscopic Findings. The cartilaginous cap, if present, is very cellular with enlarged nuclei, some of which are overtly bizarre. Binucleated cells are common. The interface with the underlying bone is irregular or jagged with variably sized aggregates of bone lying within or intermixed with cartilage. The bone is unevenly calcified, and there may be considerable osteoblastic activity. The osteoblasts, although prominent, are benign in appearance. Fibrous tissue may be intermixed, especially at the periphery of the lesion, and osteoclasts may also be seen (fig. 300).

Differential Diagnosis. Bizarre parosteal osteochondromatous proliferation is often confused, radiographically, with an osteochondroma.

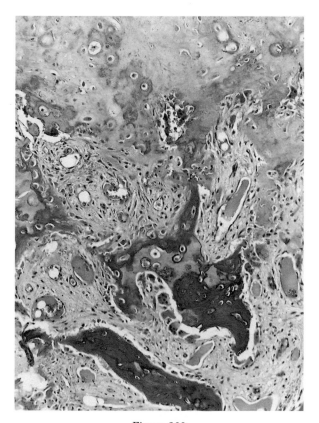

Figure 300
BIZARRE PAROSTEAL
OSTEOCHONDROMATOUS PROLIFERATION
The lesion seen in figure 299 is an irregular mixture of
bone, cartilage, and fibrous tissue without nuclear atypia.

Unlike the latter lesion, however, it appears to be "stuck on" the cortex with no cortical flaring (57). Furthermore, the degree of cellularity and cytologic atypia seen in the cartilaginous component is beyond that encountered in osteochondromas (57).

Mixtures of cartilage, bone, and fibrous tissue are common in myositis ossificans (58). However, the zonal maturation of this lesion is lacking in bizarre parosteal osteochondromatous proliferation. Florid reactive periostitis, a lesion closely related to myositis ossificans, differs, radiographically, from bizarre parosteal osteochondromatous proliferation by typically producing a variable, laminated or mature periosteal reaction. It is often poorly calcified, however, and may appear, radiographically, as a fusiform soft tissue swelling with minimal periosteal reaction. Microscopically, cartilage is uncommonly present and

does not form a surface cap. Recently, it has been suggested that bizarre parosteal osteochondromatous proliferation and florid reactive periostitis are fundamentally identical processes differing primarily in anatomic location, relation to the periosteum, and temporal interception (60).

The fibro-osseous stroma and peripheral cartilage of bizarre parosteal osteochondromatous proliferation may suggest the possibility of a parosteal osteosarcoma. The latter lesions, however, are extremely rare in the hands or feet (59). Furthermore, bizarre parosteal osteochondromatous proliferation lacks the moderate to markedly atypical fibroblasts seen in parosteal osteosarcoma.

Bizarre parosteal osteochondromatous proliferation is quite similar radiographically and microscopically to subungual exostosis. As discussed under the latter lesion, distinction is in large part definitional. Subungual exostosis is confined to the distal phalanges.

Treatment and Prognosis. Approximately half of the lesions reported by Nora et al. (57) recurred once, and half of these recurred a second time. Recurrences ranged from 2 months to 2 years after the first excision. Multiple recurrences spanned 13 years in one patient. Aside from local recurrence, no lesion was locally aggressive or metastatic.

SUBUNGUAL EXOSTOSIS

Definition. A proliferation of hyaline cartilage or fibrocartilage and bone involving the distal phalanx in a subungual or periungual location. Well-developed lesions have a fibrocartilaginous cap overlying mature bone.

General Features. Although most authors consider subungual exostosis to be a distinct clinicopathologic entity, some lump them with osteochondromas. There is no association, however, between multiple osteochondromatosis and subungual exostosis (64). The exact nature of subungual exostosis remains unclear, but several features support a reactive, rather than neoplastic process.

Clinical Features. Patients range from 4 to 77 years of age, with most in their second and third decades of life. Males and females are affected equally. Patients complain of a painful mass that elevates the nail and eventually ulcerates the nail bed. The physical findings depend

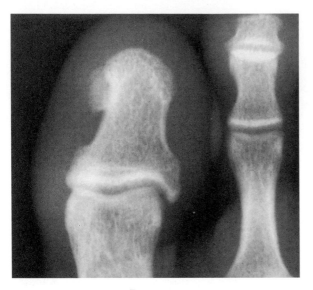

Figure 301
SUBUNGUAL EXOSTOSIS
This typical exostosis involves the distal phalanx of the great toe and protrudes medially.

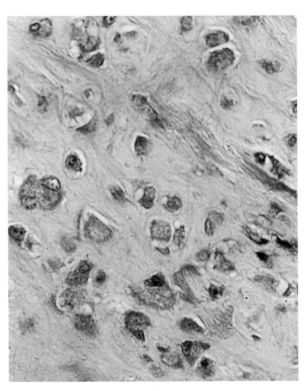

Figure 302
SUBUNGUAL EXOSTOSIS
The cartilage may be moderately cellular with considerable pleomorphism.

on the size of the lesion. Small lesions are subcutaneous masses beneath intact skin, whereas larger tumors may completely destroy the nail. Growth may be rapid, and the duration of symptoms varies from 2 months to several years. A history of significant trauma is elicited in about 25 percent of cases (64).

Sites. In a literature review of 244 cases, 189 (77 percent) involved the great toe, 25 (10 percent) were on other toes, and 30 (13 percent) were on the fingers (64). The lesions on the great toe are usually medial (61).

Radiographic Appearance. The early lesions arise as a soft tissue density without apparent attachment to the bone. There is progressive calcification and the formation of a trabecular pattern of bone. In the end stage, the trabecular bone at the base of the exostosis connects to the underlying phalanx (fig. 301). There is no periosteal reaction and no bone destruction (63). Tumors range from 5 mm to more than 2 cm.

Gross Findings. The cap is smooth and shiny unless there has been chronic ulceration, in which case it is covered by a fibrous layer or granulation tissue.

Microscopic Findings. Subungual exostosis shows considerable microscopic variation, possibly reflecting differing degrees of maturation. There is

often a proliferating fibrous tissue stroma which blurs into loosely intermixed areas of metaplastic-appearing fibrocartilage. This process can extend into the overlying dermis. In other areas, the cartilage may have a hyaline appearance and be strikingly cellular (fig. 302). Mixtures of hyaline and fibrocartilage may coexist (62). Some lesions exhibit enchondral ossification and an orderly arrangement of underlying woven and lamellar bony trabeculae (fig. 303). Others are devoid of cartilage and consist only of bone. Mitotic figures are primarily found in the fibrous stroma, where they may be numerous.

Differential Diagnosis. Clinically, subungual exostosis may be confused with a wide variety of lesions including subungual melanoma, subungual keratoacanthoma, glomus tumor, so-called pyogenic granuloma, and giant cell reparative granuloma. Microscopically, the cellular foci of cartilage in subungual exostosis may suggest the possibility of chondrosarcoma,

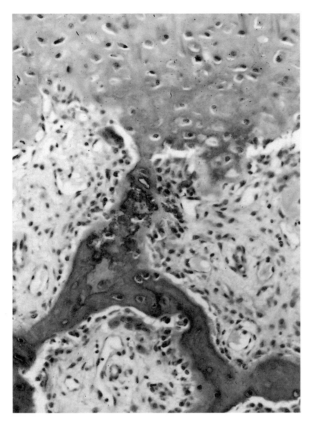

Figure 303
SUBUNGUAL EXOSTOSIS
Reactive bone with a peripheral layer of fiber cartilage is present. Note the similarity to bizarre parosteal osteochondromatous proliferation (fig. 300).

just as the cellular fibrous tissue may be confused with low-grade fibrosarcoma. Some cases have been misdiagnosed as conventional or parosteal osteosarcoma. Although the cartilaginous, fibrous, and osseous stromal elements of subungual exostosis may be disorganized, they lack severe atypia, and their haphazard pattern should not be misinterpreted as a feature of malignancy. The radiographic appearance is so characteristic that it should assure the correct diagnosis.

The histologic spectrum is similar, if not identical, to that of so-called bizarre parosteal osteochondromatous proliferation of the hands and feet (65). The latter lesion, essentially by definition, does not involve the distal phalanges, but affects the middle and proximal phalanges, metacarpals, and metatarsal bones. In the distal phalanges, such lesions would be interpreted,

radiographically and microscopically, as subungual exostoses.

Treatment and Prognosis. The reported recurrence rate of subungual exostosis has been variable. Complete excision appears to be curative, but biopsy or incomplete excision seems to stimulate further growth in about half of cases (64). Local aggressiveness or metastases have not been described.

HEMOPHILIC PSEUDOTUMOR

Definition. A non-neoplastic, destructive osseous lesion secondary to localized hemorrhage in patients with hemophilia.

General Features. Patients with hemophilia are prone to the development of intra-articular hemorrhage with reactive synovitis and secondary degenerative joint disease. Approximately 1 to 2 percent of severe hemophiliacs develop soft tissue or skeletal hemorrhagic pseudotumors. The pathogenesis is not well understood, probably because it varies with location. For example, careful studies of amputations have demonstrated pseudotumors secondary to subperiosteal hemorrhage (66), intraosseous bleeding into cancellous bone (70), and, possibly, bone erosion secondary to hemorrhage into muscles that have broad attachments to bone. Large subperiosteal hematomas may greatly elevate the periosteum and deform the underlying cortical bone, producing a radiographic appearance resembling aneurysmal bone cyst or even a neoplasm.

Clinical Features. Because of the X-linked nature of the underlying disease, hemophilic pseudotumor occurs almost exclusively in males between 20 and 70 years of age. The subperiosteal masses may enlarge and compress nerves, producing pain or neural deficits. Hemophilic pseudotumors are otherwise painless. Depending on the location and size of the lesion, a mass may be palpable.

Sites. The lesions are usually located in the pelvis, lower extremities, or buttocks. A few pseudotumors have been reported in the hands and feet of children (67).

Radiographic Appearance. Soft tissue hemophilic pseudotumors adjacent to bone may produce minimal pressure erosion of the outer cortex that can first be detected by CT scan, before becoming evident on ordinary radiographs (68).

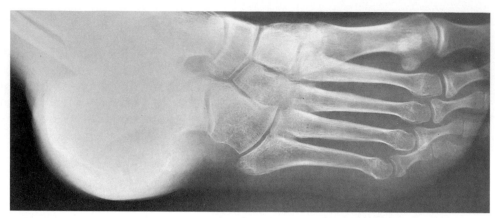

Figure 304
HEMOPHILIC
PSEUDOTUMOR
A 17-year-old hemo-
philiac has a pseudotumor
of the calcaneus that ex-
pands the bone and has
stimulated dense new
bone formation.

Subperiosteal pseudotumors may erode the entire length of a large bone such as the femur (69) or produce more localized lytic defects surrounded by reactive periosteal bone and resembling an eccentric aneurysmal bone cyst. Intraosseous pseudotumors expand the bone (fig. 304) and may be lytic or stimulate new bone formation. They may destroy the cortex and evoke a periosteal reaction.

Gross Findings. An intraosseous hemophilic pseudotumor appears grossly as either a nondescript thrombus with irregular margins, or as an organizing hematoma with variable proportions of reactive bone. If there is a subperiosteal lesion or extension into the surrounding soft tissues, a fibrous or fibro-osseous capsule formed by the periosteum demarcates the lesion.

Microscopic Findings. The periphery of the pseudotumor shows reactive bone and fibrous tissue. Blood in varying stages of degeneration is present centrally, accompanied by hemosiderin-filled histiocytes. Fibro-osseous or callus-like material extends centrally as the hematoma undergoes further organization (70).

Differential Diagnosis. Radiographically, hemophilic pseudotumor may mimic an aneurysmal bone cyst or, rarely, a neoplasm. The radiographic features in conjunction with the appropriate clinical history, however, should be diagnostic in almost all cases. The only considerations microscopically are vascular tumors, usually aneurysmal bone cysts, or possibly osteosarcoma if sections include disorganized, immature reactive bone at the periphery of the lesion. Hemophilic pseudotumor lacks the well-formed cystic spaces and delicate fibrovascular septa of aneurysmal bone cyst and the prominent osteoblastic rimming, lack of cellular anaplasia, and

zonal maturation seen in reactive osteoblastic lesions such as osteosarcoma. This distinction is discussed in greater detail in the section dealing with osteosarcoma.

Treatment and Prognosis. Pseudotumors may progressively enlarge over a long period of time. Therapy is directed at maintaining the functional integrity of the limb and varies with the presence or absence of encroachment on vital structures, destruction of joints, or pathologic fracture.

CONDENSING OSTEITIS

Definition. A reactive sclerosis affecting the medial end of the clavicle. Bilateral involvement may occur.

General Features. This uncommon reactive lesion may be confused with osteomyelitis, a neoplasm, or other reactive processes. The exact etiology is unknown, but is presumably related to mechanical stress. In some cases, there is a clear-cut history of repeated physical activity likely to have stressed the clavicle. In other instances, however, such history is absent.

Clinical Features. Almost all reported cases have been in women between 26 and 63 years old, most younger than 40 years of age (72–75). Reports of so-called condensing osteitis of the clavicle in childhood appear to represent a different entity (71). Some lesions are incidental radiographic findings. Symptomatic patients present after several months to a few years of intermittent or steady pain, localized to the medial end of the clavicle. There may be swelling over the sternoclavicular joint, but the joint per se is never involved.

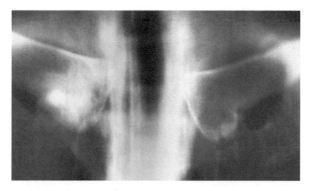

Figure 305
CONDENSING OSTEITIS
The medial one third of the right clavicle is sclerotic and slightly expanded in this tomogram. This 38-year-old woman complained of dull pain for 4 months. (Courtesy of Dr. T.E. Keats, Charlottesville, VA.)

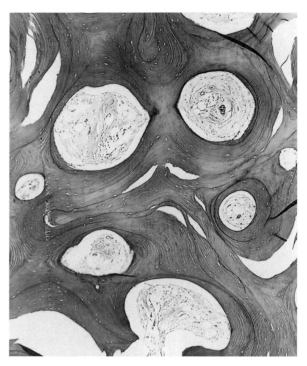

Figure 306
CONDENSING OSTEITIS
Irregularly thickened trabeculae of bone and fibrotic bone marrow are seen.

Radiographic Appearance. The medial one third of the clavicle is sclerotic and may be slightly expanded (fig. 305). Bone scans show a discrete area of increased uptake in this area (76). The sternoclavicular joint is normal. Computed tomography scans confirm the lack of an extraosseous component (73).

Microscopic Findings. The microscopic changes of condensing osteitis are not those of an ongoing inflammatory process and, hence, the term osteitis is probably a misnomer. Acute or chronic inflammation is not present. The bony trabeculae in the medullary cavity are irregularly broadened by apposition of normal lamellar bone (fig. 306). The cement lines may be slightly irregular, resembling Paget disease. Osteoblasts or osteoclasts are rarely seen, however. Small areas of the bone may be necrotic, and the intervening marrow may be focally fibrotic.

Differential Diagnosis. The radiographic differential diagnosis includes Paget disease, chronic osteomyelitis, intraosseous well-differentiated osteosarcoma, and bone infarct. These distinctions are easily made microscopically. Paget disease can be excluded by the absence of conspicuous osteoblastic and osteoclastic activity. The lack of an inflammatory component rules out osteomyelitis. Condensing osteitis lacks the cellular spindle cell stroma typical of intraosseous well-differentiated osteosarcoma. Although there may be an element of necrosis, condensing osteitis is devoid of the extensive osseous necrosis and

dystrophic marrow calcification seen in bone infarcts.

Treatment and Prognosis. Some patients are relieved with anti-inflammatory drugs. In some instances, resection of the end of the clavicle is required to alleviate severe, unremitting pain.

AMYLOID TUMOR OF BONE

Amyloid tumor of bone is a localized accumulation of intraosseous amyloid in sufficient quantity to destroy bone and be radiographically detectable.

Amyloid is a heterogeneous group of fibrillar proteins that are deposited in a "beta-pleated sheet" configuration. Virtually any organ may be involved. Amyloid deposition in the skeleton is almost always associated with multiple myeloma. However, there are a few reported cases of large intraosseous amyloid deposits in the absence of an underlying plasma cell dyscrasia. Lai and colleagues (80) described a patient with Bence-Jones proteinuria who had skeletal amyloid tumor in the absence of a detectable plasma

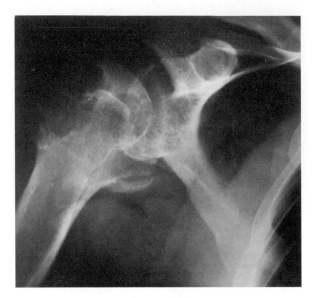

Figure 307
AMYLOID TUMOR

The head of the humerus from a 70-year-old man shows an irregular, lytic lesion with both medullary and cortical bone destruction. (Fig. 1 from Casey TT, Stone WJ, DiRaimondo CR, et al. Tumoral amyloidosis of bone of beta2-microglobulin origin in association with long-term hemodialysis: a new type of amyloid disease. Hum Pathol 1986;17:731–8.) (Figures 307 and 308 are from the same patient.)

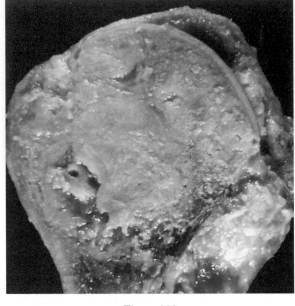

Figure 308
AMYLOID TUMOR

The humeral head seen in figure 307 is almost completely replaced by a large deposit of amyloid. (Fig. 2 from Casey TT, Stone WJ, DiRaimondo CR, et al. Tumoral amyloidosis of bone of beta2-microglobulin origin in association with long-term hemodialysis: a new type of amyloid disease. Hum Pathol 1986;17:731–8.)

cell abnormality and reviewed five previous reports of intraosseous amyloid tumor in which the type of amyloid was not further characterized. Their patient and four of the other five patients had involvement of additional organs including the heart, kidney, pancreas, and lymph nodes. Subsequently, solitary amyloid tumors of the skull or vertebra have been reported (78,79). One case had a monoclonal gammopathy without other evidence of myeloma.

Patients on long-term dialysis are at risk for amyloid tumor due to the skeletal deposit of beta2-microglobulin (82). The deposits may measure several centimeters in greatest dimension, produce lytic lesions radiographically (fig. 307), and result in fracture (77).

Grossly, tumoral amyloidosis is a solid, homogeneous, waxy yellow or tan mass (fig. 308).

Microscopically, there is amorphous, glassy eosinophilic material associated with interspersed multinucleated giant cells, mononuclear histiocytes, or plasma cells (80). Several histochemical stains have been used to identify amyloid of all protein types. The most common stain is the Congo red preparation with its characteristic red-green birefringence under cross-polarized light. The presence of plasma cells in amyloid tumor raises the possibility of a relationship with solitary myeloma, an issue that is currently unresolvable if long-term follow-up shows no progression (81).

Systemic therapy varies with the underlying disease. Local therapy is directed at repair of fractured bones or relief of pressure on vital structures.

REFERENCES

Aneurysmal Bone Cyst

1. Aho HJ, Aho AJ, Einola S. Aneurysmal bone cyst, a study of ultrastructure and malignant transformation. Virchows Arch [A] 1982;395:169–79.
2. _____, Aho AJ, Pelliniemi LJ, Ekfors TO, Foidart JM. Endothelium in aneurysmal bone cyst. Histopathology 1985;9:381–7.
3. Alles JU, Schulz A. Immunohistochemical markers (endothelial and histiocytic) and ultrastructure of primary aneurysmal bone cysts. Hum Pathol 1986;17:39–45.
4. Biesecker JL, Marcove RC, Huvos AG, Miké V. Aneurysmal bone cysts. A clinicopathologic study of 66 cases. Cancer 1970;26:615–25.
5. Clough JR, Price CH. Aneurysmal bone cyst: pathogenesis and long term results of treatment. Clin Orthop 1973;97:52–63.
6. Dabska M, Buraczewski J. Aneurysmal bone cyst. Pathology, clinical course and radiographic appearances. Cancer 1969;23:371–89.
7. Dahlin DC, Unni KK. Bone tumors: general aspects and data on 8,542 cases. 4th ed. Springfield, Ill: Charles C. Thomas, 1986:420–30.
8. Dehner LP, Risdall RJ, L'Heureux P. Giant-cell containing "fibrous" lesion of the sacrum. A roentgenographic, pathologic, and ultrastructural study of three cases. Am J Surg Pathol 1978;2:55–70.
9. Kyriakos M, Hardy D. Malignant transformation of aneurysmal bone cyst, with an analysis of the literature. Cancer 1991;68:1770–80.
10. Levy WM, Miller AS, Bonakdarpour A, Aegerter E. Aneurysmal bone cyst secondary to other osseous lesions. Report of 57 cases. Am J Clin Pathol 1975;63:1–8.
11. Lichtenstein L. Aneurysmal bone cyst. Observations on fifty cases. J Bone Joint Surg [Am] 1957;39:873–82.
12. Martinez V, Sissons HA. Aneurysmal bone cyst. A review of 123 cases including primary lesions and those secondary to other bone pathology. Cancer 1988; 61:2291–304.
13. McCarthy EF, Dorfman HD. Vascular and cartilaginous hamartoma of the ribs in infancy with secondary aneurysmal bone cyst formation. Am J Surg Pathol 1980;4:247–53.
14. Mirra JM. Bone tumors: clinical, radiologic, and pathologic correlations. Philadelphia: Lea & Febiger, 1989: 1267–311.
15. Ruiter DJ, van Rijssel TG, van der Velde EA. Aneurysmal bone cysts: a clinicopathological study of 105 cases. Cancer 1977;39:2231–9.
16. Sanerkin NG, Mott MG, Roylance J. An unusual intraosseous lesion with fibroblastic, osteoclastic, osteoblastic, aneurysmal and fibromyxoid elements. "Solid" variant of aneurysmal bone cyst. Cancer 1983;51:2278–86.
17. Sherman RS, Soong KY. Aneurysmal bone cyst: its roentgen diagnosis. Radiology 1957;68:54–64.
18. Tillman BP, Dahlin DC, Lipscomb PR, Stewart JR. Aneurysmal bone cyst: an analysis of ninety-five cases. Mayo Clin Proc 1968;43:478–95.

Cortical Irregularity Syndrome

19. Chadwick CJ. Tendinitis of the pectoralis major insertion with humeral lesions. A report of two cases. J Bone Joint Surg [Br] 1989;71:816–8.
20. Dunham WK, Marcus NW, Enneking WF, Haun C. Developmental defects of the distal femoral metaphysis. J Bone Joint Surg [Am] 1980;62:801–6.
21. Mirra JM. Bone tumors: clinical, radiologic, and pathologic correlations. Philadelphia: Lea & Febiger, 1989:1625.
22. Resnick D, Greenway G. Distal femoral cortical defects, irregularities, and excavations. A critical review of the literature with the addition of histologic and paleopathologic data. Radiology 1982;143:345–54.
23. Sklar DH, Phillips JJ, Lachman RS. Case report 683. Distal metaphyseal femoral defect (cortical desmoid; distal femoral cortical irregularity). Skeletal Radiol 1991;20:394–6.

Solitary Bone Cyst

24. Adler CP. Tumour-like lesions in the femur with cementum-like material. Does the "cementoma" of long bone exist? Skeletal Radiol 1985;14:26–37.
25. Bosecker EH, Bickel WH, Dahlin DC. A clinicopathologic study of simple unicameral bone cysts. Surg Gynecol Obstet 1968;127:550–60.
26. Campanacci M, Capanna R, Picci P. Unicameral and aneurysmal bone cysts. Clin Orthop 1986;204:25–36.
27. Capanna R, Albisinni U, Caroli GC, Campanacci M. Contrast examination as a prognostic factor in the treatment of solitary bone cyst by cortisone injection. Skeletal Radiol 1984;12:97–102.
28. Cohen J. Etiology of simple bone cyst. J Bone Joint Surg [Am] 1970;52:1493–7.
29. Grabias S, Mankin HJ. Chondrosarcoma arising in histologically proved unicameral bone cyst. A case report. J Bone Joint Surg [Am] 1974;56:1501–9.
30. Hunter WL Jr, Biersner RJ. Comparison of long-bone radiographs between U.S. Navy divers and matched controls. Undersea Biomed Res 1982;9:147–59.
31. Kragel PJ, Williams J, Garvin DF, Goral AB. Solitary bone cyst of the radius containing Liesegang's rings. Am J Clin Pathol 1989;92:831–3.
32. Mirra JM, Bernard GW, Bullough PG, Johnston W, Mink G. Cementum-like bone production in solitary bone cysts (so-called "cementoma" of long bones). Report of three cases. Electron microscopic observation supporting a synovial origin to the simple bone cyst. Clin Orthop 1978;135:295–307.

33. Moore TE, King AR, Travis RC, Allen BC. Post-traumatic cysts and cyst-like lesions of bone. Skeletal Radiol 1989;18:93–7.
34. Norman A, Schiffman M. Simple bone cyst: factors of age dependency. Radiology 1977;124:779–82.

35. Struhl S, Edelson C, Pritzker H, Seimon LP, Dorfman HD. Solitary (unicameral) bone cyst. The fallen fragment sign revisited. Skeletal Radiol 1989;18:261–5.

Subchondral Cyst

36. Glass TA, Dyer R, Fisher L, Fechner RE. Expansile subchondral bone cyst. AJR Am J Roentgenol 1982;139:1210–1.
37. Landells JW. The bone cysts of osteoarthritis. J Bone Joint Surg [Br] 1953;35:643–9.
38. Ostlere SJ, Seeger LL, Eckardt JJ. Subchondral cysts of the tibia secondary to osteoarthritis of the knee. Skeletal Radiol 1990;19:287–9.

39. Rahney K, Lamb DW. The cysts of osteoarthritis of the hip: a radiographic and pathological study. J Bone Joint Surg [Br] 1955;37:663–75.
40. Telaranta T, Solonen KA, Tallroth K, Nichels J. Bone cysts containing silicone particles in bones adjacent to a carpal silastic implant. Skeletal Radiol 1983;10:247–9.

Intraosseous Ganglion

41. Bauer TW, Dorfman HD. Intraosseous ganglion. A clinicopathologic study of 11 cases. Am J Surg Pathol 1982;6:207–13.
42. Kambolis C, Bullough PG, Jaffe HI. Ganglionic cystic defects of bone. J Bone Joint Surg [Am] 1973;55:496–505.
43. Mainzer F, Minagi H. Intraosseous ganglion—a solitary subchondral lesion of bone. Radiology 1970; 94: 387–9.

44. Pope TL Jr, Fechner RE, Keats TE. Intra-osseous ganglion. Report of four cases and review of the literature. Skeletal Radiol 1989;18:185–7.
45. Schajowicz F, Clavel Sainz M, Slullitel JA. Juxta-articular bone cysts (intra-osseous ganglia). A clinicopathological study of eighty-eight cases. J Bone Joint Surg [Br] 1979;61:107–16.

Florid Reactive Periostitis

46. Callahan DJ, Walter NE, Okoye MI. Florid reactive periostitis of the proximal phalanx. J Bone Joint Surg [Am] 1985;67:968–70.
47. Dupree WB, Enzinger FM. Fibro-osseous pseudotumor of the digits. Cancer 1986;58:2103–9.
48. Hutter RV, Foote FW Jr, Francis KC, Higinbotham NL. Parosteal fasciitis. Am J Surg 1962;104:800–7.
49. McCarthy EF, Ireland DC, Sprague BL, Bonfiglio M. Parosteal (nodular) fasciitis of the hand. A case report. J Bone Joint Surg [Am] 1976;58:714–6.
50. Mirra JM. Bone tumors: clinical, radiologic, and pathologic correlations. Philadelphia: Lea & Febiger, 1989: 1589–612.

51. Nora FE, Dahlin DC, Beabout JW. Bizarre parosteal osteochondromatous proliferations of the hands and feet. Am J Surg Pathol 1983;7:245–50.
52. Spjut HJ, Dorfman HD. Florid reactive periostitis of the tubular bones of the hands and feet. A benign lesion that may simulate osteosarcoma. Am J Surg Pathol 1981;5:423–33.
53. Yuen M, Friedman L, Orr W, Cockshott WP. Proliferative periosteal processes of the phalanges: a unitary hypothesis. Skeletal Radiol 1992;21:301–3.

Bizarre Parosteal Osteochondromatous Proliferation

54. Davies CW. Bizarre parosteal osteochondromatous proliferation in the hand. J Bone Joint Surg [A] 1985; 67:648–50.
55. de Lange EE, Pope TL Jr, Fechner RE, Keats TE. Case report 428. Bizarre parosteal osteochondromatous proliferation (BPOP). Skeletal Radiol 1987;16:481–3.
56. Jacobson SA. Early juxtacortical osteosarcoma (parosteal osteoma). J Bone Joint Surg [Am] 1958; 40:1310–28.
57. Nora FE, Dahlin DC, Beabout JW. Bizarre parosteal osteochondromatous proliferations of the hands and feet. Am J Surg Pathol 1983;7:245–50.

58. Norman A, Dorfman HD. Juxtacortical circumscribed myositis ossificans: evolution and radiographic features. Radiology 1970;96:301–6.
59. Stark HH, Jones FE, Jernstrom P. Parosteal osteogenic sarcoma of a metacarpal bone. J Bone Joint Surg [Am] 1971;53:47–53.
60. Yuen M, Friedman L, Orr W, Cockshott WP. Proliferative periosteal processes of phalanges: a unitary hypothesis. Skeletal Radiol 1992;21:301–3.

Subungual Exostosis

61. Evison G, Price CH. Subungual exostosis. Br J Radiol 1966;39:451–5.
62. Ippolito E, Falez F, Tudisco C, Balus L, Fazio M, Morrone A. Subungual exostosis. Histological and clinical considerations on 30 cases. Ital J Orthop Traumatol 1987;13:81–7.
63. Landon GC, Johnson KA, Dahlin DC. Subungual exostoses. J Bone Joint Surg [Am] 1979;61:256–9.
64. Miller-Breslow A, Dorfman HD. Dupuytren's (subungual) exostosis. Am J Surg Pathol 1988;12:368–78.
65. Nora FE, Dahlin DC, Beabout JW. Bizarre parosteal osteochondromatous proliferations of the hands and feet. Am J Surg Pathol 1983;7:245–50.

Hemophilic Pseudotumor

66. Fernandez de Valderrama JA, Matthews JM. The haemophilic pseudotumor or haemophilic subperiosteal haematoma. J Bone Joint Surg [Br] 1965;47:256–265.
67. Gilbert MS. Hemophilic pseudotumor. In: Brinkhous KM, Hemker HC, eds. Handbook of hemophilia. Amsterdam: Excerpta Medica, 1975:435.
68. Hermann G, Gilbert M. Case report 471. Hemophilic pseudotumors (presumptive diagnosis) and hemophilic arthropathy of elbow. Skeletal Radiol 1988;17:152–6.
69. _____, Yeh HC, Gilbert MS. Computed tomography and ultrasonography of the hemophilic pseudotumor and their use in surgical planning. Skeletal Radiol 1986;15:123–8.
70. Steel WM, Duthie RB, O'Connor BT. Haemophilic cysts. Report of five cases. J Bone Joint Surg [Br] 1969;51:614–26.

Condensing Osteitis

71. Appell RG, Oppermann HC, Becker W, Kratzat R, Brandeis WE, Willich E. Condensing osteitis of the clavicle in childhood: a rare sclerotic bone lesion. Review of the literature and report of seven patients. Pediatr Radiol 1983;13:301–6.
72. Brower AC, Sweet DE, Keats TE. Condensing osteitis of the clavicle: a new entity. Am J Roentgenol Radium Ther Nucl Med 1974;121:17–21.
73. Franquet T, Lecumberri F, Rivas A, Inaraja L, Idoate MA. Condensing osteitis of the clavicle. Report of two new cases. Skeletal Radiol 1985;14:184–7.
74. Greenspan A, Gerscovich E, Szabo RM, Matthews JG II. Condensing osteitis of the clavicle: a rare but frequently misdiagnosed condition. AJR Am J Roentgenol 1991;156:1011–5.
75. Kruger GD, Rock MG, Munro TG. Condensing osteitis of the clavicle. A review of the literature and report of three cases. J Bone Joint Surg [Am] 1987;69:550–7.
76. Teates CD, Brower AC, Williamson BR, Keats TE. Bone scans in condensing osteitis of the clavicle. South Med J 1978;71:736–8.

Amyloid Tumor of Bone

77. Casey TT, Stone WJ, DiRaimondo CR, et al. Tumoral amyloidosis of bone of Beta 2-microglobulin origin in association with long-term hemodialysis: a new type of amyloid disease. Hum Pathol 1986;17:731–8.
78. Dickman CA, Sonntag VK, Johnson P, Medina M. Amyloidoma of the cervical spine: a case report. Neurosurgery 1988;22:419–22.
79. Ferreiro JA, Bhuta S, Nieberg RK, Verity MA. Amyloidoma of the skull base. Arch Pathol Lab Med 1990;114:974–6.
80. Lai KN, Chan KW, Siu DL, Wong CC, Yeung D. Pathologic hip fractures secondary to amyloidoma. Case report and review of the literature. Am J Med 1984;77:037–40.
81. Lipper S, Kahn LB. Amyloid tumor. A clinicopathologic study of four cases. Am J Surg Pathol 1978;2:141–5.
82. Onishi S, Andress DL, Maloney NA, Coburn JW, Sherrard DJ. Beta 2-microglobulin deposition in bone in chronic renal failure. Kidney Int 1991;39:990–5.

LESIONS OF THE SYNOVIUM

SYNOVIAL CHONDROMATOSIS

Definition. The formation of multiple, benign cartilaginous nodules in the synovium, many of which become detached and float within the joint space. Synonyms include *synovial osteochondromatosis* and *synovial chondrometaplasia*.

General and Clinical Findings. Most authors believe that synovial chondromatosis is a reactive process of unknown pathogenesis. There is good evidence that it is self-limited and, in some cases, resolves spontaneously (6). Patients range from 14 to 67 years of age, with a peak in the fifth decade of life (7). Males are afflicted twice as often as females. Clinical findings are not distinctive and consist of various combinations of pain, swelling, and limited motion for durations of 1 month to several decades. On the average, patients are symptomatic for about 5 years.

Sites. The knee is involved in about two thirds of patients, followed by the hip and elbow. There have been isolated reports of synovial chondromatosis involving the joints of the shoulder, ankle, carpal and tarsal bones, and mandible. About 10 percent of the knee, hip, elbow, and shoulder lesions are bilateral and, rarely, three joints may be involved. Two siblings were reported with bilateral knee disease (10).

Radiographic Appearance. Radiographs strongly suggest the diagnosis if numerous calcified bodies are visualized (fig. 309). However, not all loose bodies are calcified, and in about 10 percent of patients with synovial chondromatosis no calcifications are seen.

Gross Findings. The synovium may be diffusely studded with hundreds of nodules or, less commonly, only a few square centimeters may be affected (2). The area near the synovial-cartilaginous junction tends to be most heavily involved. The surface has irregular, flat bumps, polypoid nodules of various shapes, and pedunculated masses on long delicate stalks (fig. 310). Individual nodules, whether free or attached, vary in size from less than 1 mm to 3 cm, can number over 1200, and may have a smooth or granular surface. Granularity suggests fusion of smaller nodules (fig. 311).

Extra-articular synovial chondromatosis arising in a bursa has been reported to coexist with intra-articular disease. The lack of a connection between the cartilaginous bodies in the joint and the bursa eliminates the possibility of soft tissue invasion from the joint lesion (9).

Microscopic Findings. The earliest stage of synovial chondromatosis is the formation of round, cellular islands of cartilage in the connective tissue of the joint capsule, beneath, but not involving, the synovial lining cells (fig. 312). Occasionally, the smallest microscopic foci consist of loosely arranged trabeculae of bone. Most nodules consist only of cartilage, but larger ones, including those protruding above the synovial membrane and lying free in the joint, may also contain well-formed bone with fatty marrow.

Enlarged chondrocytes with pleomorphic nuclei and binucleated cells are found focally in about two thirds of cases (fig. 313). Free-floating nodules may be covered with a layer of synovium and the cartilaginous component is usually intact, even when there is necrosis of the underlying bone and fatty marrow.

Differential Diagnosis. The most important consideration in the differential diagnosis is synovial chondrosarcoma. Bertoni et al. (1) identified several microscopic features from cases of metastasizing synovial chondrosarcoma that are indicative of true malignancy including chondrocytes arranged in sheets without a clustering architecture; crowding of cells, especially with spindle cells; myxoid change in the stroma; necrosis; and, on rare occasions, mitotic figures. Extension beyond the joint capsule should heighten the suspicion that the lesion is chondrosarcoma, although some cases of synovial chondromatosis have extra-articular extension (6).

The differential diagnosis also includes secondary synovial chondrometaplasia, which occurs when pieces of bone or articular cartilage are chipped off into the joint space due to trauma or degenerative joint disease (5). These fragments become embedded in the synovium and may stimulate a secondary cartilaginous metaplasia. The nodules differ from synovial chondromatosis by having a concentric layering of cartilage,

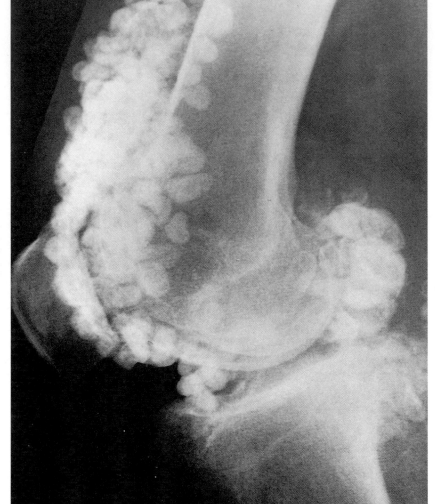

Figure 309
SYNOVIAL CHONDROMATOSIS
This radiograph shows numerous radiodense bodies in the joint and bursae of a 35-year-old man who had swelling and discomfort of the knee for several months. (Fig. 440 from Fascicle 5, 2nd Series.) (Figure 309 and 310 are from the same patient.)

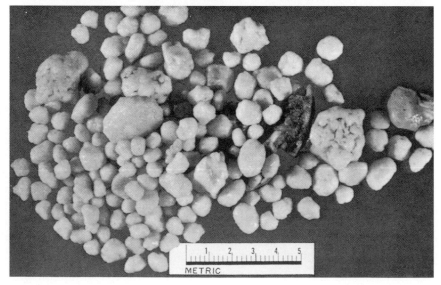

Figure 310
SYNOVIAL
CHONDROMATOSIS
Loose bodies removed from the knee have an external surface that varies from smooth to convoluted. (Fig. 441 from Fascicle 5, 2nd Series.)

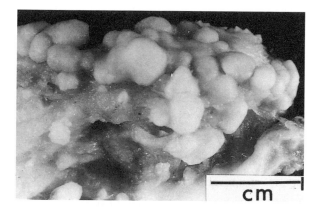

Figure 311
SYNOVIAL CHONDROMATOSIS
Intrasynovial cartilage formation includes cartilaginous bodies ranging from less than 1 mm to nearly 1 cm in size. Approximately 200 cartilaginous bodies were free in the joint space of this patient. (Fig. 1 from Fechner RE. Neoplasms and neoplasm-like lesions of the synovium. In: Ackerman LV, Spjut HJ, Abell MR, eds. Bones and joints. Baltimore: Williams and Wilkins, 1976:157–86.)

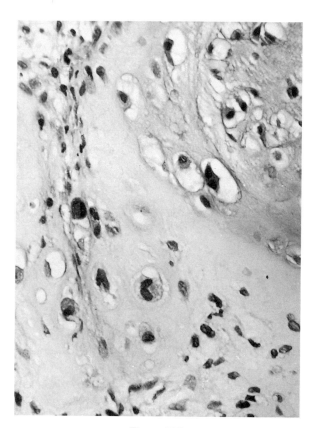

Figure 313
SYNOVIAL CHONDROMATOSIS
Cytologic variation of this degree is common in synovial chondromatosis and does not indicate malignancy. (Fig. 2 from Fechner RE. Neoplasms and neoplasm-like lesions of the synovium. In: Ackerman LV, Spjut HJ, Abell MR, eds. Bones and joints. Baltimore: Williams and Wilkins, 1976:157–86.)

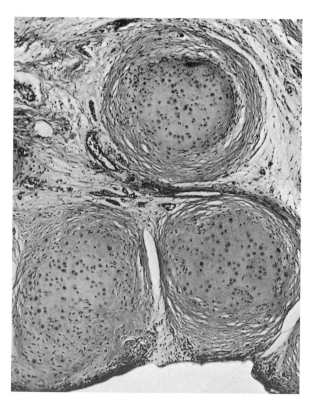

Figure 312
SYNOVIAL CHONDROMATOSIS
Three cartilaginous nodules are seen in the synovial connective tissue. They blend with the surrounding stroma. (Fig. 443 from Fascicle 5, 2nd Series.)

enchondral ossification, and a lack of nuclear atypia (11). Patients with synovial chondromatosis may have secondary degenerative joint disease and, therefore, have some nodules with features of secondary synovial chondrometaplasia. Conversely, the diagnosis of synovial chondromatosis can be made in the absence of synovial disease if the loose bodies consist of cartilage and bone lacking the concentric layering (4).

There have been a few reports of so-called intra-articular osteochondromas (8). These have been large (up to 5 cm) osteocartilaginous masses attached to the synovium by a pedicle. The surface of the lesion is covered with cartilage and the central portion is bone, in a pattern resembling an osteochondroma. It seems doubtful that these unusual lesions are related to diffuse synovial chondromatosis.

Treatment and Prognosis. The therapy usually consists of removal of loose bodies and involved synovial membrane. Many authors have pointed out that the disease appears to be self-limited, since even in the absence of total synovectomy, recurrence is uncommon.

A few cases in which one to three extra-articular masses of cartilage were easily shelled out did not recur (1,3). However, in other cases, extra-articular extensions enlarged, even in the absence of intrasynovial disease (6).

SYNOVIAL CHONDROSARCOMA

Definition. A malignant cartilaginous neoplasm arising from the synovium.

General and Clinical Findings. Synovial chondrosarcoma, either primary or secondary to synovial chondromatosis, is extremely rare. There are 24 reported cases, 15 of which have been males, suggesting a slight male predominance. Patients ranged from 28 to 70 years of age. Symptoms of pain or swelling have been present for 1 month to 25 years, and, in most patients, the duration exceeds 1 year. About half of the reported cases have evidence of concurrent, and presumably preexisting, synovial chondromatosis (17). Two patients had biopsy-proven synovial chondromatosis 24 and 25 years prior to developing a synovial chondrosarcoma (14,18).

Sites. Most synovial chondrosarcomas have involved the knee, with rare examples in the hip, elbow, or ankle.

Radiographic Appearance. Radiographically, intra-articular calcified bodies may be present that are indistinguishable from those of synovial chondromatosis. The major radiographic distinction, if present, is the finding of calcified masses lying within the joint space and also extending beyond its confines, to involve the surrounding soft tissues (16). Uncommonly, there is radiographically detectable erosion of an adjacent bone (12).

Gross Findings. The joint space contains variable numbers of loose bodies, and the synovium has the nodular appearance of synovial chondromatosis. The diagnostic gross feature, if present, is widespread extension of lobulated cartilaginous masses far beyond the joint capsule and into the surrounding soft tissues (13) or bone (14). The cartilage may be more mucinous and glistening than that of synovial chondromatosis. In one case, vein invasion was grossly evident.

Microscopic Findings. Synovial chondrosarcomas often have a lobular pattern with marked hypercellularity. Spindling of cells at the periphery of the lobules was seen in 4 of 10 cases in one series (12). The chondrocytes tend to be scattered in sheets and lack the clustered pattern that is usually present in synovial chondromatosis. Foci of myxoid change are often present and, in one case, an intrasynovial chondrosarcoma had the characteristic pattern of myxoid chondrosarcoma, as seen in soft tissues (15). Synovial chondrosarcomas range from grade 1 to grade 3, using the criteria discussed in the section on chondrosarcoma. The diagnosis of grade 1 chondrosarcoma probably should be made only in conjunction with unequivocal invasion beyond the joint capsule, in order to distinguish it from synovial chondromatosis with prominent nuclear atypia.

Differential Diagnosis. Synovial chondrosarcoma should be distinguished from synovial chondromatosis (see page 279). It should be remembered that synovial chondromatosis may show cytologic atypia and is considerably more common than synovial chondrosarcoma. Furthermore, the sarcomas often occur in a setting of prior chondromatosis. Thus, a de novo synovial cartilaginous lesion, even one exhibiting some cytologic atypia, is far more likely to represent chondromatosis, rather than sarcoma.

Treatment and Prognosis. Treatment has usually consisted of aggressive surgery in the form of amputation or extra-articular resection with reconstruction. Biopsies should be carefully planned, as poorly done procedures may contaminate tissue planes and necessitate subsequent amputation, rather than reconstruction. Nine of 24 reported patients with synovial chondrosarcoma developed pulmonary metastases, usually within 30 months following diagnosis.

PIGMENTED VILLONODULAR SYNOVITIS

Definition. A locally destructive fibrohistiocytic proliferation producing innumerable villous and nodular synovial protrusions. These structures contain large quantities of hemosiderin, giving them a grossly pigmented coloration.

General Features. Pigmented villonodular synovitis and localized nodular synovitis (next section) are often viewed as variants of the same disease. When the entire synovium is involved and there is a major villous component, the process is interpreted as pigmented villonodular synovitis. The presence of more solid, nodular masses in an otherwise predominantly villous, diffuse synovitis indicates that localized nodular synovitis and pigmented villonodular synovitis overlap both grossly and microscopically. The clefts that are seen in solid areas of some cases of localized nodular synovitis are probably remnants of spaces between fused villi. Despite these similarities, the major prognostic differences between the two lesions warrant their separation.

The cause or causes of pigmented villonodular synovitis or localized nodular synovitis are unknown. Some authors view them as benign neoplasms and one case with trisomy 7 supports this concept (32), but most pathologists interpret these as reactive proliferations. As with virtually all diseases of uncertain cause, an autoimmune pathogenesis has been suggested (19). It is of interest that both diffuse and localized forms of synovitis have been reported in several patients with rheumatoid arthritis (33). It is likely, however, that some cases of pigmented villonodular synovitis diagnosed in this setting actually represent a reactive synovial proliferation that microscopically resembles pigmented villonodular synovitis but differs from it pathogenetically. The association of pigmented villonodular synovitis with hemangioma in children raises the possibility that repeated hemorrhage from an underlying vascular malformation could be causative in some patients (20). Hemorrhage alone probably does not account for the lesion, however, because the joint changes in hemophilia differ from those of pigmented villonodular synovitis.

Clinical Features. There is a female predominance with the ratio reaching as high as 2 to 1 in one series. Patients range from 4 to 60 years of age, with most in their third or fourth decade of life. Symptoms include pain, often accompanied by intermittent or steadily progressive swelling and range of motion limitations. Two thirds of patients have a bloody effusion. Symptoms range in duration from 6 months to 25 years, with an average of 6 years.

Sites. More than 80 percent of reported cases involve the knee. The hip joint accounts for about 15 percent of cases, with a few examples reported in the ankle, foot or hand, elbow, and shoulder. Rarely, there is multiple joint involvement, which tends to be bilateral and symmetrical (22,36).

Radiographic Appearance. About 25 percent of patients have multiple cysts in the bones around the involved joint (fig. 314) (24). These contain myxoid material, fluid, or are infiltrated by the synovium with all the features of villonodular synovitis. The cysts are usually present in bones on both sides of the affected joint. Rarely, only a single bone may be involved and the appearance mimics a primary osseous neoplasm (28). Computed tomography demonstrates the extent of the disease. It is particularly useful in locating recurrent lesions and demonstrating that popliteal and posterior calf soft tissue masses are due to extensions from the knee joint itself (21).

Gross Findings. The synovium is light to dark brown with occasional, small yellow foci. It is usually diffusely involved, although small patches of normal synovium can remain, and occasionally, only a few square centimeters of synovium may be affected. The villous projections are variable in size and shape, and number in the hundreds or thousands (fig. 315). They may be filamentous, plump, or beaded. In addition, there are often broad nodules, either forming flat pads on the synovium or polypoid projections above the surface. Articular cartilage can be eroded by lesional tissue (31), and there may be extension into adjacent muscle (23). In one case involving the hip, the femoral head was invaded via the insertion of the ligamentum teres (fig. 316) (25).

Microscopic Findings. The villi are covered by reactive-appearing synovial cells containing abundant hemosiderin. The synovial layer merges imperceptibly into the underlying cellular infiltrate occupying the central core of the villi or nodules. Hemosiderin is also within macrophages or lies free in the stroma. Foamy histiocytes are common, and multinucleated giant cells are invariably seen (figs. 317, 318). Broad areas of fibrosis are occasionally present, and some villi have densely fibrotic or sclerotic cores. The solid nodules focally contain clefts lined by synovial cells. Lymphocytes may be present in the stroma, but rarely are prominent, and other

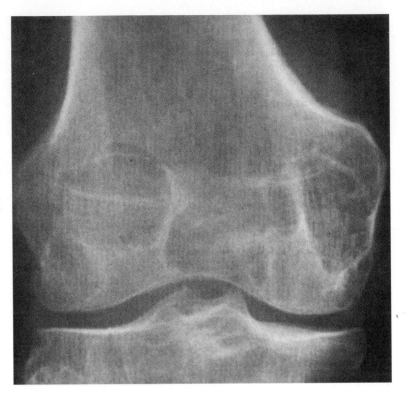

Figure 314
PIGMENTED
VILLONODULAR SYNOVITIS
Several lytic defects are present in the distal portion of the femur. These contained pigmented villonodular synovitis that had invaded bone. (Fig. 459 from Fascicle 5, 2nd Series.) (Figures 314 and 315 are from the same patient.)

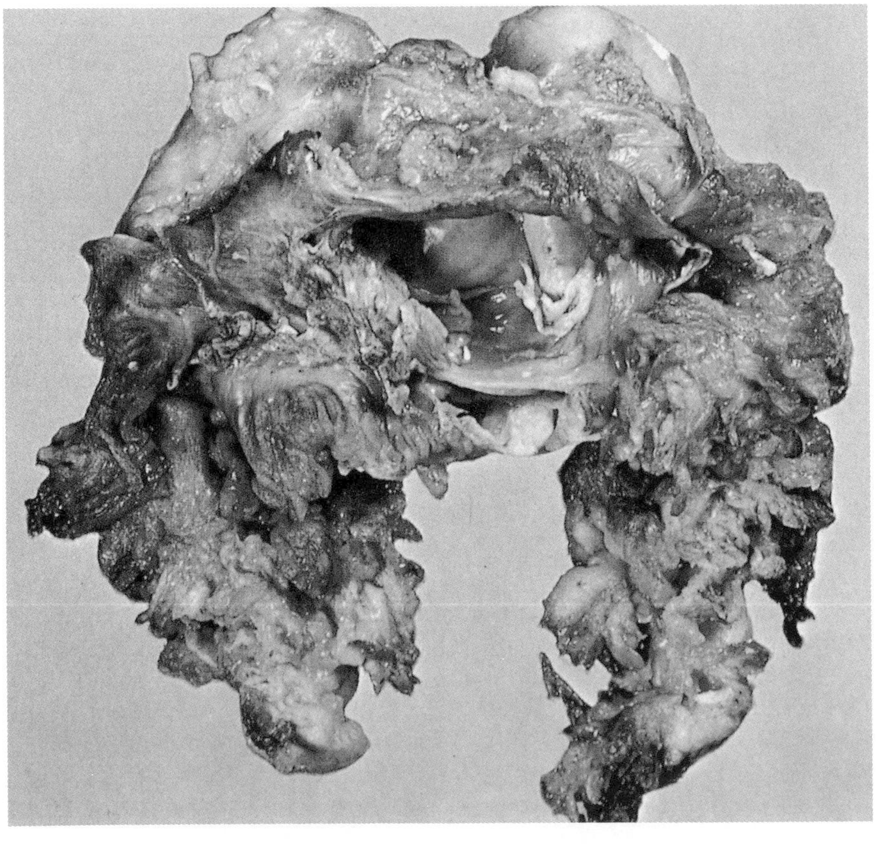

Figure 315
PIGMENTED
VILLONODULAR SYNOVITIS
This synovectomy specimen from the knee joint of a 30-year-old woman has diffuse involvement with villous areas and a few small nodules. The flat, shiny surface represents a small zone of uninvolved synovium. (Fig. 460 from Fascicle 5, 2nd Series.)

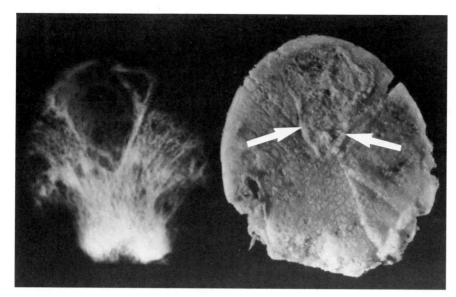

Figure 316
PIGMENTED
VILLONODULAR SYNOVITIS
This specimen radiograph of a bisected femoral head (left) shows a wedge-shaped defect due to osseous extension by pigmented villonodular synovitis at the insertion of the ligamentum teres. The area demarcated by arrows on the gross specimen (right) corresponds with the radiographic defect. (Fig. 4 from Fechner RE. Neoplasms and neoplasm-like lesions of the synovium. In: Ackerman LV, Spjut HJ, Abell MR, eds. Bones and joints. Baltimore: Williams and Wilkins, 1976:157—86.)

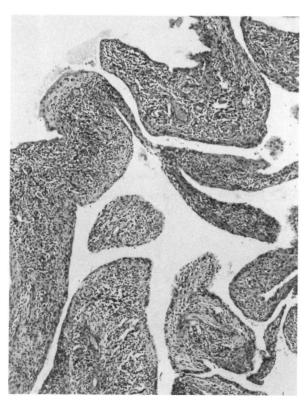

Figure 317
PIGMENTED
VILLONODULAR SYNOVITIS
Villi have cellular cores, and are of variable width and shape. (Figures 317 and 318 are from the same patient.)

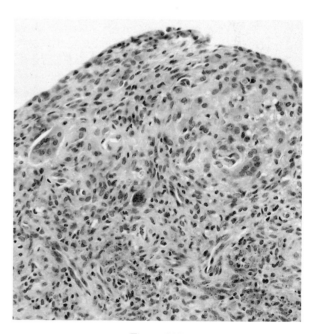

Figure 318
PIGMENTED
VILLONODULAR SYNOVITIS
The villi are lined by an attenuated layer of synovial cells. Histiocytes, giant cells, and scattered lymphocytes are present.

285

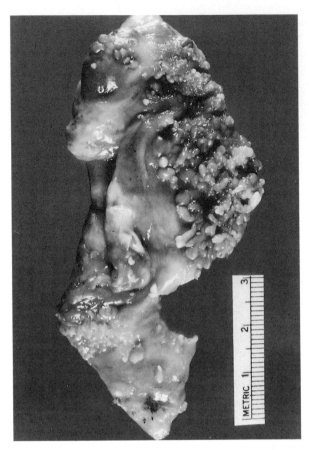

Figure 319
DETRITIC SYNOVITIS
At the time of replacement of a prosthetic knee joint, the synovium was granular, nodular, and villous. (Figures 319 and 320 are from the same patient.)

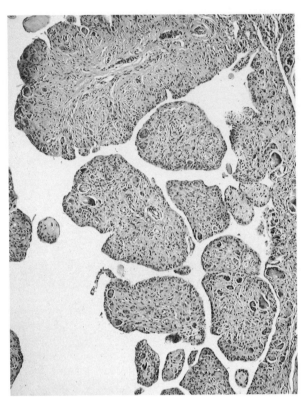

Figure 320
DETRITIC SYNOVITIS
At low power the villous architecture is indistinguishable from pigmented villonodular synovitis. Debris from the prosthesis, often engulfed by giant cells, was present throughout these villous areas.

inflammatory cells are notably absent. Mitotic figures are usually easy to find in the synovial and stromal cells, and in some cases are numerous.

Differential Diagnosis. Traumatized synovium may react by forming numerous well-formed villi. However, the synovium maintains its pink or light tan color and lacks the darker color of pigmented villonodular synovitis. Microscopically, the reactive synovium lacks the foam cells, giant cells, and hemosiderin that are conspicuous in pigmented villonodular synovitis. Joints involved with rheumatoid arthritis may also have a proliferation of villi, but these usually contain many plasma cells and lack conspicuous hemosiderin.

In hemophiliacs, intra-articular hemorrhage can elicit a villous change with large deposits of hemosiderin confined to the synovial lining cells.

The subsynovial tissue, in contrast to pigmented villonodular synovitis, is almost totally devoid of hemosiderin. The villous change is seen only in the early stages of chronic hemarthrosis, because later stages result in a flattened synovium with underlying fibrosis (34).

Villonodular hyperplasia may also occur in joints that have been replaced with prostheses (figs. 319, 320). Microscopic particles of the prosthesis are worn off and enter the joint space where they are phagocytized by histiocytes (38). The identification of foreign material easily distinguishes this *detritic synovitis* from pigmented villonodular synovitis.

A few cases of diffuse synovial neoplasms with local bone invasion and distant metastases have been reported (30). Their exact classification and relation, if any, to pigmented villonodular synovitis are unclear.

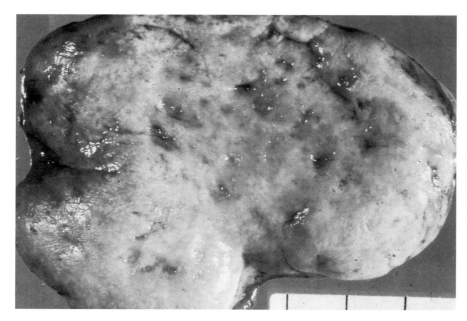

Figure 321
LOCALIZED
NODULAR SYNOVITIS
A 38-year-old man had a sensation of locking in his knee. On exploration, an 8-cm mass was found free-floating in the joint. The cut surface of the mass has a variegated appearance with areas of yellow, tan, and red coloration.

Treatment and Prognosis. Pigmented villonodular synovitis is difficult to eradicate, except in rare cases where it is localized to a portion of the synovium that can be completely excised with wide margins. Localized surgical excision is followed by recurrent symptoms in 21 to 46 percent of cases (26). Spontaneous regression is rare (27). Extensive, destructive local growth may require amputation (29). Some patients require hemiarthroplasty, total arthroplasty, or arthrodesis when there is severe joint destruction (35). Symptoms may be relieved with external beam radiation or intra-articular radiocolloid (37).

LOCALIZED NODULAR SYNOVITIS

Definition. A discrete, intra-articular mass with varying proportions of histiocytes, foam cells, giant cells, inflammatory cells, and fibrous tissue. Other terms that have been used for this lesion include *giant cell tumor (of tendon sheath), benign synovioma,* and *benign fibrous histiocytoma.*

Clinical Features. The age distribution is approximately uniform from the second to the seventh decade of life, with a slight peak between 30 and 40 years of age. Unlike pigmented villonodular synovitis, there is a 2 to 1 male predominance. A few individuals mention a specific episode of trauma. Patients invariably complain of pain. This may be severe with abrupt onset or mild

and intermittent of several years' duration. About half have signs or symptoms consistent with internal mechanical derangements such as locking or clicking of the joint (39,40).

Sites. The knee is the most commonly affected joint, with a few cases reported in the ankle, wrist, or elbow (41).

Gross Findings. At the time of surgery, the mass may be sessile, but more often it is attached to the synovium by a variably sized pedicle. Rarely, it is a loose body in the joint space, unaccompanied by synovial abnormality. Most nodules are 2 to 4 cm in size, but they have ranged from 0.9 to 8.2 cm (fig. 321). The mass is often irregularly shaped and white, bright yellow, or dark brown, depending on the cellularity, amount of lipid, and degree of hemosiderin deposition.

Microscopic Findings. Localized nodular synovitis typically consists of broad, patternless sheets of histiocytes with bland nuclei and variable cytoplasm (fig. 322). The latter may be powdery and eosinophilic, contain abundant hemosiderin, or be foamy (fig. 323). Multinucleated giant cells vary from numerous to absent. Lymphocytes may form dense, follicle-like aggregates, or be more widely scattered. Areas of the stroma may be heavily collagenized or hyalinized and sparsely cellular. Large areas of the nodule may be necrotic, presumably due to compromised vascular supply, especially in pedunculated lesions. Some examples of localized nodular synovitis contain cleft-like

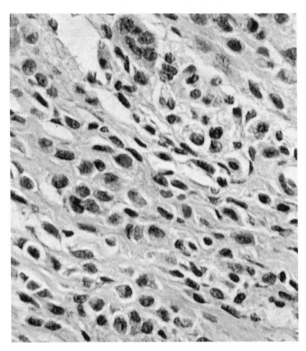

Figure 322
LOCALIZED NODULAR SYNOVITIS
Mononuclear histiocytes, a few lymphocytes, and plasma cells are scattered in a fibrous stroma. (Fig. 456 from Fascicle 5, 2nd Series.) (Figures 322 and 323 are from the same patient.)

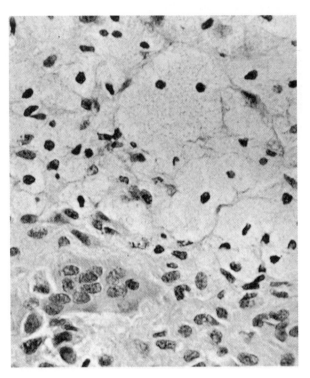

Figure 323
LOCALIZED NODULAR SYNOVITIS
Multinucleated giant cell and foamy histiocytes are present. (Fig. 457 from Fascicle 5, 2nd Series.)

spaces lined either by nondescript, flattened cells, mononuclear histiocytes, or multinucleated giant cells.

Ultrastructural studies verify the variety of cells present in localized nodular synovitis, including primitive mesenchymal cells, fibroblasts, histiocytes, and myofibroblasts. Immunohistochemical studies indicate that both the mononuclear stromal cells and multinucleated giant cells express antigens indicative of monocyte/macrophage differentiation (41,42).

Differential Diagnosis. The cleft-like structures in localized nodular synovitis may suggest the glandular or biphasic form of synovial sarcoma. The large number of giant cells and the mixture of histiocytes help to distinguish the lesion from the latter malignancy. In addition, the well-defined epithelial cells seen in biphasic or glandular synovial sarcoma are not present. In spite of its misleading name, synovial sarcoma involving a joint space is extremely rare. We have encountered only one such case and are aware of only a very small number of others.

Treatment and Prognosis. Simple excision is almost invariably curative. Only one patient has been reported to have a recurrence (41), and that may have been a new focus of localized nodular synovitis, rather than regrowth of the original lesion.

INTRA-ARTICULAR SYNOVIAL SARCOMA

Definition. A soft tissue neoplasm that has either a characteristic, biphasic mesenchymal and epithelial pattern, or consists of a monophasic proliferation of one of these elements. Although synovial sarcoma is a relatively common soft tissue tumor, its occurrence intra-articularly is extremely rare.

General Features. The term, synovial sarcoma, has come to be recognized as a misnomer for a neoplasm that shows no clear-cut synovial differentiation and quite rarely occurs in an intra-articular location. In fact, many synovial sarcomas arise in areas devoid of synovium, such

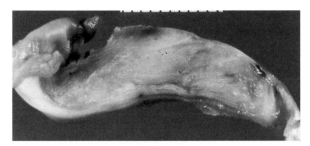

Figure 324
SYNOVIAL SARCOMA
A 43-year-old man with a normal radiograph of the knee experienced pain. A polypoid mass, 5 cm in greatest dimension, was attached to the synovium by a small base (lower right). (Courtesy of Dr. P.E. Gates and Dr. R.M. Belding, Barre, VT.) (Figures 324 and 325 are from the same patient.)

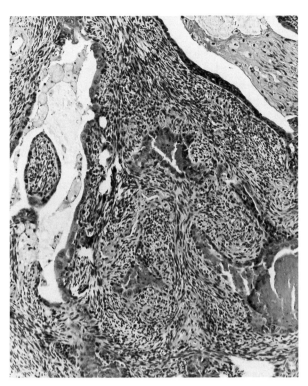

Figure 325
SYNOVIAL SARCOMA
A typical biphasic synovial sarcoma with a cellular, spindle cell stroma and gland-like epithelial spaces is seen microscopically. (Courtesy of Dr. P.E. Gates and Dr. R.M. Belding, Barre, VT.)

as the head and neck region, abdominal wall, or even within a vein (46). Synovial sarcoma does, however, often occur near joints. In one study, involvement of "the immediate structures of a joint" was reported in 18 percent of patients with synovial sarcoma, but no mention was made of any case arising within the joint (47). Zito (48) noted that 13 percent of 48 cases arose "in or close to major joints; however, no residual synovial lining was noted histologically in any of the cases." We believe that most, if not all of these cases are extra-articular synovial sarcomas that secondarily invaded the joint capsule. This would not be surprising, since synovial sarcoma is a locally aggressive lesion with 11 percent showing invasion of bone (47). The subsequent discussion deals only with synovial sarcomas that have clearly been shown to arise from articular synovium.

Clinical Features. Intra-articular synovial sarcoma is the subject of an abstract publication of six cases (43) and a case report (44). We have encountered an additional case (45). Patients range from 9 to 49 years of age. Most are in their fourth or fifth decades of life. Presenting symptoms relate to internal joint derangement (43) and, occasionally, effusion (44).

Sites. All cases have involved the knee, except for a single case arising in the elbow (43).

Radiographic Appearance. The radiographs may be entirely normal, or show nonspecific changes. In one case, there were numerous erosions into the adjacent bones (44).

Gross Findings. Typically, there is a well-defined, polypoid mass with a small point of attachment to the surrounding joint capsule (fig. 324). Alternately, there may be diffuse involvement of the synovial surface, resulting in a large volume of fragmented tissue being removed arthroscopically. In one case, following an earlier arthroscopic synovectomy, the synovium was found to be diffusely involved (44).

Microscopic Findings. Six of eight intra-articular synovial sarcomas, including our case, were biphasic tumors (fig. 325). The two remaining cases had a "predominantly" monophasic, spindle cell pattern (43). The biphasic tumors consisted of a mixture of polygonal epithelial cells and a neoplastic spindle cell component in a pattern identical to that seen in far more common extra-articular synovial sarcomas. Immunohistochemical studies, of both intra-articular and soft tissue synovial sarcomas, have demonstrated strong cytokeratin and epithelial membrane antigen positivity in the epithelial areas, as well as clear-cut positivity for these markers, along with vimentin, in the spindle cell elements.

Differential Diagnosis. Intra-articular localized nodular synovitis may have synovial-lined clefts and resemble a biphasic synovial sarcoma. However, the cells are not clearly epithelial, gland-making cells but have the appearance of histiocytes.

Treatment and Prognosis. Our patient had a polypoid lesion with a small base of attachment to the joint capsule. He was treated by local excision and is alive and well over 9 years later. Local excision of such polypoid lesions thus appears curative, although soft tissue synovial sarcomas are noted for late metastases. Diffuse synovial involvement may require ablation of the limb. In one case with diffuse synovial involvement, pulmonary metastases were found 3 months after the initial arthroscopic synovectomy, and the patient died of respiratory failure 7 months after initial diagnosis (44).

REFERENCES

Synovial Chondromatosis

1. Dunn AW, Whisler JH. Synovial chondromatosis of the knee with associated extracapsular chondromas. J Bone Joint Surg [Am] 1973;55:1747–8.
2. Fechner RE. Neoplasms and neoplasm-like lesions of the synovium. In: Ackerman LV, Spjut HJ, Abell MA, eds. Bones and joints. Baltimore: Williams and Wilkins, 1976:157–86. (IAP monograph, no. 17.)
3. Jeffreys TE. Synovial chondromatosis. J Bone Joint Surg [Br] 1967;49:530–4.
4. Milgram JW. The classification of loose bodies in human joints. Clin Orthop 1977;124:282–91.
5. _____. The development of loose bodies in human joints. Clin Orthop 1977;124:292–303.
6. _____. Synovial osteochondromatosis. A histopathological study of thirty cases. J Bone Joint Surg [Am] 1977;59:792–801.
7. Murphy FP, Dahlin DC, Sullivan CR. Articular synovial chondromatosis. J Bone Joint Surg [Am] 1962;44:77–86.
8. Sariento A, Elkins RW. Giant intra-articular osteochondroma of the knee. J Bone Joint Surg [Am] 1975;57:560–1.
9. Sim FH, Dahlin DC, Ivins JC. Extra-articular synovial chondromatosis. J Bone Joint Surg [Am] 1977;59:492–5.
10. Trias A, Quintana O. Synovial chondrometaplasia: review of world literature and study of 18 Canadian cases. Can J Surg 1976;19:151–8.
11. Villacin AB, Brigham LN, Bullough PG. Primary and secondary synovial chondrometaplasia: histopathologic and clinicoradiologic differences. Hum Pathol 1979;10:439–51.

Synovial Chondrosarcoma

12. Bertoni F, Unni KK, Beabout JW, Sim FH. Chondrosarcomas of the synovium. Cancer 1991;67:155–62.
13. Dunn EJ, McGavran MH, Nelson P, Greer RB III. Synovial chondrosarcoma. Report of a case. J Bone Joint Surg [Am] 1974;56:811–3.
14. Hamilton A, Davis RI, Hayes D, Mollan RA. Chondrosarcoma developing in synovial chondromatosis. A case report. J Bone Joint Surg [Br] 1987;69:137–40.
15. Kindblom LG, Angervall L. Myxoid chondrosarcoma of the synovial tissue. A clinicopathologic, histochemical, and ultrastructural analysis. Cancer 1983;52:1886–95.
16. King JW, Spjut HJ, Fechner RE, Vanderpool DW. Synovial chondrosarcoma of the knee joint. J Bone Joint Surg [Am] 1967;49:1389–96.
17. Manivel JC, Dehner LP, Thompson R. Case report 460. Synovial chondrosarcoma of left knee. Skeletal Radiol 1988;17:66–71.
18. Perry BE, McQueen DA, Lin JJ. Synovial chondromatosis with malignant degeneration to chondrosarcoma. Report of a case. J Bone Joint Surg [Am] 1988;70:1259–61.

Pigmented Villonodular Synovitis

19. Bhawan J, Joris I, Cohen N, Majno G. Microcirculatory change in posttraumatic pigmented villonodular synovitis. Arch Pathol Lab Med 1980:104:328–32.
20. Bobechko WP, Kostiuk JP. Childhood villonodular synovitis. Can J Surg 1968;11:480–6.
21. Butt WP, Hardy G, Ostlere SJ. Pigmented villonodular synovitis of the knee: computed tomographic appearances. Skeletal Radiol 1990;19:191–6.
22. Crosby EB, Inglis A, Bullough PG. Multiple joint involvement with pigmented villonodular synovitis. Radiology 1977;122:671–2.

23. Docken WP. Pigmented villonodular synovitis: a review with illustrative case reports. Semin Arthritis Rheum 1979;9:1–22.
24. Dorwart RH, Genant HK, Johnston WH, Morris JM. Pigmented villonodular synovitis of synovial joints: clinical, pathologic, and radiologic features. AJR Am J Roentgenol 1984;143:877–85.
25. Fechner RE. Neoplasms and neoplasm-like lesions of the synovium. In Ackerman LV, Spjut HJ, Abell MR, eds. Bones and joints. Baltimore: Williams and Wilkins, 1976:157–86. (IAP monograph, no. 17.)
26. Goldman AB, DiCarlo EF. Pigmented villonodular synovitis. Diagnosis and differential diagnosis. Radiol Clin North Am 1988;26:1327–47.
27. Granowitz SP, D'Antonio J, Mankin HL. The pathogenesis and long-term end results of pigmented villonodular synovitis. Clin Orthop 1976;114:335–51.
28. Jergesen HE, Mankin HJ, Schiller AL. Diffuse pigmented villonodular synovitis of the knee mimicking primary bone neoplasms. A report of two cases. J Bone Joint Surg [Am] 1978;60:825–9.
29. Kindblom LG, Gunterberg B. Pigmented villonodular synovitis involving bone. Case report. J Bone Joint Surg [Am] 1978;60:830–2.
30. Nielsen AL, Kiaer T. Malignant giant cell tumor of synovium and locally destructive pigmented villonodular synovitis: ultrastructural and immunohistochemi-cal study and review of the literature. Hum Pathol 1989;20:765–71.
31. Rao AS, Vigorita VJ. Pigmented villonodular synovitis (giant-cell tumor of the tendon sheath and synovial membrane). A review of eighty-one cases. J Bone Joint Surg [Am] 1984;66:76–94.
32. Ray RA, Morton CC, Lipinski KK, Corson JM, Fletcher JA. Cytogenetic evidence of clonality in a case of pigmented villonodular synovitis. Cancer 1991;67:121–5.
33. Schumacher HR, Lotke P, Athreya B, Rothfuss S. Pigmented villonodular synovitis: light and electron microscopic studies. Semin Arthritis Rheum 1982;12:32–43.
34. Stein H, Duthie RB. Pathogenesis of chronic haemophilic arthropathy. J Bone Joint Surg [Br] 1981;63:601–9.
35. Tartalgia L, Chiroff RT. Diffuse pigmented villonodular synovitis. An indication for total hip replacement in the young patient. Clin Orthop 1976;115:172–6.
36. Wagner ML, Spjut HJ, Dutton RV, Glassman AL, Askew JB. Polyarticular pigmented villonodular synovitis. AJR Am J Roentgenol 1981;136:821–3.
37. Wiss DA. Recurrent villonodular synovitis of the knee. Successful treatment with yttrium-90. Clin Orthop 1982;169:139–44.
38. Worsing RA Jr, Engber WD, Lange TA. Reactive synovitis from particulate silastic. J Bone Joint Surg [Am] 1982;64:581–5.

Localized Nodular Synovitis

39. Fraire AE, Fechner RE. Intra-articular localized nodular synovitis of the knee. Arch Pathol 1972;93:473–6.
40. Granowitz SP, Mankin HJ. Localized pigmented villonodular synovitis of the knee. Report of five cases. J Bone Joint Surg [Am] 1967;49:122–8.
41. Ushijima M, Hashimoto H, Tsuneyoshi M, Enjoji M. Giant cell tumor of the tendon sheath (nodular tenosynovitis). A study of 207 cases to compare the large joint group with the common digit group. Cancer 1986;57:875–84.
42. Wood GS, Beckstead JW, Medeiros LJ, Kempson RL, Warnke RA. The cells of giant cell tumor of tendon sheath resemble osteoclasts. Am J Surg Pathol 1988;12:444–52.

Intra-articular Synovial Sarcoma

43. Fetsch JF, Meis JM. Intra-articular synovial sarcoma [Abstract]. Mod Pathol 1992;5:6A.
44. McKinney CD, Mills SE, Fechner RE. Intraarticular synovial sarcoma. Am J Surg Pathol 1992;16:1017–20.
45. McLain R, Buckwalter J, Platz CE. Synovial sarcoma of the knee: missed diagnosis despite biopsy and arthroscopic synovectomy. A case report. J Bone Joint Surg [Am] 1990;72:1092–4.
46. Miettinen M, Santavirta S, Slaetis P. Intravascular synovial sarcoma. Hum Pathol 1987;18:1075–7.
47. Wright PH, Sim FH, Soule EH, Taylor WF. Synovial sarcoma. J Bone Joint Surg [Am] 1982;64:112–22.
48. Zito RA. Synovial sarcoma: an Australian series of 48 cases. Pathology 1984;16:45–52.

✧✧✧

INDEX*

---

* Page numbers in boldface indicate table and figure pages.

293